Trauma-Informed Principles in Group Therapy, Psychodrama, and Organizations

T0373642

This book presents trauma-informed principles for ethical, safe, and effective group work, psychodrama, and leadership.

Content will include practical guidelines, detailed instructions, and diverse examples for facilitating both trauma-informed and trauma-focused groups in treatment, community, and organizational leadership. Chapters focus on various topics including safety, empowerment, social justice, vicarious trauma, and leadership. Organizational leadership is approached through the lens of SAMHSA's guidance and the framework of group work leadership. The book includes significant focus on sociometry and psychodrama as strengths-based and experiential group approaches. Psychodrama's philosophies, theories, and interventions will be articulated through a trauma-informed lens offering psychodramatists, group workers, and organizational leaders new conceptual frameworks and action-based processes. Chapters contain a blend of theory, research, practical guidance, and examples from the author's experience.

This book will appeal to group workers, therapists, psychodramatists, creative arts therapists, organizational leaders, trainers, facilitators, supervisors, community organizers, and graduate students. This book offers group facilitators the insight and tools to lead engaging and meaningful groups. The potential for retraumatizing participants is addressed while promoting trauma-informed practice as an ethical imperative.

Dr. Scott Giacomucci, DSW, LCSW, BCD, CGP, FAAETS, TEP, is the Director/Founder of the Phoenix Center for Experiential Trauma Therapy in Media, Pennsylvania and Research Associate and Adjunct Professor at Bryn Mawr College's Graduate School of Social Work. He is author of the award-winning text, *Social Work, Sociometry, & Psychodrama* (2021).

"Scott's book is an important and necessary addition to the field about the specific aspects of psychodrama to a trauma-informed knowledge base on the uses of the dramatic arts in treatment as well as the implications of this work for organizations and for leaders." (from book foreword)

Sandra, L. Bloom, MD, *associate professor, Health Management and Policy, Dornsife School of Public Health, Drexel University, Philadelphia, PA, USA; chair of the Campaign for Trauma-Informed Policy and Practice; founder of the Sanctuary Model and Creating Presence; author of* **Creating Sanctuary** *(2013)*

"Scott Giacomucci has eloquently elucidated ways that organizations can incorporate SAMHSA's trauma-informed principles into their policies and practices. Scott has thoughtfully and skillfully integrated these important ideas with psychodrama and sociometry, creating a powerful synthesis. This book will empower leaders to put trauma-informed care into action."

Catherine D. Nugent, LCPC, TEP, *former chief, SAMHSA/CSAT Workforce Development Branch; executive director, Laurel Psychodrama Training Institute; past president, American Board of Examiners in Psychodrama, Sociometry & Group Psychotherapy*

"In this seminal book, Giacomucci skillfully explains the integration of trauma-informed care and psychodrama principles, providing a road map for theory, methodology, and psychotherapeutic applications. Readers will appreciate clearly articulated concepts and strategies that can be immediately incorporated into clinical work, group therapy, supervision, peer consultation, and trauma-informed programming across numerous settings. This volume greatly expands the intersection of psychodrama approaches and the field of traumatic stress while also incorporating leadership, ethical, and culturally-resonant practices that form the core of trauma-informed work."

Cathy A. Malchiodi, PhD, *director, Trauma-Informed Practices and Expressive Arts Therapy Institute, 2022 Cecil and Ida Green honors chair, and author of* **Trauma and Expressive Arts Therapy: Brain, Body, and Imagination in the Healing Process** *(2020), and* **Handbook of Expressive Arts Therapy** *(2022)*

"Scott Giacomucci examines the practice of group therapy, psychodrama and leadership introducing and expanding on elements of trauma-informed care in each of the practice models. Reviewing the developmental history of the three, and integrating his own significant practice and academic experience, he reminds the reader of the importance of respecting both the healing potential as well as the potential for harm in each."

Lawrence Shulman, MSW, EdD, *dean and professor emeritus, School of Social Work, University at Buffalo, State University of New York; author of* **The Skills of Helping Individuals, Families, Groups, and Communities** *(8th edition) (2018) and* **Dynamics and Skills of Group Counseling** *(2010)*

"Scott Giacomucci has produced a singularly rich work on psychodrama theory and practice. Deeply informed by the literature on trauma and its treatment in various settings, his thoughtful and imaginative guidance is so very much needed in these troubled times."

Jonathan D. Moreno, PhD, *David and Lyn Silfen University professor, University of Pennsylvania; author of* **Everybody Wants to Go to Heaven but Nobody Wants to Die: Bioethics and the Transformation of Healthcare in America** *(2020);* **The Brain in Context** *(2019); and* **Impromptu Man: J.L. Moreno and the Origins of Psychodrama, Encounter Culture, and the Social Network** *(2014)*

"This book presents the articulation of J.L. Moreno's legacy with current research in the area, making it an important contribution on the effectiveness of trauma treatment. The foundation of the basic principles of the practice, including the benefits of teletherapy, and the didactic presentation of guidelines and instructions make this textbook a necessary resource for a whole new generation of professionals dedicated to working with groups and trauma. Scott Giacomucci reached his commitment with Zerka Moreno to bring the psychodramatic method to new generations."

Heloisa Fleury, MA, *psychologist/psychodramatist in private practice, São Paulo, Brazil; president, International Association for Group Psychotherapy & Group Processes; editor-in-chief, Brazilian Journal of Psychodrama; co-editor of* **Psychodrama in Brazil (2022)** *and multiple other books.*

"Scott Giacomucci has presented a well-researched text on group therapy and psychodrama including emphases on teletherapy, ethics, and organizations. A truly needed text to have on the bookshelf of every group worker, psychodramatist, and leader."

Daniela Simmons, PhD, TEP, *president, American Society of Group Psychotherapy & Psychodrama; creator & CEO of Tele'Drama International; Dallas, Texas, USA*

"With this book, Scott Giacomucci makes a substantial contribution to the literature of group therapy and psychodrama. His integration of the principles of Trauma Informed Care with professional ethics as they apply to group therapy and psychodrama is a major advancement of the field and the treatment of clients, many of whom have histories of complex trauma. He has incorporated his extensive knowledge of the psychodrama literature and practice with contemporary advances and issues in the trauma field to offer a detailed and innovative group treatment model, applicable in many settings and organizations. His emphasis on safety and the safeguarding of clients from retraumatization and therapists from vicarious trauma is exemplary as is his emphasis on the promotion of healing through connections with others."

Christine A. Courtois, PhD, ABPP, *psychologist/consultant in private practice (retired); author of* **Healing the Incest Wound** *(1988; 2010),* **It's Not You, It's What Happened to You** *(2014; 2020); and co-editor of* **Treating Complex Traumatic Stress Disorders in Adults** *(2009; 2020)*

Trauma-Informed Principles in Group Therapy, Psychodrama, and Organizations

Action Methods for Leadership

Dr. Scott Giacomucci, DSW, LCSW, BCD, CGP, FAAETS, TEP

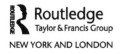

Routledge
Taylor & Francis Group

NEW YORK AND LONDON

Designed cover image: © Getty Images

First published 2023
by Routledge
605 Third Avenue, New York, NY 10158

and by Routledge
4 Park Square, Milton Park, Abingdon, Oxon, OX14 4RN

Routledge is an imprint of the Taylor & Francis Group, an informa business

© 2023 Scott Giacomucci

ISBN: 978-1-032-23478-6 (hbk)
ISBN: 978-1-032-23477-9 (pbk)
ISBN: 978-1-003-27785-9 (ebk)

DOI: 10.4324/9781003277859

Typeset in Goudy
by codeMantra

To group psychotherapists, psychodramatists, and organizational
leaders everywhere

may we never forget our sacred responsibility and professional calling

to use our knowledge and power towards the greatest good

of our clients, students, colleagues, and humankind.

Short Table of Contents

1 Introduction to Trauma-Informed Group Therapy,
Psychodrama, and Leadership   1

2 Psychodrama and Group Work as Trauma-Informed Philosophies   31

3 Trauma-Focused Psychodrama as an Effective Group
Treatment for PTSD   68

4 Trauma-Informed Experiential Sociometry Processes   103

5 Safety in Group Therapy, Psychodrama, and Leadership   133

6 Trustworthiness and Transparency in Group Therapy,
Psychodrama, and Leadership   156

7 Peer Support in Group Therapy, Psychodrama, and Leadership   174

8 Collaboration and Mutuality in Group Therapy,
Psychodrama, and Leadership   190

9 Empowerment, Voice, and Choice in Group Therapy,
Psychodrama, and Leadership   206

10 Cultural, Historic, and Gender Issues in Group Therapy,
Psychodrama, and Leadership   222

11 Trauma-Informed Organizations: From Vicarious Trauma to
Vicarious Posttraumatic Growth   248

12 Toward Trauma-Informed Ethics of Leadership in Group
Therapy, Psychodrama, and Organizations   279

Index   301

Table of Contents

About the Book   xv

Foreword   xvi

Acknowledgments   xxiv

List of Figures   xxvi

List of Tables   xxviii

About the Author   xxix

1 Introduction to Trauma-Informed Group Therapy, Psychodrama, and Leadership   1
    Chapter Summary 1
    My Journey with Psychodrama and Trauma-Informed Work 2
    Group Work and Group Therapy 8
    Introduction to Psychodrama and Sociometry 10
    Introduction to Trauma-Informed Care 13
    Trauma-Informed Leadership 19
    Trauma-Informed vs Trauma-Focused Services 21
    Three-Stage Clinical Map for Trauma Work 22
    Trauma-Informed Practice as Ethical Imperative 23
    How to Read This Book 24
    Conclusion 25
    References 25

2 Psychodrama and Group Work as Trauma-Informed Philosophies   31
    Chapter Summary 31
    Group Work as Trauma-Informed Philosophy 31
    Stages in Group Development and Trauma Therapy 40
    Morenean Philosophy as Trauma-Informed Philosophy 44

Psychodrama Theories as Trauma Theories 48
Conclusion 60
References 60

3 Trauma-Focused Psychodrama as an Effective Group
   Treatment for PTSD   68
   Chapter Summary 68
   Group Therapy's Effectiveness in Treating PTSD 68
   Psychodrama as an Effective Treatment for Trauma and PTSD 69
   Posttraumatic Growth through Psychodrama 73
   Classical Psychodrama Techniques as Trauma Interventions 77
   Therapeutic Spiral Model 83
   Relational Trauma Repair Model 88
   Trauma-Focused Psychodrama 90
   Conclusion 95
   References 95

4 Trauma-Informed Experiential Sociometry Processes   103
   Chapter Summary 103
   Experiential Sociometry as Trauma-Informed Group Processes 103
   Embodying Trauma-Informed Principles with Experiential Sociometry 104
   Dyads, Triads, and Small Groups 106
   Spectrograms 109
   Locograms 113
   Floor Checks 115
   Step-in Sociometry 118
   Hands-on-Shoulder Sociograms 121
   Circle of Strengths 126
   Conclusion 129
   References 129

5 Safety in Group Therapy, Psychodrama, and Leadership   133
   Chapter Summary 133
   Trauma as a Threat to Safety 133
   Traumatization and Retraumatization by Service Providers 135
   Trauma-Informed Leaders Prioritize Safety in the Workplace 136
   Assessment, Referral, and Screening 139
   Cultivating Safety with Group Rules and Norms 141
   Safety through Connection in Group Work 145
   Developing Safety through Roles in Psychodrama 147
   Conclusion 151
   References 152

6 Trustworthiness and Transparency in Group Therapy,
Psychodrama, and Leadership   156
Chapter Summary 156
Traumatic Disruption of Trust 156
Trusting in Clients and Community 158
*Trustworthy and Transparent Organizations, Supervisors, and
    Educators 160*
*Trustworthy and Transparent Leadership in Group Work and
    Psychodrama 163*
Trust in the Psychodrama Process 167
Conclusion 170
References 171

7 Peer Support in Group Therapy, Psychodrama, and Leadership   174
Chapter Summary 174
Trauma as Inherently Disconnecting from Self and Others 174
Reconnecting to Self through Group Therapy and Psychodrama 176
Group Work as Social Connection 178
Peer Support for Professionals, Employees, and Leaders 180
Psychodrama Centralizes the Power of Mutual Aid 183
Conclusion 186
References 187

8 Collaboration and Mutuality in Group Therapy,
Psychodrama, and Leadership   190
Chapter Summary 190
*Trauma Is Characterized by an Absence of Collaboration and
    Mutuality 190*
Mutuality as Respect for Identity and Culture 193
Finding a Place to Belong in Group 194
*Trauma-Informed Leaders Promote Collaboration, Mutuality, and
    Belonging 196*
Psychodrama as Catalyzer for Collaboration and Mutuality 198
Conclusion 202
References 203

9 Empowerment, Voice, and Choice in Group Therapy,
Psychodrama, and Leadership   206
Chapter Summary 206
Trauma is Inherently Disempowering 206
Empowered by the Group 208
Fostering Empowerment through Trauma-Informed Leadership 211

Empowerment through Psychodrama 213
Conclusion 218
References 219

10 Cultural, Historic, and Gender Issues in Group Therapy,
    Psychodrama, and Leadership   222
    Chapter Summary 222
    *Traumatic Impacts of Oppression, Discrimination, and Collective
      Trauma 223*
    Healing-Centered Engagement 225
    Anti-Oppressive Group Leadership and Cultural Humility 227
    Culture and Identity in Organizations 231
    *Addressing Impacts of Social Injustice with Psychodrama and
      Sociodrama 236*
    Conclusion 242
    References 243

11 Trauma-Informed Organizations: From Vicarious Trauma to
    Vicarious Posttraumatic Growth   248
    Chapter Summary 248
    *Vicarious Traumatization, Secondary Traumatic Stress,
      Compassion Fatigue, and Burnout 248*
    Traumatic Countertransference 252
    Vicarious Posttraumatic Growth 253
    SAMHSA's Guidance for Trauma-Informed Organizations 256
    The Sanctuary Model and Creating PRESENCE 259
    Sociometry, Psychodrama, and Sociodrama in Organizations 264
    Conclusion 273
    References 274

12 Toward Trauma-Informed Ethics of Leadership in Group
    Therapy, Psychodrama, and Organizations   279
    Chapter Summary 279
    Leadership as a Double-Edged Sword 279
    Toward a Trauma-Informed Ethics of Organizational Leadership 282
    Toward a Trauma-Informed Ethics of Group Work 285
    Toward a Trauma-Informed Ethics of Psychodrama 289
    Conclusion: Trauma-Informed Leadership in Action 294
    References 295

Index   301

About the Book

This book presents trauma-informed principles for ethical, safe, and effective group work, psychodrama, and leadership. Content will include practical guidelines, detailed instructions, and diverse examples for facilitating both trauma-informed and trauma-focused groups in treatment, community, and organizational leadership. Chapters focus on various topics including safety, empowerment, social justice, vicarious trauma, and leadership. Organizational leadership is approached through the lens of SAMHSA's guidance and the framework of group work leadership. The book includes significant focus on sociometry and psychodrama as strengths-based and experiential group approaches. Psychodrama's philosophies, theories, and interventions will be articulated through a trauma-informed lens offering psychodramatists, group workers, and organizational leaders new conceptual frameworks and action-based processes. Chapters contain a blend of theory, research, practical guidance, and examples from the author's experience. This book will appeal to group workers, therapists, psychodramatists, creative arts therapists, organizational leaders, trainers, facilitators, supervisors, community organizers, and graduate students. While group sessions and meetings have become an integral part of every treatment program, training program, organization, and social movements, the establishment of group work training is significantly inadequate – especially in graduate programs for psychologists, counselors, and social workers. This book offers group facilitators the insight and tools to lead engaging and meaningful groups. The potential for retraumatizing participants is addressed while promoting trauma-informed practice as an ethical imperative.

Scott Giacomucci
Phoenix Center for Experiential Trauma Therapy
Media, Pennsylvania, USA
www.PhoenixTraumaCenter.com
Scott@PhoenixTraumaCenter.com
Bryn Mawr College
Graduate School of Social Work & Social Research
Bryn Mawr, Pennsylvania, USA

Foreword

I am pleased to write this foreword for Scott Giacomucci's new book about group therapy and psychodrama, not only because I respect his work but because, like him, I too have despaired over the loss of expressive therapy group approaches, particularly psychodrama, to the therapeutic community. In this volume, he is integrating all he has learned professionally and personally about the power of psychodrama to propel change while integrating that knowledge with what we now understand as the basic underlying cause of most psychological, physical, and social disturbance: prolonged exposure to chronic stress, adversity, and trauma.

As I understand it, treating trauma has always been an intuitive part of the psychodramatic arts, even if the effects of trauma were not yet fully articulated and understood at the time. After all, Moreno was doing group work with sex workers as early as 1913 and in his autobiography as Scott points out, he was a trauma survivor himself in childhood and as an adult (Garcia & Buchanan, 2009; Moreno, 2019). After World War II, Maxwell Jones, considered one of the founders of the democratic therapeutic community, used drama as a fundamental part of his work with veterans and POW's starting in 1944, and then later with people who were chronically unemployed. Each week, a patient would write, produce, and perform their own drama based on their own life experience. Some of the other patients would be chosen by him as characters in the play and then everyone else became the audience in the regular Friday performance. The original idea for this format in this setting did not spring from Moreno, but later, Jones wrote, "To begin with we were quite unaware of the work of J. L. Moreno, although latterly we have borrowed freely from his works" (Jones, 1953).

In fact, the healing possibilities of dramatic performance go way, way back as pointed out by my colleague, Jonathan Shay. Jonathan is a psychiatrist and a philosopher, so his knowledge is both wide-ranging and deep. He spent his career treating Vietnam Veterans while also studying Greek philosophy. In doing so, he has developed a theory that healing from combat trauma necessitates a communal response AND that trauma disables returning veterans from participating in democratic culture. But the returning veterans he was initially referring to were not from the Vietnam era but from ancient Greece. He has developed a theory that the Greek tragedies were the methods used to reintegrate battle veterans into the community, that the chorus was comprised of young men who had not yet seen battle and represented the moral consensus of the community. The principal roles, however, were played by veterans, all mature men. It is well-known that Aeschylus and Sophocles were both battle-tested. The plays were held at the annual Athenian festival called the City Dionysia. The audience sat by military unit, with the highest rank in front and the lowest in the back. The audience, all veterans, then watched in daylight as the stories unfolded, all of which were transgressive at key moments, making it clear that what is permissible in combat is not permissible in democratic society. In doing so, the performances helped to surface and helped to heal the moral injuries that the soldiers had experienced (Shay, 1995, 2002).

In the 1970s when I was in my psychiatric residency program, art therapy groups were a standard part of treatment and my mentor, Roy Stern, the psychiatrist in charge of the inpatient psychiatric unit, would regularly turn to his art therapist first, before asking any of us our opinions, to get a deeper and less obvious understanding of the patient whose situation we were discussing. Once I got out of my residency, I went to work at a psychiatric hospital where psychodrama was a key aspect of treatment and that was when I first witnessed the power of people having the opportunity to safely relive painful memories, transform those memories through drama, and rehearse new strategies of interaction and behavior.

At that time, I became very interested in learning more about this approach to treatment, so I attended a weekend psychodrama training workshop. There I saw how dangerous and overwhelming psychodrama could be when the psychodramatist in charge was not adequately prepared for the forces she was unleashing – as if the only thing that was important was the unleashing of emotion, apparently failing to comprehend the fact that she was intentionally triggering flashbacks and traumatic memories that the participants were not prepared for and could not manage. As a result of situations such as this, as Scott explores in this book, psychodrama developed "a reputation for being overly cathartic, overwhelming, and retraumatizing for some participants." So, with this reputation and with radical changes in mental health care financing, the proverbial baby was thrown out with the bathwater and since the 1990s it has been difficult or impossible to get funding for expressive therapies.

In 1980 when I had the opportunity to turn a medical-surgical floor into a psychiatric unit in a suburban community hospital, that program ended up being one of the first inpatient treatment programs for adults who had been abused as children – long before there was anything called "trauma-informed treatment". I was in charge of the program, so I made sure we had expressive therapy groups every day – psychodrama and art therapy at first, and then movement and recreation therapy groups as well. The patients would be in groups for most of the day, with time-outs to see their therapist, have lunch, go to medical appointments, and attend family meetings as needed.

As a result, we saw what was necessary to create a true therapeutic community, established even in the brief time allotment we had for inpatient care. This helped us understand and later define what it took to create community safety in a group of people who usually entered the hospital in highly volatile states and were very fearful of being in a "loony bin" with a bunch of strangers. Since the population on the unit changed over rapidly because we had short lengths of stay, it was vitally important to orient and engage new patients quickly. The patients themselves, as a result of the group interactions, were largely responsible for quieting the fears of new patients and helping them quickly to see that there was nothing "loony" about what was happening at all. In doing so, they created the social norms that kept us all safe and helped to promote the early stages of recovery for all of them. Then as people were discharged and new people entered, the social norms around safety were passed on automatically.

At the time I was the manager for the psychiatric unit, I was also the psychiatrist for most of the patients, so I was able to learn how important it was for treatment to center on the integration of both verbal, conscious experience and knowledge with nonverbal, unconscious, enacted experience, and knowledge. As a psychodynamically trained physician, I was very capable of doing the verbal, conscious, and cognitive-emotional component of treatment, but to access the other side of the person – the other hemisphere of their brain – required specialty work that only trained psychodramatists and other creative therapists could provide. Because we always worked as a team and met together in at least two formal meetings a week to review the progress of each patient – physicians, nurses, expressive therapists, direct care staff – I was able to solicit specific help that I needed with individual patients from my expressive therapists.

I distinctly recall one person, a woman who was very depressed and suicidal and yet unable to express any anger at the abysmal situations she had been put in and the internalized anger was clearly destroying her. I asked our brilliant psychodramatist, Jean Vogel and a direct staff member, Mike – who was very good at antagonizing people and who worked the evening shift – if they could help me mobilize her anger. As expected, they were successful and in her planned psychodrama she was able to say what she needed to say to the people who had hurt her, her depression lifted, and she was sent home to outpatient therapy with far more insight than she had when she was admitted.

Sometimes, when members of our staff would be called away to deal with an acute problem of some sort, Jean would ask me to stand in as an auxiliary, while one or another of our patients triumphantly enacted their own psychodrama – an achievement that often signaled their readiness for discharge from hospital-level care. In this way, I learned first-hand the power of the dramatic arts. Even though she was dealing with very traumatized and symptomatic men and women, Jean never lost control of the psychodrama groups, while at the same time she and our patients courageously engaged with the horrors of physical abuse, sexual abuse, rape, domestic violence, industrial accidents, terrorist attacks, and all the other traumatic experiences that beset people. Like Scott, Jean too learned from and admired the work of Zerka Moreno, whose workshops she attended in New York. To my knowledge – and I was in a position to know – no one ever was retraumatized as a result of their experience with psychodrama in our program, but these groups were occurring in a context that was based on close teamwork and was itself becoming trauma-informed daily. That is what makes Scott's emphasis on training and containment so vitally important.

Long before there was anything known as "trauma-informed care" – from 1980 to 2001– we were treating people with very serious trauma histories usually beginning in childhood who had developed problems so complex and problematic that they required inpatient hospitalization in order to prevent harm to themselves or others. We only had a brief time, at most three weeks, sometimes only a few days, to help put them back together again – at least with sufficient control to enable them to function again outside a hospital and continue their therapeutic journey. In treating people with what we now call complex PTSD, we became very aware of how each person unconsciously reenacted their traumatic wounds in interactions with us. That is how my colleague, Joe Foderaro came to comment one day on the changes that we as staff had made by pointing out that we had stopped asking people "What's wrong with you?" and instead, were now asking "What happened to you?". By focusing on what had happened to them in the past and on our interactions with them in the present, we could determine that the roles of Victim, Persecutor, and Rescuer constituted the stories of their painful lives. Over and over the rotating inevitability of these roles had led to despair and hopelessness that anything in their lives ever would change for the better, and the resultant demoralization was at the heart of depression, suicidality, and all the forms of self-harming behavior that had precipitated hospitalization.

Known as the "drama triangle," first articulated by Stephen Karpman and embedded in Transactional Analysis, we came to recognize that understanding the traumatic script they were trapped in and then using our relationship with them as a way to help them out of the trap, to rescript the story, was a critical component of healing (Karpman, 1968). Using this knowledge, we achieved remarkable results, radically different from our previous approach to treatment. The Therapeutic Spiral Model in Chapter 3 carries on where Karpman left off in articulating what happens as a result of trauma. Our intensive exposure to psychodrama with all of our patients had sensitized us to understanding that behavior is language – the only language available to the nonverbal hemisphere of the brain, the part of us that many now believe is the unconscious mind. I have always wondered if what our patients actually experienced in their stay with us was a ritual passage, driven in part by the nature of our psychodrama program at the time: one week to be the audience for other people's psychodrama, another to serve as an auxiliary, and the last to do one's own transformative piece of drama. Simultaneously, as staff, we could use the first week to participate in and begin to understand their reenactment behavior, the second week to help them decide if they wanted to change that enactment, and the third week to rehearse with us that change. It was not clear to me at the time, but I think we were actually developing a therapeutic program that was integrating knowledge, feelings, sensations, and memories from the two hemispheres of the brain and I suspect that just such an integration is necessary for healing to occur.

As we became more aware of the traumatic origins of most of the psychiatric problems that we were treating, I began searching for other people who were having the same discoveries. I attended my first meeting of the International Society for Traumatic Stress Studies (ISTSS) in 1989, in San Francisco, not long after people there had experienced a significant earthquake. I was so stimulated by finding other people doing trauma work – many working with combat survivors – that I returned home and immediately suggested to the officers of the ISTSS that there needed to be a Special Interest Group for Inpatient and Partial Hospitalization. They gave me the go-ahead and in

1990, our Special Interest Group met for the first time and one of the people who joined the group was David Read Johnson. David is a psychologist AND was trained in psychodrama, so we had much to discuss. Sometime in the next couple of years at yet another ISTSS meeting, I went to a presentation that he and his partner, Hadar Lubin, a psychiatrist, gave on the dramatic enactments they did with Vietnam veterans to help them grieve the loss of their friends. Since then, David has made substantial contributions to the field in books he has co-written or co-edited about drama therapy, while Hadar and David have contributed a group therapy manual focused on women and a book focusing on trauma treatment (Johnson & Emunah, 2020; Johnson & Lubin, 2015; Lubin & Johnson, 2012; Sajnani & Johnson, 2014). Scott's book is an important and necessary addition to the field about the specific aspects of psychodrama to a trauma-informed knowledge base on the uses of the dramatic arts in treatment as well as the implications of this work for organizations and for leaders.

I read somewhere that Moreno requested that his epitaph would be "The man who brought joy and laughter to psychiatry". In my experience, he was successful at that – at least for this psychiatrist. I closed our program in 2001, so I no longer had my daily exposure to psychodrama. Wanting to experience more of participatory drama myself, I registered for several months of a workshop in Playback Theater in my local community with an all-male group except for me. I don't think I ever before or since spent so many hours laughing and enjoying the company and revelations of the group. I have also witnessed Playback Theater being used as a dramatic form of social education and activism, along the lines of what Moreno described as sociodrama as Scott reveals in this book. I live in Philadelphia, a city that is composed of about 50% white people and 50% black and brown people. I recall several years ago that Playback Theater did three sessions with audiences – one for only white people, another for only black and brown people, and the third for everyone. I was traveling a lot at the time, so I only had the opportunity to attend the first session which was for white people only. On the stage were lined up all of the members of Playback, a very diverse group of people, and when they introduced the process, they dramatically asked all of the black and brown people to leave the stage and exit the room. Each one of them walked down the steps, off the stage, walked slowly through the auditorium and left. I vividly recall the feelings of loss and sadness I felt as those members of my community were cast out. I have no words to adequately describe that absence. But that's the power of drama.

In 2010, I was honored by Creative Alternatives of New York (CANY) for my work in delineating trauma-informed care. The annual gala, *Broadway at the Boathouse*, was held at the Loeb Central Park Boathouse and was hosted by some of Broadway's finest actors. CANY, founded in 1983, spent decades providing drama therapy to vulnerable populations all over New York City, using a trauma-informed approach in the later years. CANY drew on my work as a result of my relationship with one of their long-time board members, David McCorkle. David was in the original Broadway cast of *Hello Dolly*, then went on to get a degree in social work and ended up as the facilitator for the implementation of my work into three residential programs for children owned by the Jewish Board of Family and Children's Services in New York under a grant from the National Institutes of Mental Health. Our shared love of the theater brought us together as colleagues and friends. Through CANY I also met Craig Haen, another drama therapist who was then serving as the Workshop Director for CANY and since then has contributed to the use of drama therapy especially with young people (Weber & Haen, 2004). Consistent with the despair I began this with CANY lost funding a few years ago and no longer exists.

At this point in time, when our democracy is threatened, when there are more women and children enslaved through human sex trafficking than ever before in history, when the rights of woman are scorned, when people of color still must deal with racial discrimination on a daily basis, and the rights of gender nonconforming people are threatened – as is the safety of all living things on Earth – and while we know that most people in all of our societies have experienced trauma in childhood, a book to encourage more training, research, and funding of trauma-informed expressive therapies, especially psychodrama, is timely, important, and overdue.

Sandra L. Bloom, MD
Associate Professor, Health Management and Policy,
Dornsife School of Public Health, Drexel University
Chair of the Campaign for Trauma-Informed Policy and Practice
Philadelphia, PA, USA

References

Garcia, A., & Buchanan, D. R. (2009). Psychodrama. In D. Johnson, & R. Emunah (Eds.), *Current approaches in drama Therapy* (pp. 393–423). Springfield, IL: Charles C. Thomas.

Johnson, D. R., & Emunah, R. (2020). *Current approaches in drama therapy* (3rd ed.). Springfield, IL: Charles C. Thomas.

Johnson, D. R., & Lubin, H. (2015). *Principles and techniques of trauma-centered psychotherapy*. Washington, DC: American Psychiatric Association Publishing.

Jones, M. (1953). *The therapeutic community; a new treatment method in psychiatry* (1st ed.). New York: Basic Books.

Karpman, S. B. (1968). Fairy tales and script drama analysis. *Transactional Analysis Bulletin, 7*(26), 39–43.

Lubin, H., & Johnson, D. R. (2012). *Trauma-centered group psychotherapy for women: A clinician's manual*. New York: Routledge.

Moreno, J. L. (2019). *Autobiography of a genius: Jacob L. Moreno*. United Kingdom: Northwest Psychodrama Association.

Sajnani, N., & Johnson, D. R. (2014). *Trauma-informed drama therapy: Transforming clinics, classrooms, and communities*. Springfield, IL: Charles C. Thomas.

Shay, J. (1995). 'The birth of tragedy—Out of the needs of democracy'. In *DIDASKALIA: ANCIENT THEATER TODAY*: v2.n2. https://www.didaskalia.net/issues/vol2no2/shay.html

Shay, J. (2003). *Odysseus in America: Combat trauma and the trials of homecoming*. New York: Simon and Schuster.

Weber, A. M., & Haen, C. (2004). *Clinical applications of drama therapy in child and adolescent treatment*. New York: Bruner-Routledge.

Acknowledgments

There are countless people who deserve acknowledgment in the completion of this book. I'd like to first explicitly acknowledge the clients, students, and trainees who have been harmed and retraumatized in group therapy, psychodrama, or by organizational leaders. Their feedback, experiences, and suggestions fortified a need and desire to write this book for me. I hope that this book might give voice to some of these painful experiences while offering group therapists, psychodramatists, and leaders a framework for preventing retraumatization or harm in their work going forward. This has been the primary source of motivation to write this book. My clients, students, and trainees are constantly inspiring and challenging me to refine my clinical practice, leadership, writing, teaching, and research.

I'd like to also acknowledge SAMHSA for their dedication to trauma-informed care and synthesizing trauma-informed care guidance and principles while making their publications free to the public. Without this foundation of trauma-informed care principles and philosophy, this book would have been much more difficult to write. I also extend my gratitude to my team at the Phoenix Center for Experiential Trauma Therapy, colleagues at Mirmont Treatment Center, and faculty at Bryn Mawr College Graduate School of Social Work & Social Research who have helped me to grow more fully into my own leadership and have graciously offered me feedback, affirmation, and critiques over the years. Special thanks to the many role models of leadership I have had including various therapists, colleagues, supervisors, trainers, and professors. I also extend my gratitude to my wife, Maria Sotomayor-Giacomucci for her encouragement, patience, and feedback about the book content and my writing process. Throughout the past year or so of writing, she (and our puppy Azul) provided me with love, support, and many much-needed reminders to take a break from writing.

Thank you to the team at Routledge for the warm reception of this book idea and the administrative and logistical support throughout the publishing process. I would like to thank various colleagues who read this book draft to provide feedback on the content, structure, and helped with proofreading – Edward Schreiber, Leticia Nieto, Maria Sotomayor-Giacomucci, and Lincoln Blackwell. Thank you to Sandy Bloom for her willingness to support me and write the foreword of this book. I also would like to thank the anonymous peer-reviewers who provided helpful feedback and encouragement on the book proposal. And finally, thank you reader, for your interest in this book and your demonstrated commitment to continued learning, reflection, and growth.

Figures

1.1 Jacob L. Moreno, MD, the founder of psychodrama   11

1.2 SAMHSA's six trauma-informed principles   17

1.3 SAMHSA's Ten Agency Domains for Trauma-Informed Practice   19

1.4 Trauma-informed and trauma-focused services   22

2.1 The encounter symbol (republished with permission from Giacomucci, 2021b, p. 59)   46

2.2 The three phases of a psychodrama group   49

2.3 Moreno's Canon of Creativity (republished with permission from Giacomucci, 2021b, p. 62)   50

2.4 Moreno's stages of role development   54

2.5 Roles and their relation to the biopsychosocial self   55

2.6 The social atom (republished with permission from Giacomucci, 2021b, p. 88)   57

2.7 Sociogram of a classroom (republished with permission from Giacomucci, 2021b, p. 91)   59

3.1 The five domains of posttraumatic growth   74

3.2 TSM trauma triangle role transformations (reprinted with permission from Giacomucci, 2021b, p. 138)   87

4.1 SAMHSA's six trauma-informed principles (republished with permission from Giacomucci, 2021b, p. 128)   105

5.1 Norms and rules to establish safety in group therapy   145

6.1 Relationship between transparency and trustworthiness   161

6.2 Trust in one's supervisor is fueled by a demonstration of
     benevolence, competence, and integrity   161

10.1 Cultural, historic, and gender issues in each of the ten
     agency domains   232

10.2 Jacob and Zerka Moreno in Amsterdam in 1971   237

11.1 Simplified process of traumatic countertransference fueling
     burnout   252

11.2 Five domains of posttraumatic growth (republished from
     Giacomucci, 2021, p. 170)   254

11.3 Behavioral and interpersonal variables contributing to
     vicarious posttraumatic growth   255

Tables

2.1 Strategies for integrating trauma-informed principles into group teletherapy, inspired by Gerber, Elisseou, Sager, and Keith (2020)   38

2.2 Models of group development stages   41

2.3 Three stage models of trauma therapy   43

2.4 Simplified comparison of three stage group development and trauma therapy models   44

3.1 Prescriptive roles and functions (reprinted with permission from Giacomucci, 2018, p. 117)   85

5.1 Five types of safety to consider in organizations and groups   134

11.1 SAMHSA's trauma-informed philosophy outlined in the four "R"s, six principles, and ten agency domains   257

12.1 Four main ethical paradigms for leadership (articulated by Bloom & Farragher, 2011)   284

About the Author

Dr. Scott Giacomucci, DSW, LCSW, BCD, CGP, FAAETS, TEP

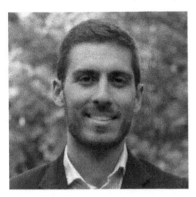

Scott is the Director/Founder of the Phoenix Center for Experiential Trauma Therapy in Media, Pennsylvania and Director of Trauma Services at Mirmont Treatment Center. He is a Research Associate and an Adjunct Professor at Bryn Mawr College's Graduate School of Social Work & Social Research teaching a course on trauma-focused psychodrama. Scott completed his Doctorate in Clinical Social Work (DSW) from the University of Pennsylvania and is recognized as a board-certified diplomate of clinical social work (BCD). He is also a Fellow of the American Academy of Experts in Traumatic Stress (FAAETS), certified EMDR Consultant, Certified Group Psychotherapist (CGP), and Board-Certified Trainer, Educator & Practitioner in Sociometry, Psychodrama, and Group Psychotherapy (TEP). He serves on the Executive Council of the American Society of Group Psychotherapy and Psychodrama (ASGPP). He is a co-chair of ASGPP's research committee, was a founding member of ASGPP's Sociatry and Social Justice Committee, and is a Co-Chief-Editor of the *Journal of Psychodrama, Sociometry, and Group Psychotherapy*.

His open-access book, *Social Work, Sociometry, & Psychodrama* (2021, Springer Nature), has been downloaded over 225,000 times and received multiple awards. He has published over a dozen peer-reviewed articles including an ongoing line of mixed-methods research on trauma-focused psychodrama. Scott is the recipient of various national and international awards, including the first recipient of the National Association of Social Workers' (NASW) Emerging Social Work Leader Award, the 2019 Group Practice Award from ACA's Association of Specialists in Group Work (ASGW), and the 2022 ASGPP David Kipper Scholar Award for his psychodrama scholarship. He presents regularly at regional, national, and international events and offers trauma-focused psychodrama training at the Phoenix Center in Pennsylvania. He co-edited the *Autobiography of a Genius* in 2019, written by psychodrama's founder, Jacob Moreno, MD. Scott also serves as co-editor of the first international psychodrama book series recently announced by Springer Nature titled, *Psychodrama in Counselling, Coaching, and Education.*

1

Introduction to Trauma-Informed Group Therapy, Psychodrama, and Leadership

Chapter Summary

Leadership in groups and organizations carries with it a significant responsibility. There is an equally great potential for harm, as well as empowerment and healing within groups, psychodrama, and organizations. The inherent power in these methods necessitates that facilitators incorporate trauma-informed principles to ensure safe, effective, and ethical practice. The goal of this book is to provide a comprehensive integration of trauma-informed principles with the practice of group work, psychodrama, and leadership. Trauma-informed principles will be presented as core ethical values while organizational leadership will be framed through the lens of group leadership. The synergy of experiential methods from psychodrama and trauma-informed approaches will be depicted as beneficial for all group workers and organizational leaders. This chapter presents an introduction to psychodrama, group work, trauma-informed philosophy, and to the author's experience with the topic.

Leaders in organizations and group work are entrusted with the well-being and care of others. Psychodrama, the creative arts therapies, and group therapy are powerful methods. They carry with them the capacity for both tremendous healing and potential harm. These potentialities become exponentially more pronounced when working with trauma survivors. As such, it is essential that all practitioners and leaders be aware of the pervasive impacts of trauma and the basics of trauma-informed principles to incorporate into our work.

DOI: 10.4324/9781003277859-1

This book is designed to promote trauma-informed practice within group work, psychodrama, and leadership but also within the creative arts therapies, group therapy, experiential psychotherapy, education, and training. Content in this book is intended to challenge practitioners and leaders to critically reflect on their practice while integrating trauma-informed principles to prevent retraumatization or adverse outcomes and ensure the highest standards for ethical practice. While chapters will be largely focused on psychotherapeutic aspects of psychodrama and group work practice, the insights and teaching of trauma-informed practice are applicable and relevant to all creative arts therapists and group workers, as well as those working outside of psychotherapy contexts such as in healthcare, education, government, activism, law, communities, and other service providers. All organizations use groups of some sort – for supervision, training, meetings, boards, or committees; therefore, organizational leaders can also benefit from learning of trauma-informed group work and experiential facilitation processes. Trauma-informed care can not only help improve clinical outcomes but also help leaders address and prevent vicarious trauma that many in the field are prone to experience. Group work and psychodrama offer trauma-informed leaders with tools to transform vicarious trauma into vicarious posttraumatic growth.

Psychodrama previously developed a reputation for being overly cathartic, overwhelming, and retraumatizing for some participants. This was the result of professionals implementing psychodrama techniques without adequate training, supervision, and without awareness of trauma-informed principles. Through this book, my hope is to provide psychodramatists and other practitioners with essential teaching related to trauma-informed practice. As psychodrama continues to spread around the world and re-establish its popularity within the United States, I believe that we have an ethical imperative to integrate trauma-informed principles into these methods. Without this crucial aspect, we risk causing potential harm to participants, neglecting vital knowledge to enhance our practice, and jeopardizing the reputation of the method.

My Journey with Psychodrama and Trauma-Informed Work

I was introduced to psychodrama and group work as an adolescent through my own personal growth journey and immediately experienced its "catching force." As a new (and resistant) psychotherapy client, the playfulness of psychodrama helped me to engage in the process while letting my guard down. At the same time, the group aspect helped me combat my sense of isolation and depression. The power of the enactment pulled me in like an emotional movie and compelled me to support my peers. The group cathar-ses and learning were shared by all. Psychodrama helped me to renegotiate traumatic loss, my relationships to drugs and alcohol, family and relationship dynamics, manage anxiety, develop social skills, and emerge as a relatively healthy adult living a life with purpose. Passion for the method, as demon-strated by the group therapists, was profound. As I matured into an adult and left home for college, I was inspired by the psychodramatists I had worked with and I wanted to have the same passion as I saw in them, for my work.

Having been a therapy client with psychodrama and gestalt therapists, I entered my Bachelor of Psychology program expecting to learn about both and was disappointed to hear almost no reference to psychodrama and little mention of group work in my four years of undergraduate study. During my freshman year, I landed a job as an overnight clinical aid at an addiction treatment center where I provided support services and began to lead my first groups. Throughout my time in undergraduate school, I also substituted as a facilitator of court-mandated Driving Under the Influence (DUI) classes and led groups on substance use in the local prisons and juvenile detention centers.

After completing my bachelor's degree, I entered a Master of Social Services/ Work program where I was disappointed again to experience little to no mention of psychodrama or even group work in general. Like many other MSW programs, my graduate program offered one optional elective on group therapy. I later learned of the historic decline of group work in social work education and its lack of representation within psychology and counseling programs. At this time, I was very involved in coordinating recovery and peer support meetings in juvenile detention centers and later prisons in Philadelphia and its surrounding counties.

My first-year internship was at the Juvenile Law Center where I worked with young people that had been sentenced to life without parole after murder convictions. Our objective was to secure resentencing for our clients and to advocate for policy changes at the state and federal levels. This field place-ment allowed me to play a small role in a movement that ultimately resulted in the 2016 US Supreme Court ruling in *Montgomery vs Louisiana*. This case upheld that sentencing youth to life without parole was unconstitutional and applied this retroactively, which gave hope to over 2,000 inmates for resen-tencing. Through my work in the prisons, the insidious impact of oppression, collective trauma, neglect, and loss became too clear to ignore. It seemed that nearly everyone I worked with in both the prison and the addiction treatment center had experienced significant trauma, childhood adversity, neglect, or loss that appeared to have had a direct impact on their mental health, substance use, relationships, behavior, as well as the crimes they committed.

My work in the prisons and courts also propelled me into other activist movements related to addiction and mental illness, the private prison system, corrupt business practices, anti-racism, immigration reform, and wars in the Middle East. Through countless discussions with my wife, Maria Sotomayor-Giacomucci – a former leader in the Pennsylvania immigration activism movement, we came to realize the lack of trauma-informed principles integrated into community work and activism. All social injustice is collective trauma; therefore, trauma-informed principles become especially helpful at preventing retraumatization while promoting safety, healing, empowerment, and corrective experiences within community and activism spaces as well.

In my early 20s, I began traveling around the world. I worked overnight shift throughout my years as a student and saved all my extra money for solo international trips which I had figured out how to plan on incredibly small budgets. I spent time in Mexico, South and Central America, Europe, North Africa, the Middle East, and Asia. Instead of spending time in tourist areas, I explored places that nobody that I knew had been to and learned enough Spanish and Arabic to get by. I slept regularly in airports, buses, train stations, and hostels. I learned of history, religion, mysticism, mythology, existentialism, and the philosophy of everyday people around the world. I often traveled to places of people who had inspired me in history – authors, teachers, psychologists, philosophers, religious leaders, poets, artists, and activists. Through my traveling, I had direct encounters with communities, cultures, religions, political systems, and social problems that I would have never been exposed to in the white, Christian, middle class suburbs I grew up in. These trips expanded my sense of self, sense of culture, and my sense of the world. Though my exposure was limited, traveling illuminated for me the extraordinary tragedy, trauma, and oppression around the globe (including in the United States), as well as the astonishing resilience, goodness, and love in the world. Traveling continues to be a meaningful part of my life today, often providing me with a sense of adventure, wonder, gratitude, and reminders of the various privileges I experience in the world. In another paper, I outline how traveling helped me develop skills that are indispensable as a trauma therapist, social worker, and psychodramatist (Giacomucci, 2018b).

My second-year internship was at Mirmont Treatment Center, also my place of employment, where I was quickly hired as an addiction counselor before my graduation. During the internship, I worked closely with the counselor who had developed the center's new trauma program just a few months prior. This placement provided me with an opportunity to help further develop and fine-tune a new trauma program while learning and practicing trauma therapy every day. My supervisors and the clinical director empowered me to contribute to the program development in meaningful ways, including beginning to introduce psychodrama and experiential therapy to the groups.

In my final year of my Master's program, I focused my clinical papers on trauma and psychodrama, while also beginning my training in another trauma therapy – Eye-Movement Desensitization and Reprocessing (EMDR). Luckily for me, the national psychodrama conference happened to be in Philadelphia that year which made it easy to attend as I lived nearby. At my first conference, I dove headfirst into the psychodrama community attending as many presentations as I could while networking and establishing what have become meaningful and lasting professional connections. Shortly after I began intensive psychodrama training in classical psychodrama with Dave Moran, sociatry and Morenean philosophy/mysticism with Ed Schreiber, and the Therapeutic Spiral Model of clinically modified psychodrama for trauma therapy with Kate Hudgins. These three trainers provided me with a unique blend of teaching and mentoring based on their roles and specialties. Kate is a trauma expert, clinical psychologist, and scholar-practitioner who created the Therapeutic Spiral Model while regularly teaching internationally. Ed is an addictions counselor, sociatrist, adjunct professor, and psychodrama historian who emphasizes the Morenean mystical and social justice traditions. Dave is a clinical social worker, treatment center senior administrator, and former president of the American Society of Group Psychotherapy and Psychodrama (ASGPP). The balanced alchemy of learning from these three mentors has continued to be invaluable throughout my professional life.

After completing my Master's program, I worked full time as an addictions counselor while co-facilitating the trauma program groups, while also offering EMDR to clients at the center. Little time had elapsed before I began receiving outpatient trauma therapy referrals, to which I decided to start a private practice. When my former supervisor left Mirmont to pursue a doctorate, I was offered a new role as the Trauma Treatment Specialist, which over time morphed into a part-time consulting role as Director of Trauma Services. This position allowed me to work closely with others in developing a robust trauma program expanding our offerings of EMDR, psychodrama, and experiential therapies to patients at the center, while providing supervision, training, and consultation to therapists throughout the entire health system and treatment continuum.

In 2016, I had the opportunity to visit the co-founder of psychodrama, Zerka Moreno just months before her death. My encounter with Zerka was deeply purposeful and spiritual. Being in her presence was a powerful and personal experience. While sharing space with her, I was inspired to articulate to her a commitment to help carry the psychodramatic method to the next generation. This visit had a profound impact on me, igniting a steadfast purpose to teach, research, and promote psychodrama. This book is fueled by this same commitment.

Within the next year, I applied and was accepted into the Doctorate of Clinical Social Work (DSW) program at the University of Pennsylvania. Here, I had the privilege to learn from internationally recognized trauma experts Sandra Bloom and Christine Courtois, as well as Lawrence Shulman an expert in social work with groups, teaching, and supervision. My doctoral dissertation focused on the decline of group work in social work education, and I developed an MSW curriculum that integrated social work with groups, psychodrama, and trauma therapy (Giacomucci, 2019, 2021c). I began teaching this course curriculum at Bryn Mawr College Graduate School of Social Work and Social Research annually since 2018. In the development of my dissertation, I discovered a huge gap in the literature related to the integration of social work and psychodrama which later inspired me to write my first book, *Social Work, Sociometry, and Psychodrama: Experiential Approaches for Group Therapists, Community Leaders, and Social Workers* (Giacomucci, 2021b – a freely available open-access publication by Springer Nature).

While in my doctorate program, I was elected to the Executive Council of the ASGPP, appointed as chair of the research committee, and served as co-editor in the publication of the founder of psychodrama's *Autobiography of a Genius* (Moreno, 2019). My DSW program also helped prepare me as a researcher, which led to an ongoing line of research on the effectiveness of trauma-focused psychodrama (see Giacomucci & Marquit, 2020; Giacomucci, Marquit, & Miller-Walsh, 2022; Giacomucci, Marquit, Miller-Walsh, & Saccarelli, 2022). As my career progressed, I began writing, teaching, and training regularly at local universities or treatment programs, national/international conferences, and creating my own ongoing psychodrama training group.

Concurrently, my clinical practice expanded quickly, driving me to expand from a solo private practice to a growing group practice called the Phoenix Center for Experiential Trauma Therapy. The Phoenix Center was not something I initially intended to create. It grew from the community demand for trauma therapy, experiential trauma therapy training, and from colleagues or former interns asking for employment opportunities. My solo private practice became a group practice largely based on the determination of a former graduate intern requesting to work with me. I declined her requests to hire her multiple times out of fear and uncertainty of how to run a larger business. After several months of being warmed-up to the idea, I changed my position and agreed to hire her under the condition that she grant me patience, grace, and time, as I figured out the mechanics of how to run a group practice. Since becoming a group practice in fall 2018, the center has grown exponentially to employ over 15 trauma therapists and 8 graduate interns. The growth of the business challenged me to fully step into leadership, and learn how to be a leader, while also learning how to run a business. In this process, I found humility, authenticity, ethics, and consultation to be indispensable. I often still joke with my staff that I'm not fully sure what I am doing as a center director/owner and that I am making it up as we go.

I intend to approach the topics in this book with a sense of humility, especially the topic of leadership, as there are many other professionals that have much more experience than I in these areas. Looking back, I am convinced that my ongoing learning to be an effective leader was/is a compilation of learning from my other roles. Ethics, integrity, and doing the right thing were ingrained into me through my own personal work and recovery process. My experience as an activist instilled a sense of passion and commitment to addressing injustice in the world. I learned how to lead others first as a group therapist, then as a trainer and educator. My competencies as a group leader made my transition to teacher/trainer much easier, approaching teaching as a form group work. In a similar way, I've also approached organizational leadership through the role of a group worker – as organizations are also groups. My training as a sociometrist and psychodramatist enhanced my understanding of sociodynamics in groups/organizations while providing spontaneity training – learning how to have adequate responses to new situations and new responses to old reoccurring situations. As an academic and researcher, I learned the importance of trying to take an unbiased perspective, see things from multiple angles, and appreciate the complexities of the world. This book is the culmination of all my professional experiences and emerges from the intersection of my professional roles as a person in long-term recovery, former therapy client, trauma expert, psychodramatist, group therapist, social worker, activist, adjunct professor, trainer, supervisor, researcher, trauma therapy center director/owner, and leader. Unfortunately, the impetus to write this book also arises from stories of retraumatization

I hear from clients participating in psychodrama and other therapies, my own experiences of witnessing psychodrama employed in ways that were potentially harmful, unethical practice in psychodrama and larger psychotherapy communities, and the continued negative reputation that some maintain about psychodrama. The mission of this book is to support psychodramatists, group workers, trauma therapists, and other professionals in integrating trauma-informed practices for ethical, safer, and effective work.

At the start of this book, I also find it important to name that this book emerges from my own personal and professional perspectives which are surely impacted by my social location in both positive and limiting ways. I am a white, cis-gender, heterosexual man. I have lived most of my life in middle class suburbs of Philadelphia – the ancestral land of the Lenape people. I am 30 years old and am a person in long-term recovery from substance use and mental illness. I am a US-born citizen and fourth generation European-American of Italian, Hungarian, and German descent. I grew up in the Catholic Church, though as a young adult I immersed myself into other religions and spiritual/philosophical traditions (including Islam, Buddhism, and shamanism), but I do not identify with any single religion. I have provided training in various countries and traveled around the world, which has had a profound impact on my perspectives, but most of my work and life has been in the United States. My life and work have been influenced by US cultural values such as individualism, independence, self-reliance, the struggle toward equality, materialism, hard work, efficiency/timeliness, and democracy. My own identity, privilege, experience, trauma, loss, and adversity undoubtedly have an impact on my thinking and practice. This book is written through the lens of my own culture, biases, limitations, beliefs, strengths, and experiences. I encourage you as readers to consider this in your reading and to critically reflect on how to adapt ideas from this book into your own practice and cultural contexts.

Group Work and Group Therapy

This book will orient primarily to group therapy and psychodrama in trauma-informed contexts. Before going further, I believe it is important to differentiate group work and group therapy while also locating psychodrama within these realms. Group therapy is primarily focused on clinical implementation of group work within treatment contexts, while group work has a much wider scope including group therapy, community work, educational groups, skill-building groups, task groups, study groups, affinity groups, groups for social action and activism, supervision groups, training groups, and organizational groups (Giacomucci, 2019). *Group therapy* is a type of *group work*; psychodrama is used in both group therapy and group work contexts. Because his work has been largely marginalized in the United States, many don't realize that psychodrama's founder, Jacob Moreno was actually the first to use the terms "group therapy" and "group psychotherapy" (Moreno & Whitin, 1932). Throughout this book, I will use the terms "group therapy" and "group psychotherapy" interchangeably.

I also find it important to note that I write this book as a professional mainly trained as a social group worker and psychodramatist, albeit I am also versed in group counseling, psychodynamic group psychotherapy, and group psychology – maintaining memberships in ACA's Association of Specialists in Group Work, APA Division 49 for Group Psychology and Group Psychotherapy, American Group Psychotherapy Association, and the International Association of Group Psychotherapy & Group Processes. While social work with groups, group counseling, group psychotherapy, group psychology, and psychodramatic group work have many fundamental similarities, there are some core differences, varying nuances, and different cultures of practice within each community.

Regardless of one's specific group orientation, group work and group therapy in general are in high demand. Every social service agency uses groups in their programs and all professional is a member of various groups (Zastrow, 2001). Therapy groups are used throughout every level of care in the treatment continuum, and all professionals participate in organizational groups, supervision groups, and training groups. The receptibility and popularity of group work is likely related to the power of groups, the increased research demonstrating its effectiveness, and its cost-efficiency in providing treatment (Giacomucci, 2019). Group therapy research has developed considerably in the past few decades, indicating that it is at least as effective as individual therapy for a multitude of clinical issues and diagnoses (Wodarski & Feit, 2012; Yalom & Leszcz, 2020). Unfortunately, while the practice of group therapy increased in the field, the group therapy education and training provided by university programs diminished significantly (Yalom & Leszcz, 2005; Drum, Becker, & Hess, 2010; Sweifach, 2014). Perhaps the most dramatic example of loss in group work education is in the social work field where group work used to be offered as an entire concentration in 76% of MSW programs in 1963. This dropped to 22% in 1981, 7% in 1992, and 2% in 2014 (Birnbaum & Auerbach, 1994; Drumm, 2006; Simon & Kilbane, 2014). While group work concentrations used to be popular, they are now nearly extinct. Simon and Kilbane (2014) also found that about 20% of MSW programs don't have a single course in group work offered to students, 58% have a required group work course, and 40% offer an optional course in group work.

One of the most famous therapists alive, Irvin Yalom, MD, warns us that:

> It is abundantly clear that, as time passes, we will rely on group approaches ever more heavily. I believe that any psychotherapy training program that does not acknowledge this and does not expect students to become as fully proficient in group as in individual therapy is failing to meet its responsibilities to the field.
>
> (2005, p. 544)

Most mental health professionals are expected to facilitate groups of some kind in their career but are not receiving the training required to do so competently (Clements, 2008; Sweifach & Heft-LaPorte, 2008; Goodman, Knight, & Khudododov, 2014; Yalom & Leszcz, 2020). This book strives to provide professionals with some of the core group work learning that may have been missing from their graduate programs. These same group work competencies are also helpful for organizational leaders as an organization is fundamentally a group. When it comes to working with trauma survivors, competence in one's area of practice becomes particularly more important due to the complexities of trauma and traumatic stress.

This publication also emerges at a unique time in the trajectory and inter-section of group work, psychodrama, and trauma work. In the past few years, interest in psychodrama has significantly increased in the United States (Giacomucci, 2021b) – especially as a treatment for trauma which has been popularized by leading trauma expert Bessel van der Kolk. At the same time, major milestones in group psychotherapy have been reached including the APA's formal recognition of group psychology and group psychotherapy as a specialty in 2018 and later in 2022 the approval of a new registry of evidence-based group therapies through APA's Division 49 of Group Psy-chology and Group Psychotherapy (Paxton & Harrison, 2022). As group psychotherapy and psychodrama continue to receive recognition in main-stream mental health dialogues, it will be essential that a foundation for trauma-informed group work and psychodrama has been established.

Introduction to Psychodrama and Sociometry

Psychodrama was developed by Jacob L. Moreno, MD, in the early 1900s (see Figure 1.1). Moreno first developed his existential, mystical, and social philosophies (see Chapter 2) in Vienna prior to immigrating to New York

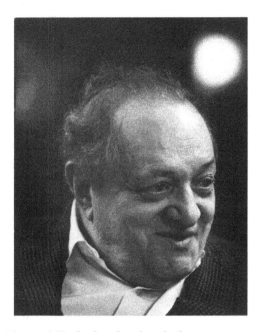

Figure 1.1 Jacob L. Moreno, MD, the founder of psychodrama.

in 1925 (Giacomucci, Karner, Nieto, & Schreiber, 2021). Psychodrama was the last of Moreno's creations, evolving from his mystical philosophy (1914, 1921), his experimental Theater of Spontaneity (1924), his group psychotherapy approach (1931), and his sociometric system (1934). Moreno writes that the first psychodrama took place on April 1, 1921, though he didn't start systematically organizing psychodrama as a psychotherapy until the opening of his New York mental health hospital in 1936 (Moreno, 2014). Moreno's methods, including his group therapy approach, psychodrama, sociometry, sociodrama, axiodrama, ethnodrama, the empty chair, and others, were inspired by his vision of Sociatry – healing for society. After studying medicine and psychiatry at the University of Vienna, he concluded that treating individuals alone was not sufficient but that a psychiatry for society, communities, and groups was needed (Moreno, 2019).

The term "psychodrama" is most regularly used to describe Moreno's entire triadic system of sociometry, psychodrama, and group psychotherapy. The practice of psychodrama is primarily employed within the context of the triadic system, which mirrors the three phases of a psychodrama group – warm-up (sociometry), action (psychodrama), and sharing (group psychotherapy) (Giacomucci, 2021b). Sociometry is defined as the study of interpersonal relationships, group dynamics, social networks, and the evolution of groups

(Moreno, 1953). Moreno believed that true group therapy was not possible until the development of group-as-a-whole assessment tools (1947). His sociometric system provides multiple tools for researching, assessing, and diagnosing the underlying dynamics within groups, communities, and social networks. The diagnostic tools for understanding the underlying dynamics of a social systems extend to the entire body of humanity as one organism; this relates to Moreno's vision of Sociatry – or healing for society. Moreno's sociometry, though largely neglected by group therapists, was adopted by sociologists, researchers, and social network theorists who credit Moreno as a forerunner of Participatory Action Research and the Social Network (Greenwood, 2015; Moreno, 2014; Treadwell, 2016). Moreno's sociometric tests and sociograms appear to have also influenced the development of the genogram and ecomaps decades later (Giacomucci, 2021b). Sociometric theory and research are mostly beyond the scope of this publication; however, Chapter 4 will present multiple experiential sociometry processes for group workers.

Psychodrama is an action-based approach for personal growth, psychotherapy, skills training, activism, and education. Some mistakenly believe that it is only used within mental health treatment contexts and, however, is also frequently employed in community, civic, and political arenas. Psychodrama utilizes aspects of role-playing and drama to help participants externalize their inner worlds or explore aspects of their social experience. Moreno defines psychodrama as a "science which explores the 'truth' by dramatic methods" (1972, p. a). The term "psychodrama" literally means "psyche in action" or "soul in action." Psychodrama is often categorized within the larger umbrellas of expressive arts therapies, creative arts therapies, experiential therapies, humanistic psychology, body- and movement-oriented approaches, or group therapies. Many mistakenly believe that psychodrama is just a set of interventions; however, the truth is that psychodrama is its own comprehensive system equipped with its own philosophy, theories, interventions, and modalities. Psychodrama was designed to be practiced as a comprehensive system but aspects of psychodrama can also be easily integrated into other systems such as social work (Giacomucci, 2019, 2021b; Giacomucci & Stone, 2019), cognitive-behavioral therapy (Treadwell, 2020), object relations (Holmes, 2015), positive psychology (Tomasulo, 2018), drama therapy (Casson, 2007; Landy, 2017), family constellations (Anderson & Carnabucci, 2011), and others.

A psychodrama enactment has five core elements – a director, the protagonist, auxiliary roles, an audience or other observing group members, and a stage (often the stage is simply the space of the group room). Psychodrama scenes vary based on the contract with the group and the protagonist but can include intrapsychic scenes, interpersonal scenes, spiritual or religious scenes, moments from the past, and future projections. Psychodrama scenes may be real or imagined. Roles in a psychodrama are also varied based on the protagonist's choices but can range from parts of self, feelings, defenses, belief systems, strengths, values, role models, archetypes, spiritual/religious figures or God, past or future versions of self, organizations, groups, and people in the protagonist's life. A psychodrama director employs a variety of interventions within a given psychodrama based on their discretion and training, which can include doubling, the mirror, role reversal, soliloquy, role training, and others. Psychodrama scenes are entirely spontaneous co-created enactments between the protagonist, the director, and the group. Enactments vary in their size, length, and number of scenes as well. While one psychodrama might include ten different roles, three scenes, and last for three hours, another psychodrama might only have one scene with two roles and last for 15 minutes.

Similar to psychodrama, Moreno also developed an approach called sociodrama. The difference between the two is that a psychodrama enacts an individual's story or topic whereas a sociodrama puts into action a collective topic or theme from the group or community (Giacomucci, 2017). Psychodrama uses personal roles ("John's mom") while sociodrama employs collective roles ("a mom") (Sternberg & Garcia, 2000). A sociodrama does not dramatize anyone's specific story but instead develops a co-created story representing the group and the group's collective response to themes and issues. This provides more aesthetic distance than a psychodrama and usually lends itself to more playfulness and emotional containment. As such, sociodrama tends to be used more in educational, community, and activist settings while psychodrama is used more often in psychotherapy. Sociodrama is structured similar to a psychodrama session with three phases, five elements, and the same options for interventions. This book will primarily orient on psychodrama enactments, but will also include sociodrama examples. Throughout future chapters, psychodrama methods will by synthesized with trauma-informed principles.

Introduction to Trauma-Informed Care

The emergence of trauma-informed care was influenced by the women's empowerment movement, the return of soldiers from the war in Vietnam, the formal recognition of posttraumatic stress disorder (PTSD) as a diagnosis in 1980 in the DSM-III, the 1994 SAMHSA Dare to Vision conference, and the Adverse Childhood Experience (ACE) studies in the 1990s (Felitti et al., 1998; Herman, 1992, Ringel & Brandell, 2011; van der Kolk, 2014). The pervasive nature of trauma and its underlying impact on a multitude of mental health and medical issues propelled professionals to give more attention to trauma. At the same time, the prevalence of retraumatization experienced by patients during their treatment processes (Wilson, Pence, & Conradi, 2013). By the early 2000s, multiple professionals were writing about trauma-informed care in organizations and treatment (Bloom, 1997; Covington, 2002; Harris & Fallot, 2001; Rivard, Bloom, & Abramovitz, 2003). These influences and developments in the field led to SAMHSA's 2014 publications synthesizing the literature on trauma-informed care and proposing best practices and principles (2014a, 2014b).

Trauma-informed care is a philosophy of providing services that accounts for the impacts that trauma has on individuals and the potential ways that service providers might aggravate pre-existing trauma, triggers, or vulner-abilities of those seeking care. Trauma-informed services are inherently strengths-based (Harris & Fallot, 2001). Trauma-informed organizations consciously avoid retraumatizing their clients while structuring the provi-sion of services to best support and meet clients where they are (SAMHSA, 2014b). Trauma-informed philosophy and principles can be incorporated into any agency including treatment centers, hospitals, social service organ-izations, universities, communities, prisons, and even entire government structures. Trauma-informed care is concerned not only with the impact of trauma upon community members and clients but also with the impact of vicarious trauma upon professionals and staff members (see Chapter 11 for more on this).

Multiple significant events took place at the end of the century from which contemporary trauma-informed care emerged. These included the continued acceptance and awareness of PTSD which was formally recognized as a diag-nosis in the DSM-III in 1980, the return of veterans from the Vietnam War and wars in the Middle East, the women's movements, the influx of new neu-roscience research on how trauma impacts the brain, the ACE study, and the 1994 Dare to Vision conference hosted by SAMHSA which focused on the prevalence of treatment consumers with trauma histories or experiencing retraumatization in treatment (Felitti et al., 1998; Herman, 1992; Ringel & Brandell, 2011; van der Kolk, 2014; Wilson, Pence, & Conradi, 2013). The intersecting momentum of each of these different movements, along with the evolution of theory, research, and practice in the trauma field, led to the emergence of trauma-informed care as we know it today.

There are many different aspects and nuances within a trauma-informed approach. In this section, some of the core ideas, assumptions, and principles will be presented. SAMHSA (2014a) outlines three "E"s of trauma – event, experience, and effect. In their process of synthesizing a workable definition of trauma, SAMHSA concludes that:

> Individual trauma results from an **event**, series of events, or set of circumstances that is **experienced** by an individual as physically or emotionally harmful or life threatening and that has lasting adverse **effects** on the individual's functioning and mental, physical, social, emotional, or spiritual well-being.
>
> (2014a, p. 7)

This definition of trauma is broad and inclusive while also reflecting the PTSD diagnostic criteria. It leaves room to consider that each individual will experience adversity in different ways and make sense of the experience differently. Specific events may be experienced as traumatic by some and not traumatic by others. This is likely impacted by culture, identity, social support, and the developmental stage of the individual. When someone experiences adversity and has a traumatic response to it, they experience negative effects from the trauma long after it has ended. Sometimes these impacts last longer than other times or their onset emerges sooner or later after the traumatic experience. The DSM-5 PTSD criteria is organized in four primary symptom clusters – intrusions and reexperiencing, arousal and reactivity, negative cognitions and mood states, and avoidance (APA, 2013). One of the simplest and most frequently used self-assessments for PTSD is the PCL-5 which is freely available online through the National Center for PTSD (www.ptsd.va.gov). While many previously believed trauma to be a rare occurrence, research suggests that 55–90% of people experience trauma in their lifetime and that many experience multiple traumatic events (Breslau, 2009; Kessler et al., 2017; Kilpatrick et al., 2013). Complex PTSD (CPTSD) has yet to be recognized in the DSM but has been established within the ICD-11. The diagnostic criteria for CPTSD builds off of PTSD symptomology with additional criteria related to emotional regulation, relational disturbances, and negative sense of self. There remains disagreement among professionals about whether CPTSD is its own separate condition or simply a more extreme and complicated version of PTSD. The International Trauma Questionnaire (ITQ) was developed as the first assessment instrument for both PTSD and CPTSD, based on ICD-11 criteria – it is available freely through The International Trauma Consortium (www.traumameasuresglobal.com). As the widespread impact and prevalence of trauma has become more recognized, there has been an increased attention to trauma-informed and trauma-focused approaches to care.

SAMHSA (2014a) describes four "R"s as key assumptions within a trauma-informed approach. A provider that operates from a trauma-informed framework implements the following four "R"s:

1) **Realizes** that trauma has extensive impacts on individuals and understands that there are multiple paths to recovering from trauma.
2) **Recognizes** the unique symptoms and manifestations of trauma or traumatic stress for individuals, groups, families, communities, and staff members.
3) **Responds** by implementing policies, procedures, and practices which are guided by trauma-informed principles.
4) **Resists Retraumatization** in all aspects of the work

These are essential, and perhaps even ethical, norms which support agencies in providing the highest quality care for the communities that they serve, especially trauma survivors.

Furthermore, SAMHSA (2014a) outlines six core principles of trauma-informed practice which serve to guide practitioners and organizations in embodying a trauma-informed care that prevents retraumatization and supports healing. SAMHSA defines trauma-informed care through these key principles (2014a):

1) **Safety:** Providers promote physical and emotional safety through the design of their facility, social interactions, and the provision of services. Providers seek to understand what safety means through the perspective and experience of those they serve.
2) **Trustworthiness and Transparency:** Decision-making at all levels is done with transparency for staff, clients, and the community in the spirit of establishing and maintaining trust.
3) **Peer Support:** Trauma survivors are incorporated as essential members of one's recovery process using their lived experiences to promote hope, safety, empathy, trust, collaboration, and meaning-making.
4) **Collaboration and Mutuality:** Power dynamics between various staff members and with clients are managed in a way that values each person, emphasizes each role as important, and distributes power and decision-making.
5) **Empowerment, Voice, and Choice:** Providers emphasize the resilience and autonomy of clients, communities, and staff. Everyone is empowered in decision-making, goal-setting, and self-advocacy. "Staff are facilitators

of recovery rather than controllers of recovery" (Brown, Baker, & Wilcox, 2012, as cited by SAMHSA, 2014a, p. 11).

6) **Cultural, Historical, and Gender Issues**: Organizations and practitioners actively address their own biases while developing practices and policies that are conducive to the needs and values related to the race, ethnicity, culture, religion, gender, sexuality, and age of those they serve and employ. The impact of historic and collective trauma or discrimination is acknowledged while mitigating the potential for reenactments of oppression and microaggressions. At the same time, the healing potential of cultural and identity values is leveraged and emphasized for clients when appropriate.

These six principles, which will this book will centralize, are depicted below (see Figure 1.2).

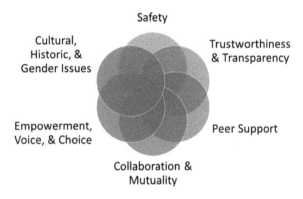

Figure 1.2 SAMHSA's six trauma-informed principles.

While these principles are presented separately, it is important to emphasize that each principle supports the others, and they exist in a state of interdependence. For example, safety can't exist without trustworthiness, transparency, mutuality, choice, and addressing cultural, historical, and gender issues; at the same time, safety promotes further trustworthiness, transparency, peer support, collaboration, mutuality, empowerment, and the elevation of unheard voices. SAMHSA's six trauma-informed principles overlap and are uniquely important. Each individual and each organization certainly operationalizes these six principles to varying degrees in the different aspects of their work. Future chapters of this book will offer a more comprehensive discussion on each of these six principles and how they can be employed by group workers, psychodramatists, and organizational leaders.

Which do you best embody in your work?

Which do you feel you have the most room to grow in?

Which does your organization best embody?

Which could your organization most grow in?

While many practitioners and organizations intuitively integrate trauma-informed principles into their work, it is also important that these principles are consciously worked on and implemented. Being trauma-informed requires critical examination and reflection by individuals and organizations. It isn't simply a buzzword to be thrown around, but a comprehensive philosophy that guides and informs policy, organizational structure, work culture, community engagement, and how services are provided.

Building upon the work of others (Bloom & Farragher, 2011; Harris & Fallot, 2001), SAMHSA (2014a) has also outlined ten organizational domains for consideration when developing a trauma-informed system. These ten domains are meant to help guide providers and practitioners implement trauma-informed principles into their work (see Figure 1.3). The articulation of these ten domains also illuminates how trauma-informed practice informs not only the ways in which treatment is provided but also every aspect of organizational structure and operations. While SAMHSA's publications on trauma-informed care are directed mostly at organizations, these principles and agency domains are also applicable to group workers. After all, an organization at its core is a group of professionals. The aforementioned ten agency domains can be extended to group workers as the ten domains of group practice as well. This guidance emphasizes that even agencies or groups that do not treat PTSD or provide psychotherapy are also working with trauma survivors and would benefit from the incorporation of trauma-informed principles into their work.

Which of the agency domains does my organization adequately integrate trauma-informed principles?

Which of the agency domains have the most room for trauma-informed growth in my organization?

---

10 AGENCY DOMAINS

1. Governance and Leadership
2. Policy
3. Physical Environment
4. Engagement and Involvement
5. Cross Sector Collaboration
6. Screening, Assessment, Treatment Services
7. Training and Workforce Development
8. Progress Monitoring & Quality Assurance
9. Financing
10. Evaluation

Figure 1.3 SAMHSA's Ten Agency Domains for Trauma-Informed Practice.

In Chapters 11 and 12, these concepts of trauma-informed organizations (and the threats to healthy organizations) will be covered in detail. Trauma-informed organizations approach not only clients but also staff with compassion, understanding, and care. It is essential that organizations and leaders are aware of the adverse impacts of traumatic countertransference, vicarious trauma, secondary traumatic stress, compassion fatigue, and burnout on staff and the organization-as-a-whole. Bloom (2013) writes that "organizations are not machines, but are living complex systems and as such are every bit as vulnerable to the impact of trauma and chronic stress as the people who receive and deliver service" (p. 14). Trauma-informed leaders approach their organization-as-a-whole as its own entity, likely with its own history of trauma, loss, resilience, and adaptation. The emergence of parallel processes between clients, staff, and the organization are examined while the needs of each are addressed.

Trauma-Informed Leadership

Trauma-informed leadership is an approach to leadership that incorporates trauma-informed care philosophy into one's approach and style of leadership. Trauma-informed leaders embody the six principles of trauma-informed care and utilize them as ethical guides for decision-making. A trauma-informed leader is an ethical professional who prioritizes the well-being of themselves, their staff, and those they work with – whether they be staff, clients, students, trainees, customers, or community members. Burnout, vicarious trauma, countertransference, and social injustice are adequately addressed while promoting self-care, peer support, trauma healing, vicarious posttraumatic growth, and social justice. The risks of retraumatization are considered in developing policy, implementing practices, and within the culture of the organization itself. In thinking about trauma-informed leadership, Brené Brown's definition of leader can guide us – "anyone who takes responsibility for finding the potential in people and processes, and who has the courage to develop that potential" (2018, p. 4). In many ways, this definition articulates the heart of being a trauma-informed professional – seeing the potential in the people (clients, staff, communities, etc.) we are working with. A trauma-informed leader implements the four R's (realize, recognize, respond, & resist retraumatization) within the ten agency domains outlined by SAMHSA, using the six trauma-informed principles as guides.

A trauma-informed leader acknowledges their own trauma, loss, countertransference, biases, privilege, limitations, weaknesses, and emotions while continuing to engage in their own personal growth. They lead with vulnerability, courage, authenticity, role modeling, and humility. They are willing to admit their faults, ask for help, discuss their limitations or weaknesses, and change their stance on issues. A trauma-informed leader emphasizes the importance of relationships and interacts with others in a way that is safe, trustworthy, supportive, collaborative, empowering, and honoring of each individual's worth and identities. A trauma-informed leader is both a nurturer and a protector. They also hold boundaries, provide containment, know when to say "no," and take a stand for what they believe in. Trauma-informed leaders recognize that they are there to serve others and are a vessel responsible for decision-making that aligns and re-aligns an organization with its mission and core values. They demonstrate humility in their leadership while helping others to become the best they can be.

My own approach to leadership is also influenced by my other roles, especially my work as a group therapist and psychodramatist. I approach leadership through the lens of group work – that many of the same responsibilities for group therapy facilitators transfer to organizational leaders. Similarly, many of the social phenomena and group interventions effective in group work are also useful knowledge and approaches within organizational leadership. As a psychodramatist, I subscribe to Jacob Moreno's core philosophy that each patient is a therapeutic agent for every other patient – and that each student is a teacher for every other student. I also strive to transfer this same philosophy in my leadership. As a leader, I hope to inspire and empower others to become leaders in their own right, based on their own strengths, preferences, and goals. My training as a psychodramatist and sociatrist also instilled within me, an awareness of the sociodynamic effect – the underlying social phenomenon that results in the unequal distribution of social wealth, resources, and privilege. I believe that trauma-informed leaders must always be aware of how the sociodynamic effect is at play within relationship, groups, organizations, communities, and society – it emphasizes the sixth trauma-informed principle considering cultural, historic, and gender issues. Trauma-informed leaders must consider their identities and socially ascribed membership in privileged or marginalized social groups while attending to the dynamic interplay of these layers of privilege and marginalization within their relationships and organizational dynamics.

I believe that trauma-informed systems require both a bottom-up approach and a top-down approach. Everyone from frontline staff to leadership must commit to trauma-informed care philosophy in a meaningful way. Without leadership's active involvement, a trauma-informed environment is almost impossible. Good leaders promote healthy work environments, mentor the next generation of professionals, and are constantly growing in both personal and professional realms. Trauma-informed leadership offers an ideal for organizational leaders, group work leaders, and psychodramatists.

The process of writing of this book was particularly transformative for me and challenged me to continue growing as a trauma-informed practitioner and leader. In the year it took to write this book, there were countless moments in my work life where I was full of anxiety and felt drawn to avoidance, inaction, or dissociation in a difficult situation. In those moments of stuckness, I often thought to myself "shit, I'm writing a book on trauma-informed leadership which means I really have to be practicing this stuff, even when it is difficult." My commitment to this book and to you as readers has made me a better leader and helped me to further embody trauma-informed principles in my own leadership.

Trauma-Informed vs Trauma-Focused Services

In discussions about trauma-informed care, it is essential that we also differentiate "trauma-informed services" and "trauma-focused services." Many mistakenly use the terms interchangeably, but there is an important difference (Giacomucci, 2021b). "Trauma-focused services" refer to practices that are directly provided for trauma survivors to address and/or treat PTSD. Trauma-informed services has a much larger scope, which includes trauma-focused services (see Figure 1.4).

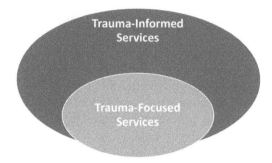

Figure 1.4 Trauma-informed and trauma-focused services.

The trauma-informed philosophy describes the processes by which services are provided and the larger context in which they are offered. Whereas trauma-focused services are dedicated to trauma-related content. One of the major differences then is that trauma-informed care highlights "process" while trauma-focused care centralizes trauma "content." Ideally, trauma-focused services are also offered within a trauma-informed framework. Unfortunately, this is not always the case as there are a multitude of examples of trauma treatment programs, practices, and providers that have been known to retraumatize participants without regard to the six trauma-informed principles. Sandra Bloom, renowned expert in trauma-informed care, suggests that "Trying to implement trauma-specific clinical interventions without first implementing trauma-informed cultural change is like throwing seeds on dry land" (Menschner & Maul, 2016, p. 2). It should be emphasized that learning to integrate and offer trauma-informed and trauma-focused services requires education, training, self-awareness, and commitment. Most trauma-focused approaches or treatments for PTSD demand extensive training and should not be offered by professionals outside the scope of their competency. Practitioners who are not aware of the limits of their practice risk retraumatizing participants, especially when attempting to implement more complex interventions. This is one of the problems that has negatively impacted the reputation of psychodrama and other complex trauma treatments.

Three-Stage Clinical Map for Trauma Work

When providing either trauma-informed or trauma-focused services, adherence to a three-stage clinical map can help ensure safety and effectiveness. Many trauma experts and trauma treatments propose three-stage clinical maps which tend to mirror each other (Chesner, 2020; Courtois & Ford,

2016; Giacomucci, 2018a; Herman, 1992; Hudgins & Toscani, 2013; Janet, 1889; Najavits, 2002; Shapiro, 2018). These clinical maps recommend pacing the content of sessions through the following three stages:

1) Safety, strengths, skills, education, connection, and containment
2) Trauma content, emotions, loss, defenses
3) Integration, transformation, posttraumatic growth, and future projections

These trajectory offers a way of cushioning the more difficult trauma content with positive content and fostering titration and pendulation in and out of the trauma. This not only promotes safety but also helps teach participants that they can consciously move in and out of trauma content rather than be pushing into it involuntarily or get stuck in it. These three stages have been written about extensively by others and can be used as a guide by group workers and psychodramatists for both trauma-informed and trauma-focused work. Hudgins and Toscani (2013) have been a driving force in integrating this clinical map into psychodrama practice through the development of Therapeutic Spiral Model. These three phases can help practitioners in structuring prompts for activities, choosing roles in psychodramatic work, and pacing content in any session including psychotherapy, community work, education, supervision, and organizational meetings (Giacomucci, 2020, 2021a, 2021b). Without the framework of a clinical map, practitioners may risk retraumatization or making decisions based on countertransference. In many ways, this three-stage clinical map helps practitioners to operationalize SAMHSA's six trauma-informed principles (see Chapter 2 for more background on the clinical map).

Trauma-Informed Practice as Ethical Imperative

Beyond arguments of effectiveness, one might also argue that consideration of trauma-informed principles is an ethical directive for practitioners and leaders of all types – especially those providing trauma-focused services. The six trauma-informed principles outlined above can also be considered ethical principles. Like other ethical principles, trauma-informed principles offer moral and practical guidance on how to make decisions for the highest good of others and society. Ethical standards are articulated for the primary purpose of informing professionals how to act while ensuring safety and protection for those they serve. Ethics help to ensure the integrity of a profession, outline norms of conduct, and provide a system of accountability for those holding positions of power.

The increased awareness of trauma's widespread impacts and prevalence highlights the need for further incorporation of trauma-informed principles as standards of practice for organizations, group workers, psychodramatists, leaders, and perhaps all professionals. I would go as far as suggesting that just about any provider or agency that works with humans is working with trauma survivors on some level. Thus, trauma-informed principles are relevant for all professionals, especially group workers and psychotherapists. Existing professional codes of ethics largely void of any explicit reference to trauma or trauma-informed philosophy, including those of the American Psychological Association (APA), National Association of Social Workers (NASW), American Counseling Association (ACA), American Group Psychotherapy Association (AGPA), International Association of Group Psychotherapy & Group Processes (IAGP), and International Association of Social Work with Groups (IASWG). Most of the codes of ethics and standards of practice of the organizations above do not mention the word "trauma." The NASW and ACA codes of ethics both briefly mention "trauma" once. The Association of Specialists in Group Work (ASGW) publications of ethics, standards, and principles seem to be slightly more informed by trauma as it is mentioned in multiple places in their group work guides.

While some of the trauma-informed principles are articulated with different language in the aforementioned codes, it is suggested that the associations listed above (and others) consider more consciously integrating trauma-informed principles into their standards of practice and codes of ethics. Further integration in this regard would concretize trauma-informed philosophy as standard practice and the norm within professional communities that are primarily treating PTSD and trauma-related conditions. Trauma survivors are largely been harmed by individuals or groups (professional and non-professional) whose actions were unethical, immoral, or simply hateful. The process of gaining the necessary trust of trauma survivors needed to engage in treatment or services demands that professionals uphold the highest of ethical principles and standards.

How to Read This Book

This book is written with a blend of history, theory, research, group examples, practice guidelines, and reflective prompts. Chapters 1–3 present much of the history, theory, and research related to group work, psychodrama, and trauma-informed care. Chapter 4 outlines experiential sociometry processes that can be employed in any group or organizational context. Chapters 5–10 are each dedicated to one of SAMHSA's trauma-informed principles outlining their relevance for trauma work, group work, psychodrama practice, and organizations. Chapter 11 is focused on vicarious trauma and organizational work using groups and Moreno's action methods. Chapter 12 is devoted to promoting a trauma-informed ethical culture of leadership in group work, psychodrama, organizations, teaching, and supervision. Each chapter is designed to stand one its own while also serving as an essential part of the book-as-a-whole.

Each chapter will include prompts or questions standing out from the text which are meant to help the reader critically consider on the topics being presented. These prompts are intended to facilitate the digestion of the content, integration of the ideas into practice, and can also serve as prompts for students, trainees, and organizations in educational spaces teaching this content. It is suggested that the reader pause and spend time honestly considering each prompt and perhaps even writing about each question. Becoming a more trauma-informed practitioner, leader, or organization will take much more than simply reading a book – it will require critical reflection, self-awareness, and action.

Conclusion

Trauma-informed principles provide a vital ingredient for programs, practices, and providers offering effective and ethical services to trauma survivors. Trauma-informed principles become particularly important for providers treating PTSD using active interventions such as psychodrama or other expressive arts therapies. While SAMHSA's trauma-informed care principles and agency domains were developed for organizations, they are all also applicable for group work. The integration of the trauma-informed philosophy and a three-stage clinical map into group work and psychodrama supports practitioners offering effective and ethical services while mitigating risks of retraumatization.

References

American Psychiatric Association. (2013). *Diagnostic and statistical manual of mental disorders: DSM-5*. Washington, DC: American Psychiatric Association.

Anderson, R., & Carnabucci, K. (2011). *Integrating psychodrama and systemic constellation work: New directions for action methods, mind-body therapies and energy healing*. London: Jessica Kingsley Publishers.

Birnbaum, M., & Auerbach, C. (1994). Group work in graduate social work education: The price of neglect. *Journal of Social Work Education, 30*(3), 325–335.

Bloom, S. L. (1997). *Creating sanctuary: Toward the evolution of sane societies.* London: Taylor & Francis.

Bloom, S. L. (2013). *Creating sanctuary: Toward the evolution of sane societies (Revised).* New York: Routledge.

Bloom, S. L., & Farragher, B. (2011). *Destroying sanctuary: The crisis in human services delivery systems.* New York: Oxford University Press.

Breslau, N. (2009). The epidemiology of trauma, PTSD, and other posttrauma disorders. *Trauma, Violence, & Abuse, 10*(3), 198–210.

Brown, B. (2018). *Dare to lead: Brave work. Tough conversations. Whole hearts.* New York: Random House.

Brown, S. M., Baker, C. N., & Wilcox, P. (2012). Risking connection training: A pathway towards trauma-informed care in child congregate care settings. *Psychological Trauma: Theory, Research, Practice, and Policy, 4*(5), 507–515.

Casson, J. (2007). Scenes from a distance: Psychodrama and dramatherapy. In P. Holmes, M. Farrall, & K. Kirk (Eds.), *Empowering therapeutic practice: Integrating psychodrama into other therapies* (pp. 157–180). London: Jessica Kingsley Publishers.

Chesner, A. (2020). Psychodrama and healing the traumatic wound. In A. Chesner, & S. Lykou (Eds.), *Trauma in the creative and embodied therapies: When words are not enough* (pp. 69–80). London: Routledge.

Clements, J. (2008). Social work students' perceived knowledge of and preparation for group-work practice. *Social Work with Groups, 31*(3–4), 329–346.

Courtois, C. A., & Ford, J. D. (2016). *Treatment of complex trauma: A sequenced, relationship-based approach.* New York: The Guildford Press.

Covington, S. S. (2002). Helping women recover: Creating gender-responsive treatment. In S. Straussner, & S. Brown (Eds.), *Handbook of women's addictions treatment* (pp. 52–72). San Francisco: Jossey-Bass.

Drum, D., Becker, M. S., & Hess, E. (2010). Expanding the application of group interventions: Emergence of groups in health care settings. *The Journal for Specialists in Group Work, 36*(4), 247–263.

Drumm, K. (2006). The essential power of group work. *Social Work with Groups, 29*, 17–31.

Felitti, V. J., Anda, R. F., Nordenberg, D., Williamson, D. F., Spitz, A. M., Edwards, V., & Marks, J. S. (1998). Adverse childhood experiences. *American Journal of Preventive Medicine, 14*(4), 245–258.

Giacomucci, S. (2017). The sociodrama of life or death: Young adults and addiction treatment. *Journal of Psychodrama, Sociometry, and Group Psychotherapy*, 65(1), 137–143. https://doi.org/10.12926/ 0731-1273-65.1.137

Giacomucci, S. (2018a). The trauma survivor's inner role atom: A clinical map for post-traumatic growth. *Journal of Psychodrama, Sociometry, and Group Psychotherapy*, 66(1), 115–129.

Giacomucci, S. (2018b). Traveling as spontaneity training: If you want to become a psychodramatist, travel the world. *International Group Psychotherapies and Psychodrama Journal*, 4(1), 34–41.

Giacomucci, S. (2019). Social group work in action: A sociometry, psychodrama, and experiential trauma group therapy curriculum. *Doctorate in Social Work (DSW) Dissertations*. 124. Retrieved from https://repository.upenn.edu/cgi/viewcontent.cgi?article=1128&context=edissertations_sp2

Giacomucci, S. (2020). Addiction, traumatic loss, and guilt: A case study resolving grief through psychodrama and sociometric connections. *The Arts in Psychotherapy*, 67, 101627. https://doi.org/10.1016/j.aip.2019.101627

Giacomucci, S. (2021a). Experiential sociometry in group work: Mutual aid for the group-as-a-whole. *Social Work with Groups*, 44(3), 204–214.

Giacomucci, S. (2021b). *Social work, sociometry, and psychodrama: Experiential approaches for group therapists, Community leaders, and social workers*: Springer Nature. https://doi.org/10.1007/978-981-33-6342-7

Giacomucci, S. (2021c). Sparc of spontaneity: Creating integration between social work, sociometry, and psychodrama. *Social Work with Groups*, 45(3–4), 278–293.

Giacomucci, S., Karner, D., Nieto, L., & Schreiber, E. (2021). Sociatry, psychodrama, and social work: Moreno's mysticism and social justice tradition. *Social Work with Groups*, 44(3), 288–303. https://doi.org/10.1080/01609513.2021.1885826

Giacomucci, S., & Marquit, J. (2020). The effectiveness of trauma-focused psychodrama in the treatment of PTSD in inpatient substance abuse treatment. *Frontiers in Psychology*, 11, 896. https://dx.doi.org/10.3389%2Ffpsyg.2020.00896

Giacomucci, S., Marquit, J., & Miller Walsh, K. (2022). A controlled pilot study on the effects of a therapeutic spiral model trauma-focused psychodrama workshop on post-traumatic stress, spontaneity and post-traumatic growth. *Zeitschrift für Psychodrama und Soziometrie*, 21(1), 171–188.

Giacomucci, S., Marquit, J., Walsh, K. M., & Saccarelli, R. (2022). A mixed-methods study on psychodrama treatment for PTSD and depression in inpatient substance use treatment: A comparison of outcomes pre-pandemic and during Covid-19. *The Arts in Psychotherapy*, 81, 101971.

Giacomucci, S., & Stone, A. M. (2019). Being in two places at once: Renegotiating traumatic experience through the surplus reality of psychodrama. *Social Work with Groups, 42*(3), 184–196. https://doi.org/10.1080/01609513.2018.1533913

Goodman, H., Knight, C., & Khudododov, K. (2014). Graduate social work students' experiences with group work in the field and the classroom. *Journal of Teaching in Social Work,* 34(1), 60–78.

Greenwood, D. J. (2015). Evolutionary systems thinking: What Gregory Bateson, Kurt Lewin, and Jacob Moreno offered to action research that still remains to be learned. In H. Bradbury (Ed.), *Handbook of action research* (3rd ed., pp. 425–433). London: SAGE Publications.

Harris, M., & Fallot, R. (2001). Using trauma theory to design service systems. *New Directions for Mental Health Services.* Hoboken: Jossey Bass.

Herman, J. L. (1992). *Trauma and recovery: The aftermath of violence—From domestic abuse to political terror.* New York: Basic Books.

Holmes, P. (2015). *The inner world outside: Object relations theory and psychodrama.* London: Routledge.

Hudgins, M. K., & Toscani, F. (2013). *Healing world trauma with the therapeutic spiral model: Stories from the frontlines.* London: Jessica Kingsley Publishers.

Janet, P. (1889). *L'Automatisme psychologique.* Paris: Félix Alcan.

Kessler, R. C., Aguilar-Gaxiola, S., Alonso, J., Benjet, C., Bromet, E. J., Cardoso, G., ... & Florescu, S. (2017). Trauma and PTSD in the WHO world mental health surveys. *European Journal of Psychotraumatology,* 8(sup5), 1353383.

Kilpatrick, D. G., Resnick, H. S., Milanak, M. E., Miller, M. W., Keyes, K. M., & Friedman, M. J. (2013). National estimates of exposure to traumatic events and PTSD prevalence using DSM-IV and DSM-5 criteria. *Journal of Traumatic Stress,* 26(5), 537–547. https://doi.org/10.1002/jts.21848

Landy, R. J. (2017). The love and marriage of psychodrama and drama therapy. *The Journal of Psychodrama, Sociometry, and Group Psychotherapy,* 65(1), 33–40.

Menschner, C., & Maul, A. (2016). *Key ingredients for successful trauma-informed care implementation.* Trenton: Center for Health Care Strategies, Incorporated.

Moreno, J. D. (2014). *Impromptu man: J.L. Moreno and the origins of psychodrama, encounter culture, and the social network.* New York: Bellevue Literary Press.

Moreno, J. L. (1914) *Einladung zu einer Begegnung.* Vienna: Anzengruber Verlag.

Moreno, J. L. (1921). *Das Testament des Vaters.* Vienna, Austria: Gustav Kiepenheuer Verlag.

Moreno, J. L. (1924). *Das Stegreiftheater.* Berlin, Germany: Gustav Kiepenheuer Verlag.

Moreno, J.L. (1931). *Application of the group method to classification.* Beacon, NY: Beacon House Inc.

Moreno, J. L. (1934). *Who shall survive? A new approach to the problems of human inter-relations.* Washington, DC: Nervous and Mental Disease Publishing Co.

Moreno, J. L. (1947). *Open letter to group psychotherapists.* Psychodrama Monograms, No. 23. Beacon, NY: Beacon House.

Moreno, J. L. (1953). *Who shall survive? Foundations of sociometry, group psychotherapy and sociodrama* (2nd ed.). Beacon, NY: Beacon House.

Moreno, J. L. (1972). *Psychodrama volume 1* (4th ed.). New York: Beacon House.

Moreno, J. L. (2019). *The autobiography of a genius* (E. Schreiber, S. Kelley, & S. Giacomucci, Eds.). United Kingdom: North West Psychodrama Association.

Moreno, J. L., & Whitin, E. S. (1932). *Application of the group method to classification.* New York: National Committee on Prisons and Prison Labor.

Najavits, L. (2002). *Seeking safety: A treatment manual for PTSD and substance abuse.* New York: Guilford Publications.

Paxton, T., & Harrison, M. (2022). *Introduction and update on the evidence-based group treatment website project.* The Group Psychologist, Spring Issue. APA Division 49. Accessed at https://www.apadivisions.org/division-49/publications/newsletter/group-psychologist/2022/03/group-treatment-project

Ringel, S., & Brandell, J. R. (Eds.). (2011). *Trauma: Contemporary directions in theory, practice, and research.* Los Angeles: SAGE.

Rivard, J. C., Bloom, S. L., Abramovitz, R., et al. (2003). Assessing the implementation and effects of a trauma-focused intervention for youths in residential treatment. *Psychiatric Quarterly, 74,* 137–154.

Shapiro, F. (2018). *Eye-movement desensitization and reprocessing (EMDR) Therapy* (3rd ed.). New York: Guilford Press.

Simon, S., & Kilbane, T. (2014). The current state of group work education in U.S. graduate schools of social work. *Social Work with Groups, 37,* 243–256.

Sternberg, P., & Garcia, A. (2000). *Sociodrama: Who's in your shoes?.* Westport: Greenwood Publishing Group.

Substance Abuse and Mental Health Services Administration. (2014a). *SAMHSA's concept of trauma and guidance for a trauma-informed approach.* HHS Publication No. (SMA) 14-4884. Rockville, MD: Substance Abuse and Mental Health Services Administration.

Substance Abuse and Mental Health Services Administration. (2014b). *Trauma-informed care in behavioral health services.* Treatment Improvement Protocol

(TIP) Series 57. Rockville, MD: Substance Abuse and Mental Health Services Administration.

Sweifach, J. (2014). Group work education today: A content analysis of MSW group work course syllabi. *Social Work with Groups, 37*(1), 8–22.

Sweifach, J., & LaPorte, H. (2008). Why did they choose group work: Exploring the motivations and perceptions of current MSW students of group work. *Social Work with Groups, 31*(3/4), 347–362.

Treadwell, T. (2016). JL Moreno: The origins of the group encounter movement and the forerunner of web-based social network media revolution. *The Journal of Psychodrama, Sociometry, and Group Psychotherapy, 64*(1), 51–62.

Treadwell, T. (2020). *Integrating CBT with experiential theory and practice: A group therapy workbook.* New York: Taylor & Francis.

Tomasulo, D. (2018). Beautiful thinking in action: Positive psychology, psychodrama, and positive psychotherapy. *The Journal of Psychodrama, Sociometry, and Group Psychotherapy, 66*(1), 49–67.

Van der Kolk, B. A. (2014). *The body keeps the score: Brain, mind, and body in the healing of trauma.* New York: Viking Press.

Wilson, C., Pence, D. M., & Conradi, L. (2013). Trauma-informed care. In *Encyclopedia of social work.* National Association of Social Work and Oxford Press. doi: 10.1093/acrefore/9780199975839.013.1063.

Wodarski, J. S., & Feit, M. D. (2012). Social group work practice: An evidenced based approach. *Journal of Evidence-Based Social Work, 9,* 414–420.

Yalom, I. D., & Leszcz, M. (2005). *The theory and practice of group psychotherapy* (5th ed.). New York: Basic Books.

Yalom, I. D., & Leszcz, M. (2020). *The theory and practice of group psychotherapy* (6th ed.). New York: Basic Books.

Zastrow, C. (2001). *Social work with groups: Using the classroom as a group leadership laboratory* (5th ed.). Pacific Grove, CA: Brooks/Cole.

2
Psychodrama and Group Work as Trauma-Informed Philosophies

Chapter Summary

Psychodrama and group work were created decades before the impacts of trauma and posttraumatic stress disorder (PTSD) were recognized in the mental health field. Nevertheless, both group work and psychodrama were both historically implemented and developed with trauma survivors and marginalized groups. Group work and psychodrama philosophies intuitively mirror trauma-informed philosophy that developed years later. Each system emphasizes person-centered, humanistic, and anti-oppressive approaches that centralize collaboration, peer support, and empowerment. Psychodrama and group work core theories and methods are non-pathologizing and honor the dignity of each person. Though they were developed over 100 years ago, both psychodrama and group work methodology are now being validated by the influx of research about the neurobiology of trauma and healing. This chapter provides an overview of group therapy and psychodrama philosophy and theories as they relate to trauma-informed care.

Group Work as Trauma-Informed Philosophy

Trauma-informed principles are organically and naturally operationalized through group work's core philosophy and approaches. The experience of participating in a group inherently emphasizes peer support, collaboration, mutuality, and empowerment though relationship. These trauma-informed principles are simply more central to group work than individual work due to

DOI: 10.4324/9781003277859-2

the fundamental difference between individual and group work. Group work, unlike one-to-one work, includes participation in a group with one's peers. This lends itself to exponentially more potentialities of relational healing, support, and empowerment. While group work philosophy embodies many aspects of trauma-informed care, it is unclear how much group workers are consciously applying trauma-informed principles in their group facilitation (Baird & Alaggia, 2021). The conscious integration of trauma-informed principles into group work practice will help prevent potential harm done in groups and enhance group work's effectiveness in treating and supporting trauma survivors.

Many trauma specialists recommend a co-leadership structure for trauma groups based on the intensity and complexity of running a trauma group (Courtois, 2010; Hudgins & Toscani, 2013). Having a co-leader provides additional benefits for group leaders that simply aren't available in a group with a single leader. Two therapists are often better than one – as long as they can effectively work together. Co-leadership of groups inherently provides a built-in sense of peer support for the professional. Co-leadership can also offer group participants more options to connect with leaders and receive direct support or feedback from leaders. This is particularly helpful in situations when a group member is overwhelmed and leaves the group room. One of the co-leaders can check-in on them while the other leader stays with the group-as-a-whole. Having two leaders also adds a layer of complexities related to transference and countertransference which can emerge and be more effectively dealt with when another therapist is present to offer reflection or facilitation. The intensity of transferential issues lessens with co-leaders, while the potential of meaningful therapeutic relationships between therapists and group members increases (Courtois, 2010). The co-leadership approach to group therapy offers increased potentials for group leaders to demonstrate trauma-informed principles in action through their collaboration, mutuality, transparency, trust, peer support, empowerment, and respect for each other's identities.

Though there are various group work models and philosophies, one of the most common and most congruent with trauma-informed principles is the mutual aid group. Mutual aid, the power of group members helping each other, is the central component in the social work with groups approach (Giacomucci, 2021a). The mutual aid groups approach emphasizes the therapeutic power of each participant rather than only the power of the leader. This redistribution of power effectively empowers participants and can help prevent retraumatization based on unhealthy power dynamics. The mutual aid model includes ten core dynamics: (1) sharing data,

(2) "all-in-the-same-boat" phenomenon, (3) the dialectical process (safe expression of perspectives and differences leading to refinement and commonality), (4) addressing taboo topics, (5) developing a universal perspective, (6) mutual support, (7) mutual demand and expectation, (8) problem solving, (9) rehearsal of new ways of being, and (10) "strength-in-numbers" phenomenon (Gitterman & Shulman, 2005; Rosenwald & Baird, 2020; Shulman, 2015). These ten mutual aid dynamics are outlined by others in detail (Shulman, 2015; Steinberg, 2014) and offer additional insight into how to promote mutual aid within groups. Mutual aid groups are inherently empowering to participants as they focus on positioning group members as therapeutic agents for each other. The mutual aid process will be described and depicted throughout other sections and examples in this book.

Rosenwald and Baird (2020) articulate a reciprocal relationship between mutual aid and trauma-informed principles:

> An integration is proposed based on mutual aid dynamics that generally serve as a catalyst to the generation of the trauma-informed practice components. In turn, the creation of a trauma-informed climate in the group further stimulates the creation of the mutual aid dynamics. Therefore, mutual aid and trauma-informed practice become conjointly reinforcing; mutual aid inspires a trauma-informed climate and a trauma-informed climate nurtures mutuality.
>
> (p. 262)

The mutual aid group approach not only embodies trauma-informed practice principles but also further promotes a trauma-informed atmosphere where retraumatization can be avoided and healing cultivated.

How am I integrating each of the ten mutual aid dynamics into my work?

Another prevalent approach to group therapy, outlined by Irvin Yalom and Molyn Leszcz (2020), proposes eleven therapeutic factors in group work, many of which mirror the ten mutual aid dynamics listed above. These curative factors are: (1) instillation of hope, (2) universality, (3) imparting of information, (4) altruism, (5) corrective recapitulation of the primary family group, (6) development of socializing techniques, (7) imitative behavior, (8) interpersonal learning, (9) group cohesiveness, (10) catharsis, and (11) existential factors. Yalom and Leszcz (2020) describe these therapeutic factors as "central organizing principles" and "the crucial aspects of the process of change" in group therapy (p. 9). They go on to articulate how each of these factors are interdependent upon the others but also are naturally differentiated from each other and operate at different levels of experience – cognitive, behavioral, and emotional. They also suggest that some therapeutic factors, such as group cohesiveness, may be better described as a therapeutic force or a precondition for change. These 11 therapeutic factors will be referenced throughout the rest of the book. While Yalom and Leszcz (2020) use the term *altruism* instead of *mutual aid*, they are also explicit in stating the group leader's primary function is to set into motion mutual aid and the therapeutic factors outlined above:

> If it is the group members who, in their interaction, set into motion the many therapeutic factors, then it is the group therapist's task to create a group culture maximally conductive to effective group interaction.
>
> (p. 157)

Ulman (2005) highlights that these 11 curative factors are particularly helpful for trauma survivors as it helps combat isolation, shame, and distorted beliefs related to the trauma while promoting support and trust between participants, management of posttraumatic stress disorder (PTSD) symptoms, validation of traumatic experiences, development of a narrative of the trauma in a safe way, expression of emotions and grief, and the reintegration of personality. Others have described how the 11 therapeutic factors help trauma survivors mobilize strengths and resources within the group needed to address the depletion of inner resources due to trauma (Foy, Unger, & Wattenberg, 2005). And in a previous publication, I have explored how Yalom's therapeutic factors relate to the practice of sociometry and psychodrama while also suggesting that they apply to community and organizational settings beyond group therapy contexts (see Giacomucci, 2021b).

How am I integrating each of Yalom's 11 therapeutic factors into my work?

Regardless of one's group work orientation, there are shared commonalities within the group experience and its healing properties when it comes to trauma and PTSD. These shared commonalities and therapeutic factors are present in both online groups and in-person groups (Gullo et al., 2022). While trauma damages relationships and communication, group work promotes interpersonal skills and healthy relationships. Trauma is characterized by control and helplessness, while group work is based on collaboration and mutuality. Trauma often takes away one's sense of safety and belonging, whereas group work promotes a sense of safety and belonging. Trauma and PTSD fuel distorted beliefs about self and others; however, group work offers reality testing and reconfiguring of distorted beliefs. Relational trauma frequently fuels reenactments in relationships or insecure attachment styles, but the therapy group serves as a safe container for corrective relational experiences and renegotiation of attachment styles. Trauma fuels defenses and walls where group work promotes vulnerability and authenticity. The group work approach is fundamentally reparative for trauma survivors.

Interpersonal Neurobiology of Group Psychotherapy

Beyond group work models, the interpersonal neurobiology research further supports the use of group therapy as a modality. Gantt and Badenoch (2013) suggest that:

> …understanding the interpersonal nature of brain development and its role in illness, healing, and recovery also helps discriminate how group therapy is different from individual therapy, and, in many instances, may be a more powerful and logical choice from a brain-based perspective.
>
> (p. xx)

In *Integrating Interpersonal Neurobiology with Group Psychotherapy*, Badenoch and Cox (2013), outline three primary group therapy components informed by interpersonal neurobiology: 1) brain development and memory, 2) group as a holding environment for emotions and sensations experienced by group members, and 3) neural integration within the following four domains – consciousness, interpersonal, vertical, and bilateral.

The impact of adverse childhood experiences and relational trauma gets coded in the brain and body as implicit memory impacting our attachment styles, emotional regulation, and sense of safety in relationships or groups (Badenoch, 2018; Cozolino, 2014; Shapiro & Applegate, 2018). The group-as-a-whole experience in group therapy initiates a right-brain to right-brain resonance between participants that can activate and renegotiate implicit and relational memory systems promoting neural integration (Siegel, 2013). These early childhood traumas, which are sometimes void of explicit memory, are difficult to access and work through in traditional therapy. The group context is unique in that the multitude of peer relationships are likely to activate, trigger, contain, and rework these implicit memories (Gantt & Badenoch, 2013) – perhaps providing neurobiology support to Yalom's therapeutic factor articulated as *the corrective recapitulation of the primary family group.* The core relational aspect of brain development supports the use of group therapy as an intervention. The social and group aspect of group therapy initiates the brain's social engagement system in a manner that creates a group holding environment and haven of regulation and safety for participants (Badenoch & Cox, 2013).

Integration of consciousness, defined as the mind's capacity to compassionately observe itself (Siegel, 2007), is achieved through the group process of storytelling, compassionate witnessing, and group cohesion (Giacomucci, 2021c). Interpersonal integration is supported through group cohesion and the multitude of therapeutic relationships between a group member and their peers, the facilitator(s), and the group-as-a-whole. Integration in the realms of the interpersonal and consciousness further support group members' experiences of bilateral and vertical integration. Vertical integration describes the process by which the body, limbic system, and neocortex become integrated in a manner that facilitates the integration of memory throughout the brain-body connection into a coherent and regulated wholeness (Badenoch & Cox, 2013). Bilateral integration, however, refers to the link between right-brain emotion and sensations with left-brain cognition. This is the process by which the visceral, emotional, and sensational experience is made sense of through narrative and cognitive meaning-making in the group process. Siegel (2013) reminds us that all forms of health are characterized by integration. Multi-leveled integration is the process that facilitates meaningful change in group therapy. He emphasizes that all systems, biological and social, are inherently programmed to move toward integration, and that the role of the group therapist is to work collaboratively with the group "to liberate the innate drive to heal" (p. 21). This inherent capacity for self-healing is further articulated in psychodrama's philosophy of the autonomous healing center within and in group work's mutual aid model. Insights from interpersonal neurobiology support the use of group work modalities and help guide practitioners in implementing trauma-informed care.

How can I use neurobiology to guide my practice?

Trauma-Informed Group Teletherapy

The coronavirus pandemic led to a widescale shift from in-person groups to online group offerings, though many were already utilizing online group formats. It is important to consider some of the implications of group tele-therapy as it relates to trauma-informed care. Group teletherapy, when implemented with some guidelines, further advances trauma-informed care by meeting clients where they are at and increasing the accessibility of services. Some studies have suggested that group teletherapy participants experience a greater sense of safety, transparency, honesty, and comfort in online sessions than in person (Azarang et al., 2019; Turgoose, Ashwick, & Murphy, 2018). Teletherapy has a distinctive advantage in reaching folks who do have barriers related to mobility, health, transportation, time, cost, or otherwise cannot physically travel to an office for a group session. In this way, group telehealth offers more potentials of mutual aid and peer support. Telehealth is also superior in its ability to provide empowerment, voice, and choice, for participants who otherwise might not have access to groups. It inherently extends a mutuality to all, regardless of ability, geographic location, or mobility. Telehealth provides exponentially more choices in group attendance than previously when individual's group options were limited to those that were within transportation distance to them. Furthermore, the increased number of group options and accessibility has inevitably led to more available groups designed for folks from marginalized communities. It is pretty clear then that the group teletherapy further advances group therapy's embodiment of trauma-informed principles. The explicit integration of trauma-informed principles into teletherapy practice is of utmost importance, especially considering practitioners' lack of training in telehealth, the unique ethical issues related to telehealth, and the increase in traumatization due to the pandemic (Gerber, Elisseou, Sager, & Keith, 2020).

Gerber, Elisseou, Sager, and Keith (2020) provide comprehensive guidance on integrating each of SAMHSA's six trauma-informed principles into telehealth practice. Table 2.1 is adapted for group teletherapy based on their guidance.

The utilization of teletherapy formats for groups is uniquely different than in person groups in some ways. For one, it requires that practitioners be aware of the telehealth practice laws and limitations related to their licensure and state license board (Weinberg, 2020). Practitioners should also be aware of their own competencies when it comes to telehealth technology and seek training or consultation. The co-leader group therapy approach is useful for telehealth groups in that one leader can attend to the technology facilitation while the other is more focused on group process. Navigating confidentiality and privacy is more complicated in online group sessions, especially when participants do not have a fully private space in their home (or elsewhere) that they can attend the session from. This creates potential

Table 2.1 Strategies for integrating trauma-informed principles into group teletherapy, inspired by Gerber, Elisseou, Sager, and Keith (2020)

Trauma-Informed Principle	Strategies for Implementation
Safety	• Obtain patients' location at the start of session • Ensure informed consent • Commitment to confidentiality, discussion of limits/risks to confidentiality • Confirm privacy/security of each patient's physical and virtual space • Discuss importance of keeping video feed on and/or communication with group leader around issues of safety, discomfort, or feelings of overwhelm • Provide local/virtual resources for support, additional treatment, or emergency care
Trustworthiness and transparency	• Utilize reliable and secure telehealth platforms • Promote transparency related to any ambient noise in environments • Suggest that each person sit far enough from their camera so others can see more of their body language • Provide clarity on telehealth and group processes
Peer support	• Promote mutual aid and cohesion through group discussion, breakout rooms, or other processes adapted for virtual group spaces • Encourage participants to unmute their microphones and contribute to the group and/or use non-verbal indicators of support such as the chat box or emojis
Collaboration and mutuality	• Clearly identify group goals and purposes to promote collaboration amongst members • Cultivate solidarity and cooperation in the online group space highlighting shared experiences
Empowerment, voice, and choice	• Discuss group norms related to keeping microphones muted or unmuted • Track all participants throughout the online group process and empower all to participate based on their comfort level • Initiate ongoing check-ins and affirmations of participants' choices throughout the process • Consider offering alternative options for sharing such as using the chat box feature or emojis

Trauma-Informed Principle	Strategies for Implementation
Cultural, historic, and gender issues	• Create group spaces that are inclusive and affirming of diverse identities
	• Consider the impact of social determinants of health (housing security, internet stability, affordability of computer equipment, access to privacy, childcare, poverty, translation, nutrition, racism, etc.)
	• Be aware of patients' comfort in revealing details of their personal space during the session
	• Encourage the use/display of gender pronouns next to each participants' name
	• Design groups that account for preferences and limitations related to different communities
	• Provide simple instructions for participants, especially those who may be less familiar with computers or telehealth video platforms

risks to confidentiality in that others may see or hear other group members. The use of headphones and screen privacy protectors, when available, can help mitigate these issues. In a review of ethical issues in teletherapy, Stoll, Müller, and Trachsel (2020) synthesized the following as the five primary ethical arguments used against online psychotherapy: 1) confidentiality, privacy, and security, 2) lack of therapist's training in telehealth, 3) communication problems related to technology, 4) lack of research, and 5) limitations and complexities in managing emergencies during teletherapy. Others have highlighted "zoom bombing" (the intrusion of zoom sessions by outsiders for joke or intentional disruption targeting specific groups) as another risk to online sessions which may retraumatize participants while also disrupting confidentiality and group process (Simmons & Wilches, 2022). Zoom bombing can be prevented through zoom features such as activating a "waiting room" or requiring a password.

While there are additional risks and concerns with group teletherapy, there are also benefits to group teletherapy which allow group workers to further embody trauma-informed principles in their work. Teletherapy provides many trauma survivors with a medium for accessing services that feels safer and more comfortable. It is more convenient for most people as it eliminates commuting time to and from the session. Teletherapy is unique in its ability to bring together a group of participants that might not be able to come together on a regular basis otherwise. Understanding the primary clinical, ethical, safety, and legal concerns related to teletherapy allows group workers to reduce risks while enhancing the benefits of group teletherapy (Weinberg, 2020, 2021). Yalom and Leszcz (2020) suggest that the same therapeutic factors for in person groups are also equally important for online groups.

How comfortable and competent am I in facilitating online groups vs in-person groups?

Have I educated myself on the ethical, legal, and clinical best practices for online group work?

Stages in Group Development and Trauma Therapy

In considering the philosophy and theories of group work and trauma work, we must also discuss the stages of group development and the commonly implemented three-stage clinical map for trauma work. These separate stage models are core components of both fields providing a framework for approaching the work. Within both the group work and trauma therapy fields, there are multiple models available for conceptualizing the different stages of the work. These will be briefly outlined below. Each of the models essentially mirrors each other and suggests similar stages of development. Which one you choose to guide your work is probably less important – what is important is that you do have a framework for conceptualizing group development.

Every group work approach, similar to every trauma work approach, appears to have an embedded process involving multiple group stages. One of the primarily problems I've seen is that different language is used to describe the different stages, particularly between social workers, psychologists, and counselors. I've often found that graduate students get confused by these different models in that the textbook used in their group work elective doesn't always use the same language for group development stages as the larger field of study they are engaged in. I've observed this happen multiple times when social work with groups courses use a group counseling or group psychotherapy textbook. Psychodramatists also have their own three-stage system to further complicate things. Table 2.2 provides an organized overview of the various group developmental stages and the authors who proposed them.

The models of group development stages above demonstrate both the similarities and differences between conceptualizations of group development. Each model articulates the trajectory of a group-as-a-whole from its

Table 2.2 Models of group development stages

Author	Primary Profession	Stages of Group Development				
Tuckman (1965)	**Psychology**	Forming	Storming	Norming	Performing	Adjourning
Corey, Corey, and Corey (2018)	**Counseling**	Forming	Initial	Transition	Working	Final
Shulman (2015)	**Social work**	Initial	Beginning	Middle		Ending
MacKenzie (1997)	**Psychiatry and group therapy**	Engagement	Differentiation	Interpersonal work		Termination
Moreno (1946)	**Psychodrama**	Warm-up – sociometry		Action – psychodrama		Sharing – group therapy

inception through its development of group cohesion into addressing the group's purpose or "work," then to its ending. Moreno's group phases are primarily used to describe the trajectory of a single session, but I find them also useful as a framework for group development. Inversely, the other proposed group phases were articulated to describe the overall development of a group's lifespan, but they are also applicable as conceptualizations for a single session. These developmental stages apply to all forms of ongoing groups (including organizations and classrooms) but are not always experienced in a linear fashion. Major changes in a group may propel a group back into an earlier stage of development as they adjust to the change. Some ongoing groups (such as inpatient groups) have a revolving door of frequently new clients and terminating clients. The stages of development will look slightly different in a group like this but are still identifiable, especially when considering that each individual in the group could be in a different stage of development with the group. For example, in an ongoing group of this nature, newer participants may be in the early stages with the group while other longer-term group members are in the middle stages and discharging clients are in the ending stage.

The differences in language and philosophy may also be representative of the originator's personality or background or the profession that they primarily work within. As indicated above, Tuckman's popular (1965) model may reflect his thinking as a psychologist, the Coreys' conceptualization (2018) may come from their shared work within the counseling profession, Shulman's (2015) simplified model reflects his social work background, MacKenzie's (1997) approach may reflect his thinking as a psychiatrist and former AGPA president, and Moreno's (1946) stages clearly operationalize his psychodramatic method and triadic system. Regardless of their differences in approach, these development stages share common ground in demonstrating how a group warms-up and forms, develops norms and cohesion while transitioning into a working stage, and ends with an integrative closure.

Which of these frameworks do I use to guide my group facilitation?

Which of the group development phases do I feel most (and least) competent and comfortable leading groups during?

How can these group phases help me structure and pace each of my group sessions?

Similar to the stages of group development, many trauma experts have proposed three-stage models for the development of trauma therapy (see Table 2.3).

The various three stage models for trauma therapy outlined below also demonstrate shared commonality with some distinct differences, partially related to specific differences in their approach or model. Generally, these approaches agree that the treatment must begin with stabilization and safety before moving into trauma processing or mourning, then ending with integration and reconnection. It can also be helpful to conceptualize the three phases of trauma therapy through the orientation of time. Phase 1 focuses on present, here-and-now; phase 2 orients on the past trauma; and phase 3 looks to the future (Herman, 1992).

Which of these clinical map phases do I feel best able to facilitate with a client/group in my work?

Which of the clinical map phases do I feel is most overlooked in my work?

How does my program or agency incorporate each of these clinical map phases into services offered?

Table 2.3 Three stage models of trauma therapy

Author	Model/ Approach	Stages of Trauma Therapy		
Janet (1889)	Stage model for treatment of traumatic stress	Stabilization	Identification	Relapse prevention
Herman (1992)	Trauma recovery	Establishing safety	Remembrance and mourning	Reconnection
Najavits (2002)	Seeking safety	Safety	Mourning	Reconnecting
Courtois and Ford (2016)	Treatment of complex trauma	Safety, stabilization, and engagement	Processing of traumatic memories	(Re)Integration
Hudgins and Toscani (2013)	TSM psychodrama	Prescriptive roles: observation, containment, and strength	Trauma-based roles: victim, perpetrator, and abandoning authority	Transformative roles: autonomy, integration, and correction
Cohen and Mannarino (2015)	Trauma-focused CBT	Stabilization	Trauma narration and processing	Integration and consolidation
Shapiro (2018) and Van der Hart et al. (2013)	EMDR	Stabilization, symptom reduction, skills training	Treatment of traumatic memories	Personality (re) integration and rehabilitation

When simplified and compared, the stages of group development and the stages of trauma therapy have some clear overlaps that can help us further integrate trauma therapy principles into the various stages of group development. As such, we can conceptualize the stage of group development also as stages of trauma therapy and recovery (see Table 2.4).

It is important to remember that these stages and phases are not entirely rigid but instead describe general stages in the process of group work and trauma work. Furthermore, though these stages, in both fields, were primarily designed to describe development of the work over the entire course of treatment, they are also useful for conceptualizing the pacing and trajectory of a single session. Interestingly, Moreno's three-stage theory is the only one above that was specifically developed to describe the stages of a single session

Table 2.4 Simplified comparison of three stage group development and trauma therapy models

	1	2	3
Group development stages	Initial/beginning stages	Middle stage	End stage
Trauma therapy stages	Safety and stabilization	Trauma processing	(Re)Integration and reconnection

rather than the entire trajectory of the treatment experience. Thinking about the impact of group development phases and the three phases of the clinical map can also be useful ideas for organizational leaders and educators to inform their leadership and teaching.

Morenean Philosophy as Trauma-Informed Philosophy

Jacob Moreno describes his philosophy as an existential and mystical philosophy emerging from his spiritual beliefs and commitment to Sociatry – healing for society (Giacomucci, Karner, Nieto, & Schreiber, 2021; Moreno, 2019). He was disappointed at the end of his life as his methods had become largely integrated into other approaches and the culture but had become disconnected from the philosophy from which they came (Moreno, 2014). He likened this to ripping children from their parents (Moreno, 1969). Moreno's philosophy was radical for its time and was rejected by many as it significantly challenged the generally accepted paradigms in the field. Though he developed his method and philosophy decades before PTSD was recognized as a diagnosis, careful examination of his philosophy reveals its congruence with modern trauma theory and trauma-informed principles. Most of the communities that Moreno directly worked with, and particularly the populations he worked with when developing his ideas, were highly traumatized and marginalized groups (Giacomucci, 2021c). His ideas of group psychotherapy emerged from his work with immigrants and sex workers, his sociometric system was generated from work with refugees, inmates, and a residential girls reform school, and his psychodramatic approach developed from work with hospitalized psychiatric patients.

Morenean philosophy is expansive and therefore difficult to summarize concisely, nevertheless, I will do my best here. Moreno starts by proposing that humans are more than biological, psychological, or social beings, but are first of all cosmic beings (Moreno, 2012). His conceptualization of human nature is fundamentally biopsychosocial-spiritual; thus, his methods are designed to address the biological, psychological, social, and spiritual/existential nuances of experience (Giacomucci, 2021b). In describing the Morenean approach, Zerka Moreno (2012) writes, "our instruments are basically spiritual and existential, pointing to and supporting the value of the human spirit" (p. 515).

In his 1912 encounter with Sigmund Freud, he articulates how his approach is different from psychoanalysis:

> Well, Dr. Freud, I start where you leave off. You meet people in the artificial setting of your office. I meet them on the street and in their homes, in their natural surroundings. You analyze their dreams. I give them the courage to dream again. You analyze and tear them apart. I let them act out their conflicting roles and help them to put the parts together again.
>
> (Moreno, 2019, p. 187)

He developed his ideas in opposition to Freud and psychoanalysis (Takis, 2020), which seems to have contributed to psychodrama's marginalization in the larger mental health system.

Moreno's approach is growth-oriented, compatible with modern strengths-based approaches and positive psychology (Giacomucci, 2021b). His humanistic perspective suggests that we should emphasize the genius and strengths of each person rather than pathology and shortcomings (Moreno, 2019). Moreno takes this as far as declaring all humans as potential geniuses, emphasizing each persons' godlikeness, and even referring to his patients as "doctors" at times. In doing so, he emphasizes each persons' dignity and worth while disrupting the inherent power dynamics within psychotherapy. He believed so much in each group members' therapeutic power that his code of ethics even suggests each group member taking the Hippocratic Oath to formalize their role as co-healers in the group therapy process (Moreno, 1957). This simple but revolutionary shift in the role expectations of therapist and group participants promotes nearly all of SAMHSA's trauma-informed principles (2014a) – particularly safety, collaboration, mutuality, empowerment, voice, trustworthiness, and peer support.

How can I further empower clients as co-healers in their treatment process?

How can I further affirm the dignity and worth of each client and professional I work with?

Moreno's spiritual philosophy promotes the idea of a Godhead, the source of all spontaneity and creativity, while suggesting that each human being is also divine. He believed in the existence of a parallel universe where all things are sacred – a place containing a "primordial nature" that fuels the life force of each new generation. Morenean philosophy suggests that this is the First Universe from which we come from and return to after birth and death in this Second Universe of form, space, and time. He believed that one could tap into the First Universe through mystical experience and that psychodrama could provide a portal into this surplus reality where all things are possible. The intersection of these two universes is depicted through the encounter symbol in Figure 2.1.

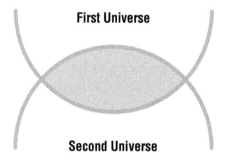

First Universe

Second Universe

Figure 2.1 The encounter symbol (republished with permission from Giacomucci, 2021b, p. 59).

Spontaneity, psychodrama's curative agent, is conceptualized as a spiritual energy, originating with the Godhead, that promotes adequate responses to new situations and new responses to old, reoccurring situations (1964, 2019). Spontaneity and creativity are conceptualized as twin-principles, foundational to psychodrama's theory of change, and underpinning all human progress (Nolte, 2014).

The Morenos articulate that the primary goal of all forms of therapy is to help a client access the *Autonomous Healing Center* within. In describing her husband's philosophy, Zerka writes that healing is attributed to a quiet process deep within the body and the self, untouched by words but stimulated through action (Moreno, 2012). The strong emphasis on the autonomous healing center demonstrates synchronicity with modern trauma theories (such as Interpersonal Neurobiology's focus on integration, the Adaptive Information Processing Model in EMDR, SELF in Internal Family Systems, and the body's ability to restore itself to goodness in Somatic Experiencing) which also underscore the self-healing nature of the human mind and nervous system (Levine, 2010; Schwartz, 2021; Shapiro, 2018; Siegel, 2020).

Moreno's philosophy emphasizes the here-and-now, even conceptualizing the past in future within the context of the present. The past is considered "memory-in-the-moment of past experiences" and the future is regarded as "here and now anticipation-in-the-moment of what might be eventually experienced" (Nolte, 2019, p. 131). This is particularly congruent with EMDR, somatic psychotherapy, and other theories of traumatic memory processing which are more concerned with the here-and-now experience of remembering trauma than the actual details of a traumatic event. Morenean philosophy teaches that spontaneity and creativity are only accessible in the moment and that each moment is wide-open with possibility. This fundamentally supports a view of human beings as active actors with agency in their life and situation rather than helpless victims of predeterminism. Psychodrama enactments are co-created in the here-and-now, acting as-if it were currently real. In this way, psychodrama provides participants with access to experiences in surplus reality that would be impossible otherwise. Furthermore, psychodrama insists on honoring the subjective reality of the protagonist based on their experience and perspective. This approach meets the client where they are through a postmodern and social constructivism lens supporting participants' unique meaning-making process rather than imposing the therapist's judgment of reality or interpretation upon them (Blatner, 2000; Oudijk, 2007).

Psychodrama, the first body-oriented therapy, is perhaps most fundamentally different from other approaches with its focus on action rather than talking. Moreno believed that "what was learned in action, must be unlearned in action" (Dayton, 2005, p. xxvii). While a traditional group psychotherapy session only involves participants sitting in their seats in discussion, every psychodrama group session involves multiple action structures initiating movement for participants. Through movement and action, psychodrama brings the body and nervous system into the treatment process. The influx of trauma research continues to support the use of body-oriented interventions to address the somatic imprint of trauma which exists within the brain and body at levels below thinking and talking (Cozolino, 2014; Levine, 2010; Malchiodi, 2020; Perry, 2006; van de Kamp et al., 2019; van der Kolk, 2014). The interpersonal neurobiologists have declared the most significant finding of the century to be that the human brain is constantly changing and evolving based on experience (Cozolino, 2014; Siegel, 2020). Psychodrama's action approach provides participants with opportunities for healing trauma through corrective experiences that would be impossible through talk therapy (Giacomucci, 2018, 2019, 2020; Giacomucci & Ehrhart, 2021; Giacomucci & Stone, 2019). Psychodrama provides a safe space for doing, undoing, and redoing in the context of renegotiating traumatic experience (Schreiber & Giacomucci, forthcoming). Redfern (2014) beautifully articulates this same process in the context of trauma healing in dramatherapy – "*a completed release (after some struggle) from a well-held pattern or structure and the embrace of a missing opposite that takes place in the arts/playspace and leaves the client significantly changed afterwards*" (p. 384).

Psychodrama Theories as Trauma Theories

Leszcz (2018) reminds us that "Theory teaches us where to head therapeutically. Technique teaches us what to do once we arrive there" (p. 285). This is important wisdom for practitioners to consider. Many contemporary practitioners seem to juxtapose various techniques together while neglecting theoretical frameworks. This is particularly true when it comes to psychodrama practice and the ways in which psychodrama techniques have been adopted by non-psychodramatists and employed without regard for their underlying philosophy and theories.

How do I use theory to guide my therapeutic approach and interventions?

Each psychodrama includes three phases and five elements. The phases begin with the warm-up, then the psychodrama enactment, and finally the sharing portion of the group (Fleury & Marra, 2022). These phases, depicted in Figure 2.2, provide a structure and a pacing for the session and each are equally important. Practitioners need to attend to each phase. Without an adequate warm-up phase, the enactment will be premature, forced, or unsafe. Without proper time for sharing and processing, we risk missing the precious integrative moments that occur after a psychodrama enactment.

In any psychodrama, there are five core elements. The five elements of a psychodrama include the director, stage, protagonist, auxiliary egos (or role players), and the audience (further described in Giacomucci, 2021b). The director is the facilitator of the psychodrama, and the protagonist is the participant whose topic and goal is to be enacted with the group's support. The

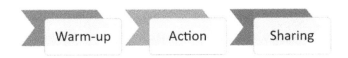

Figure 2.2 The three phases of a psychodrama group.

stage is the place where the action takes place – this is often just the space in the group room within a circle of chairs. The audience are the group members observing the process and the auxiliary egos are the roles that are being played by other group members in service of the protagonist's topic and goal. These three phases and five elements provide a structure and framework for the psychodrama session.

Psychodrama offers multiple theories that support its interventions and operationalize its philosophy. The core theories of psychodrama range from action theory (introduced above), spontaneity-creativity, role theory, developmental theory, sociometry, and catharses. Psychodrama theories are intrinsically connected to psychodrama techniques. These primary theories will be presented below while drawing connections between them and trauma theory. Psychodrama interventions and techniques will be outlined and described in Chapter 3.

Spontaneity-Creativity Theory

Moreno's theory of change is spontaneity-creativity theory, depicted through the Canon of Creativity (1953). This process shows how new cultural conserves are generated through a warming-up process which cultivates spontaneity and creativity, resulting in the creation of something new (see Figure 2.3).

Spontaneity is only accessed through a warming-up process, but once tapped into provides the readiness for new action and creation. The warming-up process helps overcome ambivalence and preparation for new action. In psychodrama theory, there is no such thing as "resistant clients," instead they are conceptualized as clients who are warmed-up to something else.

The Spontaneity Assessment Inventory Revised (SAIR) was developed by David Kipper and colleagues while validating its psychometric validity and reliability (it has also been translated into multiple languages). The SAIR has been used in multiple studies demonstrating spontaneity's

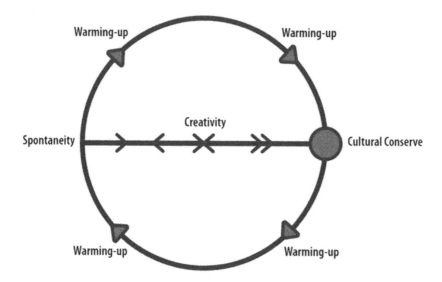

Figure 2.3 Moreno's Canon of Creativity (republished with permission from Giacomucci, 2021b, p. 62).

inverse relationship to mental health symptoms and its positive relation-ship to other measures of well-being. Nearly a century ago Moreno postu-lated that spontaneity and anxiety are inversely correlated – an idea later validated by research (Tarashoeva, Marinova-Djambazova, & Kojuharov, 2017). Moreno suggested that the warming-up process helps to mitigate anxiety while propelling one toward spontaneous action. PTSD, formerly categorized as an anxiety disorder but now a stress disorder, appears to have a similarly inverse relationship to spontaneity (Giacomucci, 2021c; Giacomucci, Marquit, & Miller Walsh, 2022). Through the lens of Moreno's spontaneity theory, we would conceptualize PTSD as a condition perpet-uated through the disconnection from healthy spontaneity (Giacomucci, 2021c). PTSD, like other psychosocial problems, would be described by Moreno as being characterized by an absence of spontaneity (immobiliza-tion or reenactment) or the presence of pathological spontaneity (novel but inadequate action). The Canon of Creativity provides us with a sim-plified map for trauma recovery and reminds us of the importance of the warming-up process which is likely to take longer for trauma survivors. The importance of warming-up is a core idea of this book which will be revisited in later sections and chapters as it relates to playfulness, internal-ized trauma roles, sociometric warm-ups, and SAMHSA's core principles of trauma-informed care.

*Do my facilitation approaches and group structures provide enough empha-
sis on the warming-up process?*

How do I warm-up myself to lead a group or meeting?

*What ways can I promote a warming-up process in my organization before
major changes?*

Traumatic stress is characterized by intrusive images or thoughts, negative
moods and beliefs, arousal and reactivity, as well as avoidance and dissociation. These symptoms provide blocks from safety, well-being, joy, and happiness. In order to access spontaneity, safety must first be established. The role
of playfulness in cultivating safety for adults is beginning to be discussed, particularly as it relates to group therapy and psychodrama (Giacomucci, 2021b;
Goldstein, 2018). Playfulness is associated with relationships, joy, and even
resilience (Trevarthen & Panksepp, 2016). Perhaps Gross (2018) provides
the most striking insights on the relationship between play and trauma in
the following passage:

> In many ways, play is the opposite experience of trauma. While play
> brings about feelings of joy, trauma brings about feelings of hopelessness
> and despair. While play serves to unite us, trauma serves to isolate us.
> While play motivates us to actively engage in the moment, trauma moti-
> vates us to fight and flee from it. And while play allows us to control our
> environment, trauma occurs when our environment controls us… play
> has the potential to serve as an antidote and powerful corrective emo-
> tional experience to trauma when integrated into treatment.
>
> (p. 369)

Playfulness then can hold an important role in the trauma recovery process as it cultivates safety, connection, engagement, control, and joy. Play
may be a core component in one's warming-up process on the Canon of
Creativity as it appears to help many access their spontaneity and creativity. Role-playing is of course, one form of play. The psychodramatic
process inherently involves play as an undercurrent through its reliance on
role-playing techniques. In a recent trauma-focused psychodrama study by
this author, after completion of a psychodrama group patients commented
on their surprise that trauma therapy could be "fun" (Giacomucci &
Marquit, 2020). A psychodrama enactment is a unique experience that
often encompasses experiences of playfulness, catharsis, and the integration of new ideas.

Catharsis

Psychodrama has developed a reputation for its potential in facilitating powerful catharsis. Catharsis is usually part of the trauma therapy process and generally something experienced during a psychodramatic role play. Moreno was perhaps one of the most prolific writers on the theory of catharsis since Aristotle, Breuer, and Freud. He expanded the concept of catharsis finding positive correlations between catharsis and spontaneity, action, and group experience (Moreno, 1940; Nolte, 2014). Moreno identified multiple distinctly different types of catharsis, most notably – audience catharsis, actor catharsis, catharsis of abreaction, and catharsis of integration. Developing on Aristotle's concept of spectator catharsis, Moreno noted how an audience's cathartic experience was enhanced when the action observed was novel (spontaneous), when the audience shared a common bond, and when the action related to the audience's own personal lives. Through his research with the *Theater of Spontaneity*, he also became acutely aware of the catharses his actors were experiencing through role-playing characters and situations that related to their personal lives. "The greater catharsis achieved through action is undeniable. The patient is able to express kinesthetically many feelings for which he has no words" (Moreno & Enneis, 1950, p. 13). Moreno differentiates between catharsis of abreaction and catharsis of integration suggesting that both are necessary, but that abreaction alone is not healing – integration is the ultimate goal (Nolte, 2014). Catharsis of abreaction describes the discharging, releasing, and expressing of built-up feelings or resistances while catharsis of integration labels the reconfiguration and inner transformation associated with meaning making and growth (Kellerman, 1984). Group therapy research supports that catharsis is only effective in promoting change when it included cognitive learning (Lieberman, Yalom, & Miles, 1973).

Zerka Moreno (2000) further adds that many of the most healing catharses occur through psychodrama scenes of experiences impossible in reality – for example, a client having a conversation for closure with a deceased family member, a childhood trauma survivor nurturing themselves as a child, or an assault survivor confronting their perpetrator and receiving an authentic amends from them. Kellerman articulately summarizes Moreno's contribution to the theory of catharsis:

> To include not only release and relief of emotions, but also integration
> and ordering; not only intense reliving of the past, but also intense liv
> ing in the here-and-now; not only a passive, verbal reflection, but also
> an active, nonverbal enactment; not only a private ritual, but also a

communal, shared rite of healing; not only an intrapsychic tension reduction, but also an interpersonal conflict resolution; not only a medical purification, but also a religious and aesthetic experience.

(1984, pp. 10–11)

Role-playing often leads to catharses, action insights and the integration of new ideas that were not previously available to an individual from the role of self. Spontaneous role-playing, in many ways, is an action-based free association method. Taking on different roles in a psychodrama offers participants a chance to step into the shoes of others, give voice to parts of self, and develop new roles or skills previous unintegrated into their sense of self. Psychodrama enactments may include a variety of roles ranging from intrapsychic roles (strengths, parts of self, visions of self, internalized trauma roles, defenses, etc.) interpersonal roles (family members, friends, colleagues, etc.) or transpersonal roles (God, ancestors, archetypes, etc.).

Role Theory

Moreno's theory of personality is role theory – which suggests that the "self" is composed of all the roles one holds in their life and that a healthy (spontaneous) personality has a wide role repertoire (Moreno, 1953). The idea of the role is a non-pathologizing way of labeling clusters of behavior, cognition, affect, somatic experience, and social phenomenon. It bridges the gap between psychiatry and the social sciences (Moreno, 1961) while offering a simple to understand language for describing behavior of clients. Psychodrama's role theory is comprehensive including a theory of role development (role taking, role-playing, and role creating), categories of roles (somatic, psychodramatic, and social), and various role dynamics and role phenomenon including role reciprocity, role lock, role fatigue, role-self congruence, role conflict, sub-roles, and others (Clayton, 1993, 1994; Giacomucci, 2021b; Telias, 2018).

One of the most important teachings from role theory is that of the three stages of role development (see Figure 2.4).

Moreno teaches that when we begin to adopt new roles into our life and our self, we are in a role taking phase. The role is new and unfamiliar at this point and there may be resistance to the role. Here we look to role models for help in learning the new role. After a role is adequately learned, we move into a role-playing phase of development which is characterized by one's ability to hold the role and start to bring themself into it. The final phase of development, role creating, is when one brings enough spontaneity and

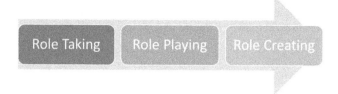

Figure 2.4 Moreno's stages of role development.

creativity into the role to transform it into something complete new. The role development theory can be particularly useful when thinking about professional development or staff development within organizations, as well as when helping clients integrate new internal or interpersonal roles related to trauma recovery.

Which phase of role development am I currently in when it comes to becoming a trauma-informed professional?

What would it look like to move to the next phase?

Role theory provides a simple language of describing parts of self which translates easily across cultures. Moreno outlines three categories of roles – somatic, psychodramatic, and social roles. Somatic roles are the first to develop in one's life at the pre-verbal stage and include the eater, the crawler, the sleeper, etc. Though somatic roles are their own category or role, both psychodramatic and social roles also have somatic aspects to them. Psychodramatic roles are the roles we play out in our mind or psyche relating to the internal dimensions of life – the dreamer, the thinker, idealized or distorted parts of self, future or past projections of self, etc. Social roles are one's we play in relation to others in our life and society, such as brother, mother, therapist, client, etc. (Moreno, 1934). Roles can be integrated parts of self, or here-and-now manifestations of behavior and experience. Moreno (1972) writes of a somatic self, psychodramatic self, and social self, composed of all the roles within each category which integrate into a singular sense of a biopsychosocial self (see Figure 2.5).

Moreno viewed human beings as role players and actors on the stage of life and that an individual's personality emerges from their roles and relationships. Roles also emerge and are embodied in situations, often with reciprocity to others. This theory of personality highlights the impacts of relationships and

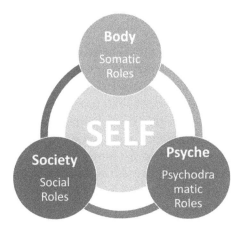

Figure 2.5 Roles and their relation to the biopsychosocial self.

social forces upon our lives and thus takes into account how relational and collective trauma may impact personality and a sense of self. Traumatic responses to adversity lead to the internalization of trauma-based roles (Giacomucci, 2018). The trauma recovery process involves transforming these trauma-based roles into roles of posttraumatic growth (Giacomucci, 2021c). Role theory provides a non-pathologizing approach to conceptualizing self that is similar to other popular trauma theories based on ego states or parts work.

Moreno's Developmental Theory

J.L. Moreno proposed a new developmental theory composed of three distinct stages which also reflect three primary psychodrama interventions – the double, the mirror, and the role reversal. Moreno's three stages of development describe a child's movement from the first universe of formlessness into the second universe. After birth, a child lives in a state of undifferentiated identity having not yet formed a sense of self or ego strength. Moreno described this as the *matrix of identity* and theorized that during this time the child experiences themselves as one with their mother, caregivers, and all of their surroundings (Moreno, 1953).

The first development stage is *doubling*, which is when caregivers and others help to give voice to a pre-verbal infant's experience and needs. Accurate doubling requires an attuned caregiver and helps the child develop a sense of self and of their needs, feelings, and experiences (Dayton, 2005). Doubling is required for healthy attachment and helps a child feel understood and seen – neurobiologically developing the internal brain circuitry for self-regulation later in life (Cozolino, 2014). When a child grows up without accurate doubling from others, "the child may feel that he is incomprehensible to others and a sort of fissure may occur within the self due to feeling misunderstood or out of sync with his external representations of self" (Dayton, 2005, p. 161). This frequently occurs in the context of childhood trauma. The second developmental stage is that of *the mirror*. This is when a child begins to develop a sense of individuality and a sense of self, to the point of being able to recognize their reflection in the mirror (Moreno, 1952). At this stage, the child develops awareness of themselves as separate from others and separate from the world (Dayton, 2005). Children whose developmental needs are not met in this stage may struggle with codependency, enmeshment, or a distorted sense of self. This is also quite common for childhood trauma survivors. The third developmental stage, role reversal, describes a stage when a child can empathize with others, see things from another's perspective, and understand that each person has their own subjective experience, feelings, and thoughts. Tian Dayton (2005) writes that "in role reversal the sense of self is intact enough so that we can temporarily leave it, stand in the shoes of another, and return safely home" (p. 439). A child experiencing trauma at this phase may not develop the capacity to consider other people's perspectives, emotions, and experiences. It may manifest as a rupture in empathy and consideration for others. These three stages of child development offer a simplified conceptualization of how traumatic disruptions at these three stages may impact an individual. The clinician's assessment in this framework then offers guidance on which of these psychodramatic interventions (doubling, mirroring, or role reversal) to emphasize (Giacomucci, 2021b).

Zerka Moreno later expanded upon Moreno's three stages, influenced by Erickson's eight psychosocial stages, outlined in *The Eight Stages of Cosmic Being in Terms of Capacity and Need to Double and Role Reverse* (2006). Zerka's expanded developmental theory goes a step further describing one's development through adulthood. It depicts how the child-caregiver roles often reverse wherein the adult child becomes the double and mirror for their aging parent, helping them as they transition from this world back to the first universe. Moreno's theories are deeply relational, highlighting the importance of relationships and social forces in each human's life. His 1914 poem, *An Invitation to an Encounter*, synthesizes the core of his interpersonal theory as well as the essence of role reversal:

> A meeting of two: eye to eye, face to face. And when you are near I will tear your eyes out and place them instead of mine and you will tear my

eyes out and place them instead of yours then I will look at you with your eyes and you will look at me with mine.

(Moreno, 1914)

Sociometric Theory

He later developed his interpersonal theory into a more comprehensive sociometric theory which became the foundation of his group therapy and psychodrama approaches. His sociometry theory offers a bridge between psychology and sociology while emphasizing a view of the person within their environment (Giacomucci, 2021b). One of the most important aspects of sociometry is the social atom, which is a visual depiction of an individual's closest relationships. Moreno's creation of the social atom appears to have also influenced the later development of the genogram and the ecomap (Dayton, 2005). The social atom is essentially a relational map showing the nature of an individual's connection to others in their life (see Figure 2.6).

The social atom is a useful assessment tool and future visioning tool for clinical work as it helps to illumination social relationships and dynamics within one's life. Having a client draw their social atom will often provide a clinician with more insight into their social life than simply interviewing

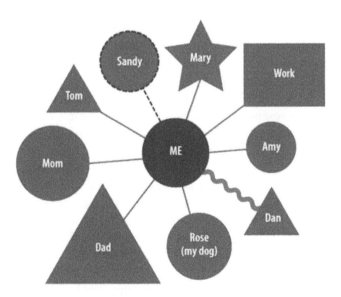

Figure 2.6 The social atom (republished with permission from Giacomucci, 2021b, p. 88).

them. In the example above, individuals in the client's life are down to scale and proximity based on closeness and the amount of social space the individual or entity occupies in their life. The line connecting the two individuals also provides information related to the nature of the connection – a straight line representing a connected relationship, dotted line to represent a lost relationship, and a squiggly line to indicate a conflictual relationship. Traditionally, circles were used for women, triangles for men, and squares for non-human roles. The social atom has been further developed in the past several years by modern psychodramatists to offer options for non-gender conforming and transgender folks such as the use of a star or simply giving participants the option of using any shape for any person on the social atom (as suggested by this writer's former graduate student Jordan Briem) (Giacomucci, 2021b). The social atom can be used in a variety of different ways including as an assessment tool, as a treatment planning or evaluation tool, for self-examination, or as a warm-up for a psychodrama.

While the social atom is a person-centered view of one's relationships, Moreno also developed a tool called the sociogram, which is a group-centered exploration of relationships and sociodynamics. Moreno's sociograms, generated through a sociometric test, depict the distribution of choices, preferences, connections, and social wealth within a group of any size (see Figure 2.7).

Sociograms can be done drawn on paper, generated by computer programs (Raimundo & Raimundo, 2021), or done experientially through "hands-on-shoulder sociometry" which will be described in Chapter 4. The sociogram was one of Moreno's earlier sociometric tools and illuminated the presence of two core sociometric phenomenon – *tele* and the *sociodynamic effect*. Tele describes "the socio-gravitational factor, which operates between individuals, drawing them to form more positive or negative pair-relations…than on chance" (Moreno, 1947, p. 84). Moreno further explains tele as a type of two-way empathy, as the opposite of transference, as a knowing and insight into another person, and as the foundation for all wholesome relationships (1953, 1959). Tele appears to be related to non-verbal, right-brain to right-brain communication and intuition that promotes synchronicity and unexpected connection (Dayton, 2005, Giacomucci, 2021b, Yaniv, 2014). On the other hand, the sociodynamic effect, is a term labeling an underlying social force in all groups that leads to the unequal distribution of connection, choices, preferences, and social wealth (Moreno, 1943). This effect leads to the presence of social stars and social isolates in every group while also underlying most social problems in the world such as collective trauma, poverty,

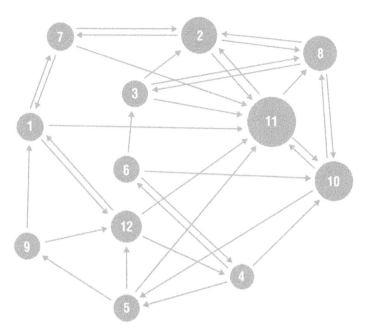

Figure 2.7 Sociogram of a classroom (republished with permission from Giacomucci, 2021b, p. 91).

discrimination, racism, and inequality. The sociodynamic effect is also at the core of many (or most) experiences of trauma, neglect, and abandonment. Trauma-informed practitioners have a responsibility to maintain awareness of the sociodynamic effect while working to mitigate and reverse its negative impact in groups, organizations, communities, and society (Giacomucci, 2017; Giacomucci et al, 2018; Korshak & Shapiro, 2013; Schreiber, 2018).

If we were to generate a sociogram of my group, community, organization, or team, who would be in the positions of the "social star" and the "isolate"?

How can I contribute to reversing the sociodynamic effect in the areas listed above?

Moreno's sociometry theory and particularly his sociograms were of great interest to sociologists and became the foundation for later social network theories and Participatory Action Research as well as aspects of the therapeutic community and milieu therapy (Greenwood, 2015; Landy, 2008; Moreno, 2014). His sociometric tests and sociograms were used in the military and in various organizations to assess and improve cohesion (Moreno,

2014). Beyond work with small groups, Moreno also applied and developed his sociometric theory with all of society:

> A truly therapeutic procedure cannot have less an objective than the whole of mankind. But no adequate therapy can be prescribed as long as mankind is not a unity in some fashion and as long as its organization remains unknown.
>
> (1934, p. 3)

He believed that working one on one was simply not enough and that we needed to promote healing and change on a larger scale. His philosophy of viewing the group as its own entity also translated into his view of human-kind as having an organic unity – that all humans are bound together by a core commonality that transcends all differences (Moreno, 1934). His sociometric system, he believed, was an essential pre-requisite for assessing groups, communities, and society in order to offer adequate interventions for change. Moreno's sociometry on a macro level is designed to address, miti-gate, and prevent social injustice while promoting equity and equality in all spheres of life.

Conclusion

Though he is most recognized for his psychodrama group therapy approach, Moreno's methods transcend group therapy and also offer tools creating change within non-clinical groups, individuals, communities, organizations, and all of society. In this way, his philosophy and theories are not only trauma-focused treatments but also provide a framework congruent with trauma-informed care that is applicable to work with individuals, groups, communities, organizations, and all of society. As noted at the start of this chapter, Moreno's theories and philosophy are quite expansive. This chapter offers an introduction to his ideas as they relate to trauma-informed care. A more comprehensive exploration of Moreno's philosophy and theory is available through other publications (see Dayton, 2005; Giacomucci, 2021b; Hale, 1981; Moreno, 1953, 1972, 2019; Nolte, 2014; von Ameln & Becker-Ebel, 2020).

References

Azarang, A., Pakyurek, M., Giroux, C., Nordahl, T. E., & Yellowlees, P. (2019). Information technologies: An augmentation to post-traumatic stress disorder treatment among trauma survivors. *Telemedicine and e-Health, 25*(4), 263–271.

Baird, S. L., & Alaggia, R. (2021). Trauma-informed groups: Recommendations for group work practice. *Clinical Social Work Journal, 49*(1), 10–19.

Badenoch, B. (2018). *The heart of trauma: Healing the embodied brain in the context of relationships*: New York: W.W. Norton & Company.

Badenoch, B., & Cox, P. (2013). Integrating interpersonal neurobiology with group psychotherapy. In S. P. Gantt, & B. Badenoch (Eds.), *The interpersonal neurobiology of group psychotherapy and group process* (pp. 1–18). London: Karnac Books Ltd.

Blatner, A. (2000). *Foundations of psychodrama: History, theory, and practice* (4th ed.). New York City: Springer Publishing Company.

Clayton, M. (1993). *Living pictures of the self. Applications of role theory in professional practice and daily life*: Caulfield: ICA PRESS.

Clayton, M. (1994) Role theory and its application in clinical practice. In P. Holmes, M. Karp, & M. Watson (Eds.), *Psychodrama since Moreno: Innovations in theory and practice* (pp. 121–144): London: Routledge.

Cohen, J. A., & Mannarino, A. P. (2015). Trauma-focused cognitive behavioral therapy for traumatized children and families. *Child and Adolescent Psychiatric Clinics of North America, 24*(3), 557.

Corey, M. S., Corey, G., & Corey, C. (2018). *Groups: Process and practice* (10th ed.). Boston, MA: Cengage Learning.

Courtois, C. A. (2010). *Healing the incest wound* (2nd ed.). New York: W. W. Norton & Company.

Courtois, C. A., & Ford, J. D. (2016). *Treatment of complex trauma: A sequenced, relationship-based approach*. New York: The Guildford Press.

Cozolino, L. J. (2014). *The neuroscience of human relationships* (2nd ed.). New York: W.W. Norton & Company.

Dayton, T. (2005). *The living stage: A step-by-step guide to psychodrama, sociometry, and experiential group therapy*. Deerfield, FL: Health Communications Inc.

Fleury, H. J., & Marra, M. M. (2022). Theoretical and methodological foundations of socionomy. In H. J. Fleury, M. M. Marra, & O. H. Hadler (Eds.), *Psychodrama in Brazil* (pp. 17–29). Singapore: Springer.

Foy, D. W., Unger, W. S., & Wattenberg, M. S. (2005). Module 4: An overview of evidence-based group approaches to trauma with adults. In B. Buchele, & H. Spitz (Eds.), *Group interventions for treatment of psychological trauma* (pp. 116–166). New York City: American Group Psychotherapy Association.

Gantt, S. P., & Badenoch, B. (2013). *The interpersonal neurobiology of group psychotherapy and group process*. London: Karnac Books Ltd.

Gerber, M. R., Elisseou, S., Sager, Z. S., & Keith, J. A. (2020). Trauma-informed telehealth in the COVID-19 era and beyond. *Federal Practitioner, 37*(7), 302.

Giacomucci, S. (2017). The sociodrama of life or death: Young adults and addiction treatment. *Journal of Psychodrama, Sociometry, and Group Psychotherapy, 65*(1): 137–143. https://doi.org/10.12926/0731-1273-65.1.137

Giacomucci, S. (2018). The trauma survivor's inner role atom: A clinical map for post-traumatic growth. *Journal of Psychodrama, Sociometry, and Group Psychotherapy, 66*(1): 115–129.

Giacomucci, S. (2019). *Social group work in action: A sociometry, psychodrama, and experiential trauma therapy curriculum.* Doctorate in Social Work (DSW) Dissertations, 124. https://repository.upenn.edu/cgi/viewcontent.cgi?article=1128&context=edissertations_sp2

Giacomucci, S. (2020). Addiction, traumatic loss, and guilt: A case study resolving grief through psychodrama and sociometric connections. *The Arts in Psychotherapy, 67,* 101627. https://doi.org/10.1016/j.aip.2019.101627

Giacomucci, S. (2021a). Experiential sociometry in group work: Mutual aid for the group-as-a-whole. *Social Work with Groups, 44*(3), 204–214.

Giacomucci, S. (2021b). *Social work, sociometry, and psychodrama: Experiential approaches for group therapists, community leaders, and social workers.* Singapore: Springer Nature.

Giacomucci, S. (2021c). Traumatic stress and spontaneity: Trauma-focused and strengths-based psychodrama. In J. Maya, & J. Maraver (Eds.), *Psychodrama advances in psychotherapy and psychoeducational interventions* (pp. 1–44). New York: Nova Science Publishers.

Giacomucci, S., & Ehrhart, L. (2021). Introduction to psychodrama psychotherapy: A trauma and addiction group vignette. *Group, 45*(1), 69–86.

Giacomucci, S., Gera, S., Briggs, D., & Bass, K. (2018). Experiential addiction treatment: Creating positive connection through sociometry and therapeutic spiral model safety structures. *Journal of Addiction and Addictive Disorders, 5,* 17. http://doi.org/10.24966/AAD-7276/100017

Giacomucci, S., Karner, D., Nieto, L., & Schreiber, E. (2021). Sociatry, psychodrama, and social work: Moreno's mysticism and social justice tradition. *Social Work with Groups, 44*(3), 288–303. https://doi.org/10.1080/01609513.2021.1885826

Giacomucci, S., & Marquit, J. (2020). The effectiveness of trauma-focused psychodrama in the treatment of PTSD in inpatient substance abuse treatment. *Frontiers in Psychology, 11,* 896. https://dx.doi.org/10.3389%2Ffpsyg.2020.00896

Giacomucci, S., Marquit, J., & Miller Walsh, K. (2022). A controlled pilot study on the effects of a therapeutic spiral model trauma-focused psychodrama workshop on post-traumatic stress, spontaneity and post-traumatic growth. *Zeitschrift für Psychodrama und Soziometrie, 21*(1), 171–188.

Giacomucci, S., & Stone, A. M. (2019). Being in two places at once: Renegotiating traumatic experience through the surplus reality of psychodrama. *Social Work with Groups, 42*(3), 184–196. https://doi.org/10.1080/01609513.2018.1533913

Gitterman, A., & Shulman, L. (2005). *Mutual aid groups, vulnerable and resilient populations, and the life cycle* (3rd ed.). New York: Columbia University Press.

Goldstein, B. (2018). Cultivating curiosity, creativity, confidence, and self-awareness through mindful group therapy for children and adolescents. In T. Marks-Tarlow, M. Solomon, & D. J. Siegel (Eds.), *Play & creativity in psychotherapy* (pp. 338–358). New York: W.W. Norton & Company.

Greenwood, D. J. (2015). Evolutionary systems thinking: What Gregory Bateson, Kurt Lewin, and Jacob Moreno offered to action research that still remains to be learned. In H. Bradbury (Ed.), *Handbook of action research* (3rd ed., pp. 425–433). London: Sage Publications.

Gross, S. (2018). The power of optimism. In T. Marks-Tarlow, M. Solomon, & D. J. Siegel (Eds.), *Play & creativity in psychotherapy* (pp. 359–375). New York: W.W. Norton & Company.

Gullo, S., Lo Coco, G., Leszcz, M., Marmarosh, C. L., Miles, J. R., Shechtman, Z., … & Tasca, G. A. (2022). Therapists' perceptions of online group therapeutic relationships during the COVID-19 pandemic: A survey-based study. *Group Dynamics: Theory, Research, and Practice, 26*(2), 103.

Hale, A. E. (1981). *Conducting clinical sociometric explorations: A manual for psychodramatists and sociometrists.* Roanoke, VA: Royal Publishing Company.

Herman, J. L. (1992). *Trauma and recovery: The aftermath of violence—From domestic abuse to political terror.* New York: Basic Books.

Hudgins, M. K. & Toscani, F. (2013). *Healing world trauma with the therapeutic spiral model: Stories from the frontlines.* London: Jessica Kingsley Publishers.

Janet, P. (1889). *L'Automatisme psychologique.* Paris: Félix Alcan.

Kellerman, P. F. (1984). The place of Catharsis in psychodrama. *Journal of Group Psychotherapy, Psychodrama, and Sociometry, 37*(1): 1–13.

Korshak, S. J., & Shapiro, M. (2013). Choosing the unchosen: Counteracting the sociodynamic effect using complementary sharing. *Journal of Psychodrama, Sociometry, and Group Psychotherapy, 61*(1): 7–15.

Landy, R. J. (2008). *The couch and the stage: Integrating words and action in psychotherapy*. Lanham, MD, US: Jason Aronson.

Leszcz, M. (2018). The evidence-based group psychotherapist. *Psychoanalytic Inquiry*, 38(4), 285–298.

Levine, P. A. (2010). *In an unspoken voice: How the body releases trauma and restores goodness*. Berkeley, CA. North Atlantic Books.

Lieberman, M. A., Yalom, I. D., & Miles, M. (1973). *Encounter groups: First facts*. New York: Basic Books.

MacKenzie, K. R. (1997). Clinical application of group development ideas. *Group Dynamics: Theory, Research, and Practice*, 1(4), 275–287.

Malchiodi, C. A. (2020). *Trauma and expressive arts therapy: Brain, body, and imagination in the healing process*: New York: Guilford Publications.

Moreno, J. D. (2014). *Impromptu man: J.L. Moreno and the origins of psychodrama, encounter culture, and the social network*. New York: Bellevue Literary Press.

Moreno, J. L. (1914) *Einladung zu einer Begegnung*. Vienna: Anzengruber Verlag.

Moreno, J. L. (1934). *Who shall survive? A new approach to the problems of human interrelations*. Washington, DC: Nervous and Mental Disease Publishing Co.

Moreno, J. L. (1940). Mental catharsis and the psychodrama. *Sociometry*, 3, 209–244.

Moreno, J. L. (1943). Sociometry and the cultural order. *Sociometry*, 6(3), 299–344.

Moreno, J. L. (1946). *Psychodrama volume 1*. Beacon, NY: Beacon House Press.

Moreno, J. L. (1947). Progress and pitfalls in sociometric theory. *Sociometry*, 10, 268–272.

Moreno, J. L. (1952). Psychodramatic production techniques. *Group Psychotherapy, Psychodrama, & Sociometry*, 4, 273–303.

Moreno, J. L. (1953). *Who shall survive? Foundations of sociometry, group psychotherapy and sociodrama* (2nd ed.). Beacon, NY: Beacon House.

Moreno, J. L. (1957). Code of ethics of group psychotherapists. *Group Psychotherapy*, 10, 143–144.

Moreno, J. L. (in collaboration with Z.T. Moreno) (1959). *Psychodrama second volume, foundations of psychotherapy*. Beacon, NY: Beacon House.

Moreno, J. L. (1961). The role concept, a bridge between psychiatry and sociology. *American Journal of Psychiatry*, 118(6), 518–523.

Moreno, J. L. (1972). *Psychodrama volume 1* (4th ed.). Beacon, NY: Beacon House Press.

Moreno, J. L. (2019). *The autobiography of a genius* (E. Schreiber, S. Kelley, & S. Giacomucci, Eds.). United Kingdom: North West Psychodrama Association.

Moreno, J. L., & Enneis, J. M. (1950). *Hypnodrama and psychodrama.* New York: Beacon House.

Moreno, Z. T. (1969). Moreneans: The heretics of yesterday are the orthodoxy of today. *Group Psychotherapy, 22,* 1–6.

Moreno, Z. T. (2000). The Function of 'Tele' in human relations. In J. Zeig (Ed.), *The evolution of psychotherapy: A meeting of the minds* (pp. 289–301). Phoenix, AZ: Erickson Foundation Press.

Moreno, Z. T. (2006). *The Quintessential Zerka* (T. Horvatin, & E. Schreiber Eds.). New York: Routledge.

Moreno, Z. T. (2012). *To dream again: A memoir.* New York: Mental Health Resources.

Najavits, L. (2002). *Seeking safety: A treatment manual for PTSD and substance abuse:* New York: Guilford Publications.

Nolte, J. (2014). *The philosophy, theory, and methods of J.L. Moreno: The man who tried to become god.* New York: Routledge.

Nolte, J. (2019). *JL Moreno and the psychodramatic method: On the practice of psychodrama.* New York: Routledge.

Oudijk, R. (2007). A postmodern approach to psychodrama theory. In C. Baim, J. Burmeister, & M. Maciel (Eds.), *Psychodrama: Advances in theory and practice* (pp. 139–150). London: Routledge.

Perry, B. D., & Szalavitz, M. (2006). *The boy who was raised as a dog and other stories from a child psychiatrist's notebook: What traumatized children can teach us about loss, love, and healing.* New York, US: Basic Books.

Raimundo, C. A., & Raimundo, M. (2021). RCompass, a digital sociometry. What would Moreno think about it? Celebrating 100 years of Moreno's psychodrama and 60 years of Rojas-Bermúdez psychodrama. *Journal of the Psychodrama, Sociometry, and Group Psychotherapy, 68*(1), 39–62.

Redfern, M. (2014). Safe spaces and scary encounters: Core therapeutic elements of trauma-informed dramatherapy. In N. Sajnani, & D. R. Johnson (Eds.), *Trauma informed drama therapy: Transforming clinics, classrooms, and communities* (pp. 365–388): Springfield: Charles C Thomas Publisher.

Rosenwald, M., & Baird, J. (2020). An integrated trauma-informed, mutual aid model of group work. *Social Work with Groups, 43*(3), 257–271.

Schreiber, E. (2018). Sociatry part 2: Moreno's mysticism. *Psychodrama Network News, Winter 2018,* 24–25. American Society of Group Psychotherapy and Psychodrama.

Schwartz, R. C. (2021). *No bad parts: Healing trauma and restoring wholeness with the internal family systems model*. Boulder, CO: Sounds True.

Schreiber, E. W., & Giacomucci, S. (forthcoming). Psychodrama, sociodrama, sociometry, & sociatry. In B. J. Sadock, V. A. Sadock, & P. Ruiz (Eds.), *Kaplan & Sadock's comprehensive textbook of psychiatry* (11th ed., p. XXXX). Philadelphia, PA: Lippincott Williams & Wilkins publishers.

Shapiro, J. R., & Applegate, J. S. (2018). *Neurobiology for clinical social work: Theory and practice* (2nd ed.). New York: W.W. Norton & Company.

Siegel, D. J. (2007). *The mindful brain: Reflection and attunement in the cultivation of well-being*. New York: W.W. Norton & Company.

Siegel, D. J. (2013). Reflections on mind, brain, and relationships in group psychotherapy. In S. P. Gantt, & B. Badenoch (Eds.), *The interpersonal neurobiology of group psychotherapy and group process* (pp. 19–23). London: Karnac Books, Ltd.

Siegel, D. J. (2020). *Developing mind: How relationships and the brain interact to shape who we are* (3rd ed.). New York: Guilford Press.

Simmons, D., & Wilches, A. (2022). TELE'DRAMA—International sociometry in the virtual space. *Zeitschrift für Psychodrama und Soziometrie, 21*(1), 119–129.

Shapiro, F. (2018). *Eye-movement desensitization and reprocessing (EMDR) therapy* (3rd ed.). New York: Guilford Press.

Shulman, L. (2015). *The skills of helping individuals, families, groups, and communities* (8th ed.). Boston, MA: Cengage Learning.

Steinberg, D. M. (2014). *A mutual-aid model for social work with groups*: London: Routledge.

Stoll, J., Müller, J. A., & Trachsel, M. (2020). Ethical issues in online psychotherapy: A narrative review. *Frontiers in Psychiatry, 10*, 993.

Substance Abuse and Mental Health Services Administration. (2014a). *SAMHSA's concept of trauma and guidance for a trauma-informed approach*. HHS Publication No. (SMA) 14-4884. Rockville, MD: Substance Abuse and Mental Health Services Administration.

Takis, N. (2020). Reflections on Moreno's ambivalent view on Sigmund Freud and psychoanalysis. *Journal of Psychodrama, Sociometry, and Group Psychotherapy, 67*(1), 9–18.

Tarashoeva, G., Marinova-Djambazova, P., & Kojuharov, H. (2017). Effectiveness of psychodrama therapy in patients with panic disorders: Final results. *International Journal of Psychotherapy, 21*(2), 55–66.

Telias, R. (2018). *Moreno's personality theory and its relationship to psychodrama: A philosophical, developmental and therapeutic perspective*. New York: Routledge.

Trevarthen, C., & Panksepp, J. (2016). In tune with feeling. In S. Hart (Ed.), *Inclusion, Play and Empathy: Neuroaffective Development in Children's Groups* (pp. 29–54). London: Jessica Kingsley Publishers.

Tuckman, B. W. (1965). Developmental sequence in small groups. *Psychological Bulletin, 63*, 384–399.

Turgoose, D., Ashwick, R., & Murphy, D. (2018). Systematic review of lessons learned from delivering tele-therapy to veterans with post-traumatic stress disorder. *Journal of Telemedicine and Telecare, 24*(9), 575–585.

Ulman, K. H. (2005). Module 1: Group interventions for treatment of trauma in adults. In B. Buchele, & H. Spitz (Eds.), *Group interventions for treatment of psychological trauma* (pp. 13–59). New York City: American Group Psychotherapy Association.

van der Hart, O., Groenendijk, M., Gonzalez, A., Mosquera, D., & Solomon, R. (2013). Dissociation of the personality and EMDR therapy in complex trauma-related disorders: Applications in the stabilization phase. *Journal of EMDR Practice and Research, 7*(2), 81–94.

van de Kamp, M. M., Scheffers, M., Hatzmann, J., Emck, C., Cuijpers, P., & Beek, P. J. (2019). Body-and movement-oriented interventions for posttraumatic stress disorder: A systematic review and meta-analysis. *Journal of Traumatic Stress, 32*(6), 967–976.

van der Kolk, B. A. (2014). *The body keeps the score: Brain, mind, and body in the healing of trauma*. New York: Viking Press.

von Ameln, F., & Becker-Ebel, J. (2020). *Fundamentals of psychodrama*. Singapore: Springer Nature.

Weinberg, H. (2020). Online group psychotherapy: Challenges and possibilities during COVID-19—A practice review. *Group Dynamics: Theory, Research, and Practice, 24*(3), 201.

Weinberg, H. (2021). Obstacles, challenges, and benefits of online group psychotherapy. *American Journal of Psychotherapy, 74*(2), 83–88.

Yalom, I. D., & Leszcz, M. (2020). *The theory and practice of group psychotherapy* (6th ed.). New York: Basic Books.

Yaniv, D. Z. (2014). Tele and the social atom: The oeuvre of J. L. Moreno from the perspective of neuropsychology. *Zeitschrift für Psychodrama und Soziometrie, 13*(1): 107–120.

3

Trauma-Focused Psychodrama as an Effective Group Treatment for PTSD

Chapter Summary

The clinical research on the effectiveness of group therapy and psychodrama continues to evolve with compelling data to support group therapy as at least as effective as individual therapies in treating various mental health disorders. Group work in its various forms is regularly implemented in hospitals and treatment centers at all levels of care to address posttraumatic stress disorder (PTSD) and trauma. Psychodrama's evidence base, though smaller, suggests it is a promising treatment for PTSD. Psychodrama practitioners and participants highlight its unique power in providing corrective emotional experiences, promoting safety and empowerment, and cultivating posttraumatic growth. This chapter presents classical psychodrama interventions as well as two trauma-focused psychodrama models – the Relational Trauma Repair model and the Therapeutic Spiral Model. Trauma-focused psychodrama is summarized with a clinical vignette.

Subsections on Therapeutic Spiral Model and Relational Trauma Repair Model are reprinted from Giacomucci, 2021b with permission.

Group Therapy's Effectiveness in Treating PTSD

Group therapies help trauma survivors normalize their feelings and experiences while realizing that they are not alone. The peer support and mutual aid within a group effectively reduces isolation, shame, stigma, hopelessness, and self-judgment often associated with posttraumatic stress disorder (PTSD).

DOI: 10.4324/9781003277859-3

The group becomes a holding environment or a healing matrix providing a safe container for traumatic memories to be explored, desensitized, renegotiated, and reprocessed (Klein & Schermer, 2000). The safety of the group and relationships within it help a trauma survivor to trust again, to change their sense of self, and challenge distorted beliefs about the world. Opportunities during the group process to help others create a sense of empowerment, meaning making, and posttraumatic growth (PTG) in that trauma survivors can turn their traumatic experiences into a source of inspiration and positive change for others in a practical way. Group work and group therapy operationalize trauma-informed principles in ways that individual therapy simple doesn't have the same opportunities for – particularly when it comes to the principles of trustworthiness, peer support, collaboration, mutuality, empowerment, and cultural, history, and gender issues related to group or community identities.

Group therapy has become more and more popular as a treatment for trauma and PTSD and its evidence base continues to grow. Group therapy offers unique opportunities for relational healing that individual therapy simply can't replicate. The multitude of relationships within a group setting can provide correction and growth beyond a single therapeutic relationship – if one is traumatized by a group, it often makes sense healing would come through a group. At the same time, there are, of course, some prefer individual therapy to group therapy or situations when an individual may benefit from one-to-one therapy more so than group work. The research on group therapy demonstrates that it is at least as effective as individual therapy for a variety of mental health and psychosocial issues (Burlingame & Krogel, 2005; Wodarski & Feit, 2012; Yalom & Leszcz, 2020) including PTSD (Sloan et al., 2013; Schwartze et al., 2019). Group work is also more financially viable and more efficient than individual work in that multiple clients can receive therapy at the same time. This makes it particularly appealing for providers and funders, especially insurance companies. While the majority of PTSD group therapy research has been with cognitive behavioral or exposure therapies, other group interventions including psychodrama are continuing to strengthen their research base.

Psychodrama as an Effective Treatment for Trauma and PTSD

The empirical evidence supporting psychodrama as an effective treatment for PTSD continues to grow and evolve. Current research positions psychodrama as a promising modality but more research is needed, particularly research trials with rigorous study designs (Orkibi & Feniger-Schaal, 2019). Multiple studies have already been published that demonstrate psychodrama's effectiveness in significantly reducing PTSD symptoms or trauma-related issues in various populations including military veterans (Cowden, Chapman, Houghtaling, & Worthington, 2021; Perry, Saby, Wenos, Hudgins, & Baller, 2016), patients in addiction treatment (Giacomucci & Marquit, 2020; Giacomucci, Marquit, Miller Walsh, & Saccarelli, 2022), mass shooting survivors (Cowden et al., 2022), child survivors of natural disasters (Hamidi & Sobhani Tabar, 2021; Tabar, Hamidi, & Tahmasebipour, 2020), women victims of intimate partner violence (Damra, 2022; Ron & Yanai, 2021; Mondolfi Miguel & Pino-Juste, 2021), abused women (Avinger & Jones, 2007; Bucuță, Dima, & Testoni, 2018), men with varied trauma histories (Giacomucci, Marquit, & Miller Walsh, 2022) and other forms of interpersonal trauma (Seppälä, 2020). Furthermore, psychodrama has been included in the literature bases of other larger categories of modalities that have significant evidence of effectively treating PTSD and trauma such as the experiential psychotherapies (Benish, Imel, & Wampold, 2008; Elliott, Greenberg, & Lietaer, 2004; Elliott et al., 2013), the creative arts therapies (Baker et al., 2018; Feniger-Shaal & Orkibi, 2020; Malchiodi, 2020), and the body- and movement-oriented interventions (van de Kamp et al., 2019).

In the qualitative component of my own ongoing research on trauma-focused psychodrama (N = 85), participants overwhelmingly reported finding the groups helpful (95.29%), feeling safe in the groups (96.47%), and that they would recommend the psychodrama trauma group to others (94.12%) (Giacomucci & Marquit, 2020). Actually, in each of these areas, every participant (100%) that answered the question did so positively; not a single person reported that it was unhelpful, unsafe, or that they wouldn't recommend to others. The difference between the percentages above and 100% is accounted for a few participants who did not answer the question at all in the survey. Furthermore, in this study, participants commented on psychodrama being not only a tolerable treatment but also fun at times. These themes are particularly significant in the context of high dropout rates for many other treatments for PTSD (Imel, Laska, Jakupcak, & Simpson, 2013). Here are some of the patient's comments about the group (from Giacomucci & Marquit, 2020):

> "I always thought trauma groups had to be painful – I found that not to be truthful."

> "I was able to release and let go of my trauma without reliving it."

"I liked that it was also a fun experience."

"Psychodrama was cool!"

These patient responses come from an inpatient trauma-focused psychodrama group that emphasized strengths-based psychodramas and PTG rather than re-enacting scenes of trauma. While many assume that trauma-focused psychodrama would involve re-enacting trauma scenes, and thus being potentially unsafe and retraumatizing, this is not true in most cases. There are times when revisiting the trauma scene would be therapeutic for a protagonist and can be done safely with support and strengths-based roles, but trauma-focused psychodrama is also used with a focus on restoration, strengths-based roles, PTG, and intrapsychic roles (Giacomucci, 2021c).

Neuroscience of Trauma-Focused Psychodrama

In addition to the empirical research, the constantly evolving neuroscience research also supports psychodrama as an effective treatment for trauma and PTSD. Moreno has suggested nearly 100 years ago that the body remembers what the mind forgets. This wisdom is echoed throughout the core philosophies of many of the foremost trauma experts today who regularly emphasize the somatic imprints of trauma and how the body keeps the score (Levine 2010; van der Kolk, 2014):

> Prone to action, and deficient in words, these patients (trauma survivors) can often express their internal states more articulately in physical movements or in pictures than in words. Utilizing drawings and psychodrama may help them develop a language that is essential for effective communication and for the symbolic transformation that can occur in psychotherapy.
>
> (van der Kolk, 1996, p. 195)

Our understanding of the neuroscience of trauma is constantly evolving. The research points to how trauma impacts the brain at levels below thinking, cognition, and talking. Trauma leaves an imprint on the nervous system and within the body – even when the traumatic experience is not consciously remembered by the survivor. In the case of repressed traumatic memories, the body continues to keep the score and respond to stimuli or triggers related to the traumatic event. Research shows that when someone remembers a traumatic experience, the left hemisphere of the brain is largely inactive (including the Broca's area which is dedicated to speech and language), while the right hemisphere is overactive (Rauch et al., 1996; van der Kolk, 2014).

This finding strongly challenges the use of talk therapies alone in the treatment of PTSD and trauma-related issues. Bessel van der Kolk, MD describes how the limbic system is impacted, "the imprint of trauma doesn't sit in the verbal, understanding part of the brain…but in much deeper regions – amygdala, hippocampus, hypothalamus, brain stem – which are only marginally affected by thinking and cognition" (as cited in Wylie, 2004, pp. 30–41). These neuroscience findings provide further validation for trauma survivors who so often report that it is difficult to talk about their trauma or that they struggle to remember it and describe it in words (Malchiodi, 2020). The voicelessness that commonly results from trauma can now be understood partially as a neurobiological process. Psychodrama's emphasis on symbolic representation, body movement, action, relationship, and other right-brain processes positions it as an ideal trauma treatment in that it can access and renegotiate trauma in the places it is stored within the mind, body, and brain.

The limbic system of the brain is significantly involved in attachment and relationships. So much of trauma is experienced in the context of relationship and results in later complications in one's social life. Cozolino articulates how "our brains are structured and restructured by interactions with our social and natural environments" (2014, pp. 77–78). After birth, human beings are entirely dependent on caregivers and attachment figures longer than any other species on the planet. Early childhood experiences and attachments provide the psychological and neurobiological architecture for a sense of self, template of relationship, core belief systems, and abilities for self-regulation later in life (Cozolino, 2014; Shapiro & Applegate, 2018; Wallin, 2007). Throughout the first several months of life all communication is non-verbal and through action such as facial expression, body language, posture, pointing, and gesturing. As a child develops, their communication evolves to include language and words while continuing to also be largely composed of action and non-verbal language. The emphasis on action, interaction, and non-verbal communication in psychodrama further validates its effectiveness in addressing childhood adversity and relational trauma. In addition to thought and cognition, the brain's primary languages are action and relationship. Louis Cozolino (2014) informs us that the field of "interpersonal neurobiology assumes that the brain is a social organ built via experience" (p. xvii).

Perhaps the most groundbreaking neuroscience finding of the century is that the brain changes through experience and maintains its neuroplasticity throughout the entire lifespan (Siegel, 2012). This highlights how adversity and traumatic experiences change the brain, but also points to the power of new positive experiences in promoting neurobiological change (Shapiro & Applegate, 2018). The surplus reality of the psychodrama stage provides an avenue for new experiences that are otherwise impossible in real life (Giacomucci & Stone, 2019). Though the psychodramatic role-play is different from a real experience, when the group is fully warmed-up and acting as-if in the here-and-now, it appears that the brain/body process the psychodrama experience in the same way any other experience is processed. Psychodrama participants often comment on how real the role-play felt for them which further validates this idea. Psychodrama offers the potential of changing both psychological and somatic impacts of past adversity by activating one's traumatic neural network in the safety of the group; the traumatic memory is renegotiated through new corrective experiences on the psychodrama stage (Giacomucci, 2021b). Previously incomplete survival responses from the moment of the trauma can be resolved. A client immobilized or frozen in their trauma, stuck in a chronic freeze response (dorsal vagal), can be released through the safe activation of a fight or flight response (sympathetic nervous system), and a resulting return to social engagement (as described in Polyvagal theory). In this way, the nervous system can discharge pent up somatic energy related to the trauma and be restored to a state of equilibrium (Levine, 2010; Porges, 2011, 2017). For example, a survivor of complex childhood abuse who perpetually is stuck in a freeze response long into adulthood, could engage in a series of psychodrama scenes that involve building up the strengths, support, and safety to face the trauma; nurturing and validating their younger self; address any abandoning authorities that failed in their responsibility to prevent or stop the abuse; have an embodied experience of successfully defending themselves and fighting off their perpetrator or successfully fleeing from their perpetrator; experience correction and the fulfillment of unmet developmental needs through scenes of repair with a perpetrator or idealized/archetypal parent figure; and engage in future projection scenes that involve role training aspects of PTG.

How can I incorporate body-oriented interventions into my work with trauma?

In what ways can I provide corrective emotional experiences to the clients I serve?

Posttraumatic Growth through Psychodrama

PTG is the phenomenon of growing after trauma or as a direct result of adversity (Calhoun & Tedeschi, 2014). It is estimated that as many as 90% of the population report some growth through major life difficulties (Calhoun & Tedeschi,

2012). Furthermore, nearly half of trauma survivors report moderate-to-high growth after trauma (Wu et al., 2018). When we compare these numbers to the 25% or so of folks who develop PTSD as a result of trauma, we can find significant hope in these statistics (Giacomucci, 2021b). PTG and PTSD often exist together, many trauma survivors experience aspects of traumatic stress and growth at the same time. Nevertheless, higher rates of PTG are related to lower rates of PTSD. These findings point to the importance of PTG when working with trauma and an emphasis on not overlooking the third phase of the clinical map outlined in Chapter 2.

Tedeschi and Calhoun, the pioneers of PTG research, have organized PTG into five domains based on results of research and thousands of surveys of trauma survivors (see Figure 3.1):

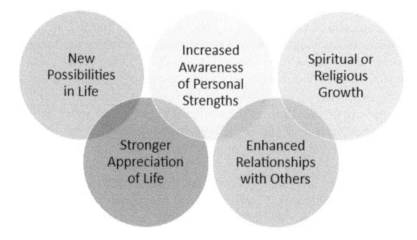

Figure 3.1 The five domains of posttraumatic growth.

1) **New Possibilities in Life** – trauma turns our life upside down and challenges us to develop new perspective. Many trauma survivors uncover opportunities in life that they hadn't considered previously.
2) **Increased Awareness of Personal Strengths** – survivors are often surprised by the incredible strength they tap into while surviving and bouncing back from trauma. They often come to realize that they are much stronger than they had previously thought and/or develop new personal strength due to adversity.
3) **Enhanced Relationships with Others** – coping with trauma is most often something done through relationships, groups, and community. When trauma is relational in nature, it can also prompt one to place increased value in the healthy relationships in their life.

4) **Stronger Appreciation of Life** – trauma is a threat to one's life and frequently reminds us how fleeting and precious life is. Having experienced some of the deepest tragedy and suffering, many trauma survivors are also able to later experience joy, gratitude, and happiness to a stronger degree.

5) **Spiritual or Religious Change** – many trauma survivors seek support from spiritual or religious resources, figures, or communities – especially when the trauma was relational in nature. Many make sense of the existential nature of trauma through spiritual or religious belief systems.

PTG can be measured using the Posttraumatic Growth Inventory which is available online in full, shortened, and translated versions.

It is important to note that professionals working with trauma also experience these five domains through vicarious PTG. As professionals, we not only are at risk of experiencing vicarious trauma, but we also are likely to experience vicarious PTG. The concept of vicarious PTG with be covered in detail in Chapter 11 with reference to the research and ways to cultivate it in practice.

Which of these domains do I notice the most in my clients?

Which of these have I grown the most in myself as a professional working with trauma?

Psychodrama is unique in its capacity to cultivate PTG through action. One of my recent research findings pointed to a positive relationship between spontaneity and PTG for psychodrama participants (Giacomucci, Marquit, & Miller Walsh, 2022). Using psychodramatic techniques, especially role-playing, we are able to provide clients with avenues for exploring areas of PTG experientially rather than simply talk about it. On the psychodrama stage we can act out scenes embodying PTG in the above domains while helping a client internalize these new roles, experiences, behaviors, perspectives, and beliefs. These domains of PTG offer clients a template for future growth and the rewards of trauma recovery. PTG offers clients a vision of a future where their traumatic stress is transformed into growth. As such, these domains can be helpful for instilling hope, treatment planning, and guiding the progress of one's recovery.

> For example, Nadine, a 35-year-old complex trauma survivor has been struggling with seeing a future for herself beyond her trauma. After

adequate warming-up and resourcing Nadine in the scene, the facilitator asks her to choose someone to play the role of future Nadine living in posttraumatic growth. This initiates a dialogue between Nadine today and future Nadine. Throughout this interaction, Nadine envisions herself in the future having transformed her trauma into growth and gets to ask questions about the process of getting there. The facilitator instructs Nadine to reverse roles with herself in the future and respond to her own questions, now repeated by the other role player. Now embodying the role of herself in posttraumatic growth, Nadine speaks from this place to herself struggling today offering inspiration, advice, and insight. This exchange is entirely spontaneous. Nadine speaks from the role and experiencing multiple action insights through the process of validating, nurturing, and guiding herself. When stuck, the director or other group members offer Nadine support to help her stabilize in the role and continuing producing from the role. After some time, the director invites Nadine to role reverse back to the role of herself today receiving and taking in all the messages now being repeated to her from the role of herself in the future.

This deceptively simple role-play provides Nadine (and the rest of the group) with a powerful experience of encountering a vision of self in the future having transformed trauma into PTG. In my clinical work, I find that most clients haven't heard of this concept of PTG before but that it provides a strong sense of hope. It concretizes and gives language to trauma recovery. Trauma-focused psychodrama allows us to bring trauma recovery to life and embody PTG through role-playing.

The emerging research on PTG also points to a significant role that creativity plays in the transformation from traumatic stress to PTG. Forgeard (2013) was the first to uncover a connection in their research, concluding that "posttraumatic growth may be manifested through perceptions of increased creativity" (p. 245). Follow-up studies further contribute to our understanding of the ways in which creativity predicts PTG. Tolleson and Zeligman (2019) conducted a study with folks with chronic illness/disability and concluded that creativity predicted both traumatic stress and PTG. Orkibi and Ram-Vlasov (2019) uncovered that exposure to more trauma was related to higher scores in creative self-efficacy, emotional creativity, and divergent thinking. They also discovered that emotional creativity and creative self-efficacy, but not divergent thinking, "mediated the positive association between exposure and PTG as well as the negative association between exposure and mental health symptoms" (p. 416). A more recent study, focused on the impact of COVID-19 concludes that perceived social support plays a mediating role in a positive relationship between PTG and emotional creativity and that perceived social support also mediates a negative association between emotional creativity and various mental health symptoms and conditions (Zhai et al., 2021). These studies point to emotional creativity as having an important role in promoting PTG after traumatic experiences. This is a particularly interesting finding in the context of psychodrama practice, which is entirely rooted in spontaneity-creativity theory as a theory of change.

Classical Psychodrama Techniques as Trauma Interventions

Many of the methodological elements within classical psychodrama can be framed as trauma-informed interventions that are applicable within both psychodrama practice and can be utilized within other approaches. There are numerous interventions that the psychodramatist can employ in their facilitation, which provides a greater ability to slowly and safely move into traumatic content (Sajnani & Johnson, 2014). Outlined here are some of those interventions and how they fit within a trauma-informed framework (see Chapters 13 and 16 in Giacomucci, 2021b for more in-depth coverage of these interventions). See Chapter 4 for sociometric interventions and how to use them in trauma-informed and trauma-focused ways.

The first three interventions outlined below, the double, the mirror, and the role reversal correspond to Moreno's developmental stages. These three interventions may be particularly useful for healing trauma that an individual experienced within the corresponding developmental phase (see Giacomucci, 2021b for detailed exploration of this). For example, a client who grew up without accurate doubling from caregivers may find that accurate doubling from the therapist and group members helps to repair their developmental wounds related to this period in childhood.

> And so we may say that the double, the mirror, and the reversal are like three stages in the development of the infant which have their counterpart in the therapeutic techniques which we can use in the treatment of all human relations problems.
>
> (Moreno, 1952, p. 275)

The Double

This is an intervention where the director or another group member positions themselves next to the protagonist and offers a statement attempting to further articulate something unspoken for the protagonist. Doubling provides the client with a sense of feeling seen, heard, and understood by the therapist and the group while deepening their experience within the role, the psychodrama, and the experience. When a doubling statement is accurate, the protagonist is instructed to repeat it in their own words; when the doubling is inaccurate, they are instructed to correct it. Doubling effectively helps trauma survivors find words to express their feelings, sensation, and experiences (Baratka & Martin, 2021). This intervention can help cultivate insight, integration, cognitive processing, and the creation of a coherent narrative related to the experience. Doubling can be done with a short statement from a group member or director, or a double can be enrolled as a role that stays with the protagonist throughout the entire psychodrama scene. Doubling provides consistent attunement, empathy, support, and reflection for the protagonist. The latter use of a double role is most representative of how the Morenos worked, which has been replicated in the Therapeutic Spiral Model (TSM)'s use of the body double and containing double as roles to establish safe trauma processing for trauma survivors (this will be expanded on later in this chapter). There are various other doubles that have emerged in psychodrama practice such as the somatic double (Aaron, 2013), the cognitive double (Kipper, 2002), and others.

The Mirror

The mirror intervention provides the protagonist with the opportunity to see themselves in action from a third-person perspective. This is done by having the group replay a scene while the protagonist observes it from the audience stand point. The mirror position is particularly useful when a protagonist is guarded, in denial, stuck in a role or response, or unaware of how their behavior is experienced by others. The mirror position is a helpful intervention when a client may be unable to experience a scene first-hand due to the intensity of it. This intervention then becomes very useful when practicing trauma-focused psychodrama as it gives the director an intervention that can effectively titrate the emotional experience of the protagonist by providing distance from the action. Experiencing the scene from the mirror position provides distance, safety, perspective, compassion for self, and perhaps desensitization while warming up the protagonist to enter the scene or change the scene for healing. The mirror position can also be helpful as an integrative intervention where the protagonist is able to see a moment of healing from another perspective and therefore more fully internalize it (Giacomucci, 2021b).

The Role Reversal

This is perhaps the most important of all psychodrama interventions; Zerka Moreno describes role reversal as the *sine qua non* of psychodrama (Dayton, 2005). Role reversal allows an individual to step into another person's shoes and see things through their eyes. During a role reversal, the protagonist leaves their sense of self and assumes the role of another, often experiencing new insight, catharsis, and integration. This experience often leads to an expansion of self, ego strength, spontaneity, understanding, empathy, awareness, social skills, and closure (Dayton, 2005; Kellermann, 1992). The process of reversing roles and integrating the embodied perspective of another person or role promotes new perspectives, integrations, and a deepened understanding of the self, the other, and the situation. The cyclical movement in the role reversal facilitates the consolidation of change and growth – from the fixed identity of the self to the embodied role of the other and back to the self.

When working with trauma, there are clinical guidelines to consider when using role reversal to avoid retraumatization. It helps to keep in mind that role reversal is the final developmental stages and thus is safest when used after adequate doubling and mirroring interventions have been employed. Doubling and mirroring help the protagonist and the group to stabilize within the scene, accurately observe without dissociation, label undifferentiated affect, and release unexpressed feelings. After these goals have been accomplished, role reversal promotes new insight, integration, and understanding. In classical psychodrama, it is common to immediately role reverse a protagonist with a new role in the scene which is problematic when it comes to antagonist, perpetrator, or victim roles. A director should ensure that the protagonist can successfully engage with these trauma-based roles from their own role before role reversing them. If a role reversal is attempted prematurely with a trauma survivor, it is likely to cause dissociation, provoke other defenses, diminish spontaneity, and could cause psychological harm. A trauma-informed psychodrama director has a sufficient understanding of defense mechanisms, particularly those related to trauma (which often feel like "resistance") and helps the group to honor those defenses while establishing the safety needed to continue the work without them. The ego strength of the protagonist, each individual participant, and the group-as-a-whole must be taken into account before proceeding with trauma-based scenes. Even when a protagonist has the willingness and resources to engage in a trauma-based psychodrama scene, it will only be effective and responsible to continue if the rest of the group is able to safely go with the protagonist and support them (Giacomucci, 2021b).

When directing trauma-based scenes, it is essential to begin with strengths-based roles that can help resource the protagonist and the group while establishing safety, spontaneity, and support. After enrolling strengths and support into the scene, if appropriate to continue to a trauma-based role, it can help to use an empty chair or an object to represent the role instead of a role-player. This limits the activity of the role providing a greater sense of control and enhanced safety. Another option, when possible, is to use a trained staff member other than the therapist to hold the trauma-based role (Hudgins & Toscani, 2013). A trained staff member would know how to pace their production within the trauma-based role as not to overwhelm the group. When working with trauma roles and scenes, it is essential to facilitate the scene to closure and integration including a thorough de-roling of the difficult roles. There are various ways to de-role difficult roles including verbal de-roling, symbolically de-roling, de-roling with movement, and de-roling through the use of an empty chair or object to differentiate the role-player and the role.

Soliloquy

The soliloquy intervention is borrowed from the classical theater and is used to help a protagonist access expression or catharsis by verbalizing an internal monologue as if nobody were listening (Moreno, 1972). The soliloquy provides the protagonist with an opportunity to further access insight from the role and within the scene. It can be used in conjunction with the role reversal to give a protagonist a deepened experience of another role (Nolte, 2020). This intervention is often used when a protagonist seems stuck or resistant – it can give the director important information about what the protagonist might be experiencing. The soliloquy is a helpful trauma-informed technique as it deepens the experience and provides transparency for the director about how to continue the work in a safe way.

Concretization

Psychodrama is based on the use of surplus reality and the externalization of internalized elements of self. The psychodrama stage becomes a bridge between the inner reality of the client and the external reality emerging on the stage. Surplus reality and concretization "allow the protagonist to experience physically what has been experienced psychologically" (Watersong, 2011, p. 21). Concretization is the process by which nonphysical elements, parts of self, or entities are symbolically represented by objects or role-players in psychodrama. For example, we could concretize the protagonist's grief with a black scarf so that it can be held, made conscious, and spoken to. Or the forgiveness a client craves from their higher power could be concretized and presented to them symbolically during the role-play. The intrapsychic fragmentation and undifferentiation resulting from trauma can be made sense of, reorganized, differentiated, and integrated through psychodrama in that it is externalized, concretized, reorganized, and finally internalized it in a new way. Concretization allows a trauma survivor to take back control and hold the internal residue of trauma that has had a hold on them for so long. Concretization can also be used with positive aspects such as strengths which will be covered in more detail in Chapter 4.

Empty Chair

The empty chair is a versatile technique which can be used for a warm-up, for a psychodrama, for de-roling a role, in groups or individual settings, and with a single chair or multiple chairs representing different roles. The empty chair is essentially a form of concretization in that it is holding space and representing a role. Though Fritz Perls' Gestalt Therapy popularized the use of the empty chair, he later affirmed that he had taken the technique from Moreno's psychodrama (Moreno, 2014; Perls, 1969). The primary difference between its use in Gestalt and in psychodrama is that Gestalt uses it for the client to talk to a role while psychodrama takes it further employing doubling, role reversal, and other interventions in conjunction (Knittel, 2009). While the empty chair is a powerful intervention, it is important to consider trauma-informed principles when employing it as it can be overwhelming or retraumatizing for clients when used inappropriately or prematurely in one's recovery process. Many of the same clinical considerations outlined in the subsection on role reversal above apply to the use of the empty chair in clinical work. The empty chair can be used in both psychodramatic and sociodramatic contexts; examples of a multiple empty chair sociodramatic process are described in Chapter 10 (on racism and slavery) and Chapter 11 (on PTSD and vicarious trauma).

Psychodramatic Sculpting

Sculpting is the process of concretizing relationships between roles, parts of self, or relationships through auxiliary role-players (Blatner, 2000). Sculpting is a useful intervention for groups that may not be familiar with psychodrama, warmed-up enough for psychodrama, or spontaneous enough yet. Sculpting is essentially a slower-paced psychodrama without nearly as much movement, messages, or intensity. In this process, the director helps a protagonist position role-players to represent aspects of the scene using physical proximity, positioning, posture, minor movements, and perhaps short messages. It creates a concretized and workable expression of a system's structure (Cruz et al., 2018). Other interventions such as doubling, mirroring, and role reversal are also used in a psychodramatic sculpture. Sculpting offers a contained way of using psychodrama for trauma survivors who might not be ready for a full psychodrama. Tian Dayton has advocated sculpting as a method of externalizing frozen moments of internalized trauma so that they can be renegotiated for trauma healing (Dayton, 2015).

Psychodramatic Letter Writing and Journaling

Psychodramatic letter writing and journaling are other alternatives to a full psychodrama that can be employed in groups or individual settings. In psychodramatic letter writing, the client is instructed to write a letter to someone, something, or a part/version of self. This can also be followed-up with another psychodramatic letter where the client writes a response letter from the recipient. For example, a client struggling with self-blame and closure related to the death of a friend could write a letter to their friend expressing their emotions, then be instructed to write a letter from their deceased friend to themselves in response. This letter provides the client with a contained role reversal and an opportunity for renegotiating their self-blame and moving toward closure. Psychodramatic letter writing is often used to write letters to parts of self, versions of self in the past or future, other people where there is unresolved business, to express gratitude, to make an amends, to set a boundary, or to express anger/hurt. In mental health treatment it can be helpful to have clients write letters to their addiction, depression, anxiety, trauma, grief, chronic pain, personal strengths, defense mechanisms or other internal aspects of self.

Psychodramatic journaling is essentially a contained role reversal followed by a written soliloquy (Dayton, 2015). A client could be instructed to write a psychodramatic journal entry from the role of themselves 1 year sober from alcohol, from their younger self at the time of trauma, from a fly on the wall during a significant event, or from another person's perspective after an experience. This intervention provides an opportunity for expression, catharsis, integration, and deepened insight into a role.

Role Training

Role training is a process that is employed to provide a protagonist with opportunities to practice or rehearse for future situations (Blatner, 2000). It can be used as a warm-up, as the central component of a role-play, or as a final scene in a psychodrama. A role training segment offers the group the chance to replay a situation and demonstrate or experiment with different responses to the situation. Role training is particularly useful in education and when developing competencies in a given area. This intervention helps a protagonist develop or internalize a new role and can be useful for roles related to trauma recovery or PTG. Psychodrama scenes of role training could include having difficult conversations, setting boundaries, managing overwhelming feelings, practicing social skills, responding to cravings or negative thoughts (see Giacomucci, 2021b for a more comprehensive overview with examples). A clinical example of role training is depicted in Chapter 10 related to a non-binary client practicing conversations about gender pronouns with a parent; another role training example is described in Chapter 11 in the context of exploring new intervention approaches to a difficult client situation an ongoing training group with mental health professionals.

Therapeutic Spiral Model

The TSM is a clinically modified psychodrama model rooted in clinical psychology, attachment theory, and neurobiology; it underlines the importance of safety, containment, and strengths (Hudgins & Durost, 2022; Hudgins & Toscani, 2013). TSM comes equipped with a comprehensive clinical map called the Trauma Survivor's Inner Role Atom (TSIRA) which provides a framework for working with trauma using the simplicity of role theory (Giacomucci, 2018; Hudgins, 2019). It facilitates the safety needed to establish a therapeutic alliance and group cohesion while keeping clients in their window of tolerance and transforming internalized trauma-based roles into roles of PTG (Giacomucci, 2018; Hudgins, 2017). Over the past two decades, TSM has increased in popularity in the psychodrama world and contributed to the movement toward trauma-focused and strengths-based approaches in psychodrama (Giacomucci & Marquit, 2020).

While classical psychodrama most often explores interpersonal roles and relationships, TSM is an entirely intrapsychic model. It developed from the realization that before one could interface with others in the world in a healthy way, they needed to do their own personal work and reorganize their internal role atom (Hudgins & Toscani, 2013). The Trauma Survivors Inner Role Atom provides a template of 18 inner roles that contribute to stability, integration, and growth. The simplest way to describe the TSIRA is using a visual of a spiral with three strands – prescriptive roles, trauma-based roles, and transformative roles (Giacomucci, 2017). The first strand represents prescriptive roles which focus on developing the ability for non-judgmental observation, containment, and strengths. The term prescriptive is used to reflect that these roles are directives from a professional and are necessary for the change to occur, just like a prescription from a medical doctor. The second spiral symbolizes the internalization of the trauma. And the transformation that emerges between the interaction of prescriptive and trauma-based roles is represented by the final strand of the spiral. The TSIRA provides a template with intervention steps that target the development of specific psychological functions necessary for healthy functioning after trauma (Hudgins, 2017, 2019).

Prescriptive Roles and Safety Structures

The clinical map includes eight prescriptive roles with the functions of observation, containment, and restoration/strength (see Table 3.1).

In addition to the prescriptive roles, the TSM model includes six experiential safety structures to establish connection, containment, and safety in any group (Giacomucci et al., 2018). Some of these safety structures pull from classical sociometry (including spectrograms, step-in sociometry, and hands-on-shoulders sociometry), one safety structure is an art project, and two of the safety structures are inherently new to TSM and concretize prescriptive roles. These will be covered in further detail in Chapter 4.

The TSM model employs types of psychodrama doubles – the *containing double* and the *body double*, which are often combined into one role in clinical settings. In some places, classical psychodrama doubling has evolved to often be employed as one sentence of doubling, the body double and containing double are roles assigned to group members which stay with the protagonist at all times throughout the entire group. This method of giving the double a stable and centralized role in a psychodrama, as opposed to only employing doubling statements, more closely resembles Zerka Moreno's teaching on doubling which continues to be utilized by many classical psychodramatists as well (Moreno, 1965/2006). The body double mirrors body movements/postures while making grounding statements to prevent dissociation

Table 3.1 Prescriptive roles and functions (reprinted with permission from Giacomucci, 2018, p. 117)

Function	Prescriptive Roles
A. Observation	1. Observing ego
	2. Client role
B. Containment	3. Containing double
	4. Body double
	5. Manager of defenses
C. Restoration/strength	6. Intrapsychic strengths
	7. Interpersonal strengths
	8. Transpersonal strengths

and enhance somatic processing (Burden & Ciotola, 2001; Carnabucci & Ciotola, 2013). The body double reconnects the trauma survivor with awareness of their own body, thus strengthening vertical neural integration and providing grounding (Lawrence, 2011).

The containing double offers statements anchoring the protagonist in the present moment by expanding or containing feelings or thinking, depending on what is clinically appropriate. The containing double adapts based on the needs of each protagonist. For a protagonist with overwhelming feelings, the containing double would contain the feelings while helping to label internal experience; but for a protagonist prone to intellectualizing or overthinking, the containing double would contain the thinking while helping him access his feelings and physical sensations. One might say that it serves as the corpus callosum, connecting the left and right hemispheres of the brain and providing a balance between cognition and emotion (Hug, 2013).

The Triangle of Trauma Roles

The second phase of TSM's clinical map is only used once the protagonist and the group has adequately accessed their prescriptive roles. The trauma triangle is an evolution of Karpman's (1968) interpersonal drama triangle of victim, perpetrator, and rescuer. In one's experience of trauma, however, there was no rescuer, otherwise the trauma would not have occurred. So TSM teaches that a trauma survivor unconsciously internalizes the roles of *victim, perpetrator,* and *abandoning authority* (Hudgins & Toscani 2013; Toscani & Hudgins,

1995). These three trauma-based roles are the TSM operational definition of PTSD symptomology in action (Giacomucci, 2018).

These three internal roles – victim, perpetrator, and abandoning authority, create a triangulation of role reciprocity. TSM theory conceptualizes the trauma as living within the survivor in terms of these roles, which can be thought of as the introjections of the spoken and unspoken messages from the perpetrator and abandoning authority at the time of the trauma. Although the actual trauma is over, it lives within the survivor and is reexperienced through the surplus reality of flashbacks, night terrors, negative cognitions and feeling states, avoidance, dissociation, and insecure attachments (American Psychiatric Association, 2013).

The interaction of the prescriptive roles with the trauma-based roles is exactly what creates the intrapsychic change according to TSM theory. TSM defines its prescriptive roles as the operational definition of spontaneity in action (Hudgins, 2017) which, when interacting with the trauma-based roles, allows the protagonist to respond in a new, adequate way instead of resorting to the repetitive trauma triangle patterns (Giacomucci & Stone, 2019). The alchemy of prescriptive roles interacting with trauma-based roles is precisely what creates transformative roles – the final stage of the TSIRA clinical map.

Transformative Roles of Posttraumatic Growth

PTG refers to phenomenon of positive transformation that is often experienced after a traumatic life event (Calhoun & Tedeschi, 2014). The TSIRA's transformative roles are the operational definition of PTG in action and embodied in the simplicity of role theory. The TSIRA's transformative roles include eight labeled roles organized on the three poles of transformative functions – autonomy, integration, and correction. These functions can be conceptualized of as the opposite sides of the trauma triangle roles constituting role transformations from abandonment to integration, victimhood to autonomy, and perpetration to correction (Giacomucci, 2018) (see Figure 3.2).

One of the most important transformative roles on the TSIRA clinical map is the *appropriate authority*, which is necessary to help remove one's self from cycling around the internal trauma triangle (Hudgins & Toscani 2013). The appropriate authority is an internal role that intervenes in the repetition of continued abandonment, victimization, and perpetration of the self. TSM's

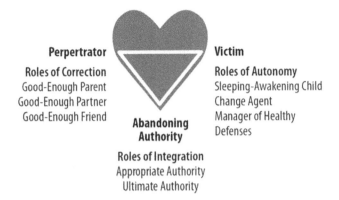

Perpetrator

Roles of Correction
Good-Enough Parent
Good-Enough Partner
Good-Enough Friend

Abandoning Authority

Victim

Roles of Autonomy
Sleeping-Awakening Child
Change Agent
Manager of Healthy Defenses

Roles of Integration
Appropriate Authority
Ultimate Authority

Figure 3.2 TSM trauma triangle role transformations (reprinted with permission from Giacomucci, 2021b, p. 138).

other role of integration, the *ultimate authority*, is the integration of all eight of the transformative roles having been internalized, enacted in the protagonist's intrapsychic world, then their interpersonal world, and finally out in the world. This role is, in a spiritual sense, awakening to the fact that one is a co-creator and co-responsible for mankind (Z.T. Moreno, 2012).

The *sleeping-awakening child* is another role unique to TSM. Many trauma survivors indicate that they feel as though they have lost their innocence, spontaneity, creativity, or inherent goodness. The sleeping-awakening child role reframes these beliefs and offers a new construct; this is the role that holds all of the innocence, goodness, uniqueness, creativity, and spontaneity. It was never lost or taken, it simply went to sleep at the time of the trauma and waits for the protagonist to make their life safe enough to be awoken (Hudgins 2017). It is a truly beautiful moment in a TSM psychodrama to experience an auxiliary play the role of the sleeping child as the protagonist awakens this part of self, and in doing so, taps into a source of inner goodness.

The Transformative roles of corrective connection, which are *good-enough parents*, *good-enough significant other*, and *good-enough spirituality*, are significant in their ability to provide protagonists with corrective emotional experiences that have the power to repair the negative influence of prior experiences (Alexander & French, 1946; Cozolino, 2014). TSM psychodrama allows participants to embody the roles of transformation and PTG in the safety of a psychodrama, effectively role-training them to hold the roles in other arenas of their lives. While the TSIRA provides a template for transforming trauma, these templated roles are sure to materialize differently in each psychodrama, and especially from culture to culture. TSM has been taught and practiced in over 40 countries with its clinical map consistently providing a framework for inner change (Hudgins, 2017).

Relational Trauma Repair Model

The Relational Trauma Repair (RTR) model, developed by Tian Dayton, sometimes referred to as *NeuroPsychodrama*, is another clinically modified approach for using psychodrama and other action methods for work with trauma. RTR is also grounded in the interpersonal neurobiology research and attachment literature offering a variety of Socio Metric group processes ranging from experiential psychoeducation, action-based sociometry tools, and psychodramatic enactments (Dayton, 2015; Giacomucci & Marquit, 2020). A major strength of RTR is that it can be adapted for clinical use in shorter groups and offers a potent alternative to full psychodrama sessions while employing psychodrama interventions. A common RTR group includes a series of an action-based sociometry exercises followed by a small, but precise, psychodrama vignette. While a TSM or classical psychodrama would often include multiple roles and scenes, an RTR psychodrama most often only has two or three roles but still has the option of growing into a larger psychodrama.

The RTR model has two levels. Level 1 is present moment focused and helps to identify group themes, provide psychoeducation, cultivate interpersonal connection in the group, and warm-up participants for deeper work. RTR level 1 addresses trauma survivors' disconnection from self and others through group processes that encourage inner reflection and social communication which effectively treats both PTSD symptoms and the underlying trauma. Level 2 is more oriented on the past and involves experiential regression work through the surplus reality psychodrama in addition to role training for the future. RTR's first level is primarily psychoeducational and sociometric processes, while the second level involves both sociometry and psychodrama (Dayton, 2014).

Level 1: Socio Metrics

The first level was designed to engage, educate, and enhance group cohesion and safety. It was originally developed by Tian Dayton for use in treatment with addictions, trauma, and grief-related issues but has been incorporated into a wide variety of group treatment settings in addition to one-to-one sessions. The facilitation of processes from RTR level 1 requires less psycho-drama training than level 2 as it emphasizes educational exercises, sociometry processes, and psychodramatic journaling or letter writing. This phase of treatment includes sociometry processes such as the spectrogram, locograms, and floor checks, as well as writing exercises involving timelines, journaling, and psychodramatic letter writing. RTR's trauma timeline is a notable contribution to the field which helps contextualize, clarify, and provide coherence to trauma survivors' often fragmented narratives of the past (Dayton, 2014). Advanced level one practice also includes some simple empty chair work using letter writing to keep the process contained.

One of RTR's biggest contributions to the field is the *floor check* structure, which takes the traditional sociometric locogram and expands it into a more dynamic group tool (Dayton, 2014). This process will be covered extensively in Chapter 4. RTR developed with an emphasis on experiential processes "that could put healing in the hands of the process itself rather than exclusively in the hands of the therapists" (2015, p. 10). The RTR model uses mutual aid as its lynchpin by positioning group members as therapeutic agents for each other (Giacomucci, 2019, 2021a). These psychosocial processes are congruent with 12-step principles focused on sharing and identification; and are widely employed into addictions treatment programs at both inpatient and outpatient levels of care (Dayton, 2014; Giacomucci, 2020).

Level 2: Reconstructive Role-Plays

The second level of RTR practice focuses on traumatic "role reconstructions" and "frozen moments," in addition to strengthening positive, resilient roles, which does require more psychodrama training. Dayton (2014) describes it as "surgical role reconstruction" which allows trauma survivors to renegotiate internalized trauma scenes for moments of repair. The various processes described in this phase include social atom exercises, family sculpting, creating moving sculptures of painful or healing moments, and short psychodrama vignettes.

RTR's therapist handbook (2014) outlines various ways of creating a social atom including basing it on a point in the past, the present, or the future. Level two RTR work brings these pen-to-paper exercises to life using sculpting – an experiential process by which a group member uses other group members to stand-in as the roles depicted on the social atom. Sculpting is different from psychodrama in that it often only involves body posturing, short and prescribed movement, and/or short messages from the roles. Sculptures provide living scenes of past or internal experiences – they are simple and effective processes that can be moved into further action by a trained facilitator. The protagonist can talk to themselves or others from outside the scene, role reverse with roles the scene, or offer doubling statements for roles. After exploring the scene, it can be recreated in a new way to provide corrective emotional experiences and role training – effectively making up for what was missing, lost, or craved-for in the original experience. In sculpting, the protagonist takes a more active role co-directing the scene and often observing it from a mirror position. Some action sculptures may only involve placing role-players on the stage using proximity and posture without words or movement. Sculpting is versatile in that it can be used to concretize internal parts, the family system, the social atom, or other social situations in the past or future.

RTR's "frozen moment sculptures" describe the process of identifying a *frozen moment* for the protagonist – an experience in which a trauma occurred, and the protagonist feels stuck. These frozen moments might be instances from the past when one resorted to a freeze response due to the danger at hand or when one felt helpless or simply stuck and unable to take action. In describing the RTR process of sculpting, Dayton writes:

> We are helping clients to revisit moments from their past that block them from moving forward and to resolve them through a process of making their split-off emotions conscious and then translating them into words and processing them rather than defending against feeling them.
> (2016, p. 49)

These specific moments are reconstructed using sculpting or role-playing with the purpose of empowering the protagonist with an opportunity to alter the situation for closure or transformation. The same process can also be used as an integrative experience whereby positive memories or celebratory moments from time are sculpted (Dayton, 2014).

Trauma-Focused Psychodrama

In my experience, I find that there are benefits and limitations to classical psychodrama, the Therapeutic Spiral Model, and the RTR model. My practice tends to integrate aspects of all three of these approaches, along with SAMHSA's trauma-informed philosophy. While classical psychodrama methodology is flexible, the actual practice of many classical psychodramatists isn't always guided by trauma-informed principles. Some of the classical psychodrama practice norms that have emerged may include risks of retraumatization. Though Zerka and others expanded classical psychodrama into intrapsychic realms, J. L. Moreno's psychodrama practice focused on interpersonal roles. Classical psychodrama provides the framework from which other clinically modified models emerged. The philosophy of classical psychodrama is highly congruent with trauma-informed care philosophy, but some of the practice norms may need to shift in order to align with contemporary best practices in trauma-focused and trauma-informed services. In my experience, the primary concerns are the over emphasis on catharsis, confrontation, unconditionally following the protagonist without first employing strength-based roles, and a need for more attention to ethical standards (this will be discussed further in Chapter 12).

The TSM model was developed to remedy some of these limitations of classical psychodrama in that it prescribes strength-based roles, integrates a clinical map as a structure to follow the protagonist within, and emphasizes intrapsychic roles. While TSM offers significant contributions to the practice of trauma-focused psychodrama, I also find it limiting in that it is an entirely intrapsychic model focused on internal roles. TSM is a comprehensive model with increased complexities that also makes it more difficult to integrate into real treatment settings where group lengths are only 1–2 hours and trained assistant leaders or auxiliary egos are not available.

The RTR model was designed as a trauma-focused experiential approach that could be more easily taught to professionals without requiring hundreds of hours of training to employ safely and effectively. This is one of the big benefits of RTR, especially in comparison to TSM and classical psychodrama which have training requirements requiring hundreds of hours of training, supervision, and practicums. At the same time, RTR's simplicity is also a limitation in that it primarily is based on sociometry processes, psychodrama-like interventions, and short psychodrama vignettes. It rarely includes longer, more dynamic psychodrama enactments involving several roles, which tend to characterize classical psychodrama and TSM practice. I also find that classical psychodrama and RTR, which both emphasize strength-based warming-up processes and sociometry, are sometimes lacking in their attention to strength-based roles in the psychodrama enactment.

Furthermore, SAMHSA's six trauma-informed principles offer additional guidance for practitioners of classical psychodrama, TSM, and RTR. These principles are already largely embodied in each model, nevertheless there is always more room to grow in embodying these principles throughout the theory, practice, and training programs. Both TSM and RTR models significantly shift psychodrama practice toward trauma-informed and trauma-focused approaches; yet, neither seem to make any explicit reference to SAMHSA's trauma-informed care publications, the six trauma-informed principles, and/or any other standards articulated by SAMHSA in their guidance on implementing trauma-informed care. SAMHSA's six trauma-informed principles, provide psychodrama, TSM, and RTR practitioners with six core ethical and clinical values to guide practice and training. In the United States psychodrama community, perhaps the principle most lacking is SAMHSA's final trauma-informed value – cultural, historic, and gender issues (this will be covered in detail in Chapter 10).

One of the limitations I've come to notice in my practice of trauma-focused psychodrama is that the strong emphasis on strengths-based roles, safety, warm-up, and gradually moving into trauma work requires considerable time. While it ensures that more participants and protagonists are having a safe experience, it also means that some psychodramas are not nearly as efficient or quick as they could be without multiple layers of precautions for potentially retraumatizing someone.

In a general and literal sense, the term "trauma-focused psychodrama" simply refers to the application of psychodrama as a treatment for PTSD and trauma-related conditions. My own flavor of trauma-focused psychodrama is a blend of classical psychodrama, TSM, and RTR, build upon the foundational framework of SAMHSA's trauma-informed principles and philosophy. The various chapters of this book will offer multiple clinical vignettes depicting trauma-focused psychodrama in action within the contexts of group therapy and organizations. The example below comes from my work with an ongoing inpatient trauma group.

> Javier is chosen by the group based on his topic of traumatic loss related to the death of his father who was a firefighter responding to the September 11th 2001 terrorist attack in New York City. He shares of how he idolizes his father who had his own problems with alcoholism but gave his life to save others. Javier is a firefighter like his father but developed his own drinking problem in response to the pain from his traumatic grief. He shares about feeling numb when thinking about his father today and that his goal for the psychodrama is related to moving towards closure with his father's death, not blaming himself for being unable to save his father, and finding ways to honor his father. The psychodrama commences with the enrollment of a double to support Javier in his process. He chooses another firefighter in the group to play this role for him and begins to prepare himself emotionally for the scene to come. As the director, I ask the group to call out strengths that they experience in Javier, inviting Javier

to choose one or two strengths that could be helpful in his psychodrama. He chooses purpose and resilience and invites other group members to play these roles for him. In his psychodramatic dialogues with purpose, he begins to develop an existential commitment to his trauma healing work and a steadiness to move forward in the scene. The dialogue with resilience was particularly powerful for Javier. In the role reversal with resilience, multiple group members volunteered to offer doubling statements (from resilience to Javier) which effectively helped him enlarge and enliven his sense of his own resilience. From the role of resilience, he spoke to himself – "you are stronger than you realize," "what doesn't kill you only makes you stronger," and "you survived and are here for a purpose; your family and the world need you". Fortified by the strength-based roles and support from the group, Javier indicates he is ready to continue to address his traumatic loss.

He is invited to choose someone to play the role of his deceased father and to begin talking to his father as if he were here in front of him. Javier begins the dialogue but appears emotionally disconnected and cut off, even after deepening statements from the double. I remember Javier in the previous group sharing about growing up bilingual and his experience as a Puerto Rican in New York. I ask him to speak Spanish with his father in the psychodrama, just as he would have conversed when his father was still alive. Soon after he begins speaking to his father in Spanish, his eyes fill with tears, and he begins to express his grief. Even though the rest of the group doesn't speak Spanish, they are all clearly attuned and invested in Javier's psychodrama. Javier expresses himself, sharing about his feelings of self-blame and loss – soon after offering the group an English summary of what he said. As the director, I prompt him to reverse roles with his father and to respond to himself in Spanish, addressing the feelings of loss, grief, and blame as his father. In the role of his father, I instruct him to speak to his son about the self-blame, to share with his son about his feelings towards him today, and to provide his son with his hopes for him going forward into the future. In the role of his father, catharsis shifts from intense expression of grief to a gradual and quieter emotional experience. He tells himself to stop feeling guilty and blaming himself for the death – "son it is not your fault. It was my time to die, and you couldn't have done anything to prevent it. It pains me to see you blame yourself, to drink yourself to death, and to struggle like this." He continues and translates for the group – "I am proud of the man you are becoming and your willingness to seek treatment for your drinking and trauma. You have a purpose in life, and I want you to honor me by maintaining your recovery and breaking our family's generational cycle of alcoholism." Javier offers a final message to himself from the role of his father and is instructed to reverse roles back. The group member playing the role of his father repeats the messages in English as Javier takes it in. I instruct him to imagine hearing the same messages in Spanish in his father's voice. In this process, the role player becomes emotional too which contributes to the realness of the experience for all. Javier integrates the messages from his father and makes a final commitment to him about maintaining recovery and teaching his own children a new way of life going forward.

This psychodrama enactment depicts the power of the process using a mix of intrapsychic and interpersonal roles, guided by trauma-informed principles. The use of intrapsychic strengths provides Javier with the support, grounding, and safety needed to access his traumatic grief. The doubling from the group helped him feel supported by his peers. The cultural awareness and suggestion to speak Spanish with his father gave him the opportunity to access the memory and familial relationship in the context of his native language. He had felt numb and disconnected from his grief partially because he was speaking about it in English in other therapy sessions. The fact that nobody in the group directly understood his messages didn't matter because the group was attuned to his emotions and non-verbal communication with his father. In psychodrama theory, we would conceptualize his powerful grief catharsis as an abreactive catharsis – and the catharsis he experienced while playing the role of his father as an integrative catharsis. The expression of powerful emotions only leads to lasting change if it is followed by integration and meaning making, which in this case, came through the role reversal. Reversing roles with his father allowed him the opportunity to challenge his self-blame and renegotiate the traumatic grief by considering how his father would feel about him blaming himself for his death. As his father, he was able to articulate multiple ways of making meaning of the loss and honoring the death, namely through breaking the generational cycle of alcoholism in the family.

Later in the sharing phase of the group, the group member who played the role of his father shared about his own grief and loss related to a parent's death. He expressed how playing the role for Javier allowed him the opportunity to access his own feelings and work toward closure himself. This experience of tele in the psychodrama enactment becomes heightened when the topic is sociometrically chosen by the group based on identification with a shared topic and issue. Other group members also shared about how the process helped him imagine having similar discussions with their deceased loved ones, and how it assisted them in considering integrative ways of honoring their losses through their recovery. There are various advanced psychodrama directing techniques which allow the director to use clinical role assignments for other group members based on roles that may help them in their own healing while supporting the psychodrama of the protagonist (more on that in Giacomucci, 2021b). In my clinical experience, psychodrama is one of the most effective methods of renegotiating traumatic and complicated grief (Giacomucci, 2020). To further explore this clinical observation, I currently collecting data in this same ongoing psychodrama group to measure changes in traumatic grief and explore its relationship to spontaneity (as a continuation, replication, and expansion of previous studies – Giacomucci & Marquit, 2020; Giacomucci, Marquit, Miller Walsh, & Saccarelli, 2022).

Conclusion

There are unique benefits to engaging in trauma treatment through group work rather than individual therapy alone. Trauma-focused psychodrama is emerging as an effective treatment for PTSD and other trauma-related conditions. While the research is still growing, there appears to be sufficient evidence to support psychodrama as an effective trauma treatment. Beyond the empirical research, the neurobiology research further supports the use of psychodrama in that it helps renegotiate trauma's somatic and non-verbal impacts. The surplus reality of psychodrama allows for experiences of developmental repair, correction, and PTG that may be impossible otherwise. While classical psychodrama interventions are suitable as trauma-informed techniques, multiple clinically modified psychodrama models emerged to specifically focus on its safe and effective use with trauma survivors. The literature and practice of trauma-focused psychodrama provides clinicians with a variety of interventions to keep the action-based process safe and effective.

References

Aaron, S. G. (2013). The somatic double—A key role in psychodramatic body-work®. *The Journal of Psychodrama, Sociometry, and Group Psychotherapy, 61*(1), 29–41.

Alexander, F., & French, T. (1946). *Psychoanalytic therapy: Principles and application.* New York: Ronald Press.

American Psychiatric Association. (2013). *Diagnostic and statistical manual of mental disorders: DSM-5.* Washington, DC: American Psychiatric Association.

Avinger, K., & Jones, R. (2007). Group treatment of sexually abused adolescent girls: A review of outcome studies. *American Journal of Family Therapy, 35*, 315–326.

Baker, F. A., Metcalf, O., Varker, T., & O'Donnell, M. (2018). A systematic review of the efficacy of creative arts therapies in the treatment of adults with PTSD. *Psychological Trauma: Theory, Research, Practice, and Policy, 10*(6), 643.

Baratka, C., & Martin, N. (2021). Using psychodrama to aid sensory integration in the treatment of early childhood trauma. *Journal of the Psychodrama, Sociometry, and Group Psychotherapy, 68*(1), 75–88.

Benish, S. G., Imel, Z. E., & Wampold, B. E. (2008). The relative efficacy of bona fide psychotherapies for treating post-traumatic stress disorder: A meta-analysis of direct comparisons. *Clinical Psychology Review, 28*(5), 746–758.

Blatner, A. (2000). *Foundations of psychodrama: History, theory, and practice* (4th ed.). New York City: Springer Publishing Company.

Bucuţă, M. D., Dima, G., & Testoni, I. (2018). "When you thought that there is no one and nothing": The value of psychodrama in working with abused women. *Frontiers in Psychology, 9*, 1518.

Burden, K., & Ciotola, L. (2001). *The body double: An advanced clinical action intervention module in the therapeutic spiral model to treat trauma.* Retrieved from http://www.healing-bridges.com/psychodrama.html

Burlingame, G., & Krogel, J. (2005). Relative efficacy of individual versus group psychotherapy. *International Journal of Group Psychotherapy, 55*(4), 607–611.

Calhoun, L. G., & Tedeschi, R. G. (2012). *Posttraumatic growth in clinical practice.* New York: Routledge.

Calhoun, L. G., & Tedeschi, R. G. (Eds.). (2014). *Handbook of posttraumatic growth: Research and practice*: New York: Psychology Press.

Carnabucci, K., & Ciotola, L. (2013). *Healing eating disorders with psychodrama and other action methods: Beyond the silence and the fury.* London: Jessica Kingsley Publishers.

Cowden, R. G., Chapman, I. M., Houghtaling, A., & Worthington Jr., E. L. (2021). Effects of a group experiential therapy program on the psychological health of military veterans: a preliminary investigation. *Person-Centered & Experiential Psychotherapies, 20*(2), 119–138.

Cowden, R. G., Captari, L. E., Chen, Z. J., De Kock, J. H., & Houghtaling, A. (2022). Effectiveness of an intensive experiential group therapy program in promoting mental health and well-being among mass shooting survivors: A practice-based pilot study. *Professional Psychology: Research and Practice, 53*(2), 181.

Cozolino, L. J. (2014). *The neuroscience of human relationships* (2nd ed.). New York: W.W. Norton & Company.

Cruz, A., Sales, C., Alves, P., & Moita, G. (2018). The core techniques of Morenean psychodrama: A systematic review of literature. *Frontiers in Psychology, 9*, 1263. https://doi.org/10.3389/fpsyg.2018.01263

Damra, J. K. (2022). The effects of psychodrama intervention on intimate partner violence and quality of life: Trial of Syrian refugee abused women. *Journal of International Women's Studies, 23*(1), 33.

Dayton, T. (2005). *The living stage: A step-by-step guide to psychodrama, sociometry, and experiential group therapy.* Deerfield, FL: Health Communications Inc.

Dayton, T. (2014). *Relational trauma repair (RTR) therapist's guide* (revised ed.). New York: Innerlook, Inc.

Dayton, T. (2015). *NeuroPsychodrama in the treatment of relational trauma: A strength-based, experiential model for healing PTSD.* Deerfield Beach, FL: Health Communications, Inc.

Dayton, T. (2016). Neuropsychodrama in the treatment of relational trauma: Relational trauma repair—An experiential model for treating posttraumatic stress disorder. *The Journal of Psychodrama, Sociometry, and Group Psychotherapy, 64*(1), 41–50.

Elliott, R., Greensberg, L., & Lietaer, G. (2004). Research on experiential psychotherapy. In M. Lambert, A. Bergin, & S. Garfield (Eds.), *Handbook of psychotherapy and behavior change* (pp. 493–539). New York: Wiley.

Elliott, R., Watson, J., Greenberg, L. S., Timulak, L., & Freire, E. (2013). Research on humanistic-experiential psychotherapies. In M. J. Lambert (Ed.), *Bergin & Garfield's handbook of psychotherapy and behavior change* (6th ed., pp. 495–538). New York: Wiley.

Feniger-Schaal, R., & Orkibi, H. (2020). Integrative systematic review of drama therapy intervention research. *Psychology of Aesthetics, Creativity, and the Arts, 14*(1), 68.

Forgeard, M. J. (2013). Perceiving benefits after adversity: The relationship between self-reported posttraumatic growth and creativity. *Psychology of Aesthetics, Creativity, and the Arts, 7*(3), 245.

Giacomucci, S. (2017). The sociodrama of life or death: Young adults and addiction treatment. *Journal of Psychodrama, Sociometry, and Group Psychotherapy, 65*(1), 137–143. https://doi.org/10.12926/0731-1273-65.1.137

Giacomucci, S. (2018). The trauma survivor's inner role atom: A clinical map for post-traumatic growth. *Journal of Psychodrama, Sociometry, and Group Psychotherapy, 66*(1): 115–129.

Giacomucci, S. (2019). *Social group work in action: A sociometry, psychodrama, and experiential trauma therapy curriculum.* Doctorate in Social Work (DSW)

Dissertations, 124. Retrieved from https://repository.upenn.edu/cgi/viewcontent.cgi?article=1128&context=edissertations_sp2

Giacomucci, S. (2020). Addiction, traumatic loss, and guilt: A case study resolving grief through psychodrama and sociometric connections. *The Arts in Psychotherapy*, 67, 101627. https://doi.org/10.1016/j.aip.2019.101627

Giacomucci, S. (2021a). Experiential sociometry in group work: Mutual aid for the group-as-a-whole. *Social Work with Groups*, 44(3), 204–214.

Giacomucci, S. (2021b). *Social work, sociometry, and psychodrama: Experiential approaches for group therapists, community leaders, and social workers*: Springer Nature. https://doi.org/10.1007/978-981-33-6342-7

Giacomucci, S. (2021c). Traumatic stress and spontaneity: Trauma-focused and strengths-based psychodrama. In J. Maya, & J. Maraver (Eds.), *Psychodrama advances in psychotherapy and psychoeducational interventions* (pp. 1–44). New York: Nova Science Publishers.

Giacomucci, S., & Marquit, J. (2020). The effectiveness of trauma-focused psychodrama in the treatment of PTSD in inpatient substance abuse treatment. *Frontiers in Psychology*, 11, 896. https://doi.org/10.3389%2Ffpsyg.2020.00896

Giacomucci, S., Marquit, J., & Miller Walsh, K. (2022). A controlled pilot study on the effects of a therapeutic spiral model trauma-focused psychodrama workshop on post-traumatic stress, spontaneity and post-traumatic growth. *Zeitschrift für Psychodrama und Soziometrie*, 21(1), 171–188.

Giacomucci, S., Marquit, J., Walsh, K. M., & Saccarelli, R. (2022). A mixed-methods study on psychodrama treatment for PTSD and depression in inpatient substance use treatment: A comparison of outcomes pre-pandemic and during Covid-19. *The Arts in Psychotherapy*, 81, 101971.

Giacomucci, S., & Stone, A. M. (2019). Being in two places at once: Renegotiating traumatic experience through the surplus reality of psychodrama. *Social Work with Groups*, 42(3), 184–196. https://doi.org/10.1080/01609513.2018.1533913

Giacomucci, S., Gera, S., Briggs, D., & Bass, K. (2018). Experiential addiction treatment: Creating positive connection through sociometry and therapeutic spiral model safety structures. *Journal of Addiction and Addictive Disorders*, 5, 17.

Hamidi, F., & Sobhani Tabar, S. (2021). Effect of psychodrama on post-traumatic stress disorder symptoms in primary school students living in earthquake-stricken areas. *Iranian Journal of Psychiatry and Clinical Psychology*, 26(4), 400–417.

Hudgins, M. K. (2017). PTSD unites the world: Prevention, intervention and training in the therapeutic spiral model. In C. E. Stout, & G. Want (Eds.), *Why global health matters: Guidebook for innovation and inspiration* (pp. 294–325): Self-Published Online.

Hudgins, K. (2019). Psychodrama revisited: Through the lens of the internal role map of the therapeutic spiral model to promote post-traumatic growth. *Zeitschrift für Psychodrama und Soziometrie, 18*(1), 59–74.

Hudgins, K., & Durost, S. W. (2022). *Experiential therapy from trauma to post-traumatic growth: Therapeutic spiral model psychodrama.* Singapore: Springer Nature.

Hudgins, K., & Toscani, F. (Eds.) (2013). *Healing world trauma with the therapeutic spiral model: Stories from the front-lines.* London: Jessica Kingsley Publishers.

Hug, E. (2013). A Neuroscience perspective on trauma and action methods. In K. Hudgins, & F. Toscani (Eds.), *Healing world trauma with the therapeutic spiral model* (pp. 111–131). London: Jessica Kingsley Publishers.

Imel, Z. E., Laska, K., Jakupcak, M., & Simpson, T. L. (2013). Meta-analysis of dropout in treatments for posttraumatic stress disorder. *Journal of Consulting and Clinical Psychology, 81*(3), 394.

Karpman, S. (1968). Fairy tales and script drama analysis. *Transactional Analysis Bulletin, 7*(26), 39–43.

Kellermann, P. F. (1992). *Focus on psychodrama: The therapeutic aspects of psychodrama.* London: Jessica Kingsley.

Kipper, D. A. (2002). The cognitive double: Integrating cognitive and action techniques. *Journal of Group Psychotherapy Psychodrama and Sociometry, 55*(2–3), 93–107.

Klein, R. H., & Schermer, V. L. (Eds.). (2000). *Group psychotherapy for psychological trauma*: New York: Guilford Press.

Knittel, M. G. (2009). *Counseling and drama: Psychodrama a deux.* Tuscan, AZ: Author.

Lawrence, C. (2011). *The architecture of mindfulness: Integrating the therapeutic spiral model and interpersonal neurobiology.* Retrieved from http://www.drkatehudgins.com

Levine, P. A. (2010). *In an unspoken voice: How the body releases trauma and restores goodness.* Berkeley, CA. North Atlantic Books.

Malchiodi, C. A. (2020). *Trauma and expressive arts therapy: Brain, body, and imagination in the healing process*: New York: Guilford Press.

Mondolfi Miguel, M. L., & Pino-Juste, M. (2021). Therapeutic achievements of a program based on drama therapy, the theater of the oppressed, and psychodrama with women victims of intimate partner violence. *Violence against Women, 27*(9), 1273–1296.

Moreno, J. D. (2014). *Impromptu man: J.L. Moreno and the origins of psychodrama, encounter culture, and the social network.* New York: Bellevue Literary Press.

Moreno, J. L. (1952). Psychodramatic production techniques. *Group Psychotherapy, Psychodrama, & Sociometry, 4*, 273–303.

Moreno, J. L. (1972). *Psychodrama volume 1* (4th ed.). New York: Beacon House.

Moreno, Z. T. (1965/2006). Psychodramatic rules, techniques, and adjunctive methods. In T. Horvatin, & E. Schreiber (Eds.), *The quintessential Zerka* (pp. 104–114). New York: Routledge.

Moreno, Z. T. (2012). *To dream again: A memoir.* New York: Mental Health Resources.

Nolte, J. (2020). *J.L. Moreno and the psychodramatic method: On the practice of psychodrama.* New York: Routledge.

Orkibi, H., & Feniger-Schaal, R. (2019). Integrative systematic review of psychodrama psychotherapy research: Trends and methodological implications. *PLoS One, 14*(2), e0212575.

Orkibi, H., & Ram-Vlasov, N. (2019). Linking trauma to posttraumatic growth and mental health through emotional and cognitive creativity. *Psychology of Aesthetics, Creativity, and the Arts, 13*(4), 416.

Perls, F. (1969). *In and out the garbage pail.* Lafayette, CA: Real People Press.

Perry, R., Saby, K., Wenos, J., Hudgins, K., & Baller, S. (2016) Psychodrama intervention for female service members using the therapeutic spiral model. *The Journal of Psychodrama, Sociometry, and Group Psychotherapy*: Spring 2016, 64(1), 11–23.

Porges, S. W. (2011). *The polyvagal theory: Neurophysiological foundations of emotions, attachment, communication, and self-regulation.* New York: W. W. Norton & Company.

Porges, S. W. (2017). *The pocket guide to the Polyvagal theory: The transformative power of feeling safe.* New York: W.W. Norton & Company

Rauch, S. L., van der Kolk, B. A., Fisler, R. E., et al. (1996). A symptom provocation study of posttraumatic stress disorder using positron emission tomography and script-driven imagery. *Archives of General Psychiatry, 53*(5), 380–387.

Ron, Y., & Yanai, L. (2021). Empowering through psychodrama: A qualitative study at domestic violence shelters. *Frontiers in Psychology, 12*, 1017.

Sajnani, N., & Johnson, D. R. (2014). *Trauma-informed drama therapy: Transforming clinics, classrooms, and communities*: Springfield: Charles C Thomas Publisher.

Schwartze, D., Barkowski, S., Strauss, B., Knaevelsrud, C., & Rosendahl, J. (2019). Efficacy of group psychotherapy for posttraumatic stress disorder: Systematic review and meta-analysis of randomized controlled trials. *Psychotherapy Research, 29*(4), 415–431.

Seppälä, K. M. (2020). *A thematic analysis: How dramatic techniques can be applied in therapy to facilitate clients in regaining an integrated sense-of-self after experiencing interpersonal trauma* (Doctoral dissertation). FCHS (DCPC) – Dissertações de Mestrado, Repositório Institucional da Universidade Fernando Pessoa.

Shapiro, J. R., & Applegate, J. S. (2018). *Neurobiology for clinical social work: Theory and practice* (2nd ed.). New York: W.W. Norton & Company.

Siegel, D. (2012). *Developing mind: How relationships and the brain interact to shape who we are.* New York: Guilford Press.

Sloan, D. M., Feinstein, B., Gallagher, M. W., Beck, J. G., & Keane, T. M. (2013). Efficacy of group treatment for posttraumatic stress disorder: A meta-analysis. *Psychological Trauma: Theory, Research, Practice, and Policy, 5*, 176–183.

Tabar, S., Hamidi, F., & Tahmasebipour, N. (2020). Effectiveness of psychodrama in reducing the psychological nervous problems of students with post-traumatic stress disorder. *Neuropsychology, 6*(1), 121–146.

Tolleson, A., & Zeligman, M. (2019). Creativity and posttraumatic growth in those impacted by a chronic illness/disability. *Journal of Creativity in Mental Health, 14*(4), 499–509.

Toscani, M. F., & Hudgins, M. K. (1995). *The trauma survivor's intrapsychic role atom.* Workshop Handout. Madison, WI: The Center for Experiential Learning.

van de Kamp, M. M., Scheffers, M., Hatzmann, J., Emck, C., Cuijpers, P., & Beek, P. J. (2019). Body-and movement-oriented interventions for posttraumatic stress disorder: A systematic review and meta-analysis. *Journal of traumatic stress, 32*(6), 967–976.

van der Kolk, B. A. (1996). The body keeps the score: Approaches to the psychobiology of posttraumatic stress disorder. In B. A. van der Kolk, A. C. McFarlane, & L. Weisaeth (Eds.), *Traumatic stress: The effects of overwhelming experiences on mind, body, and society* (pp. 214–241). New York: Guilford Press.

van der Kolk, B. A. (2014). *The body keeps the score: Brain, mind, and body in the healing of trauma.* New York: Viking Press.

Wallin, D. J. (2007). *Attachment in psychotherapy:* New York: Guilford Press.

Watersong, A. (2011). Surplus reality: The magic ingredient in psychodrama. *Journal of the Australian and Aotearoa New Zealand Psychodrama Association, 20*, 18–27.

Wodarski, J. S., & Feit, M. D. (2012). Social group work practice: An evidenced based approach. *Journal of Evidence-Based Social Work, 9*, 414–420.

Wu, X., Kaminga, A. C., Dai, W., Deng, J., Wang, Z., Pan, X., & Liu, A. (2019). The prevalence of moderate-to-high posttraumatic growth: A systematic review and meta-analysis. *Journal of Affective Disorders, 243*, 408–415.

Wylie, M. S. (2004). The limits of talk: Bessel van der Kolk wants to transform the treatment of trauma. *Psychotherapy Networker, 28*, 30–41.

Yalom, I. D., & Leszcz, M. (2020). *The theory and practice of group psychotherapy* (6th ed.). New York: Basic Books.

Zhai, H. K., Li, Q., Hu, Y. X., Cui, Y. X., Wei, X. W., & Zhou, X. (2021). Emotional creativity improves posttraumatic growth and mental health during the COVID-19 pandemic. *Frontiers in Psychology, 12*, 600798.

4
Trauma-Informed Experiential Sociometry Processes

Chapter Summary

This chapter outlines multiple experiential sociometry processes and Thera-peutic Spiral Model safety structures as practical trauma-informed tools that can be adapted for any group. These action-based methods are presented with instructions for new and experienced facilitators to quickly incorpo-rate into their work while adapting them for various populations, topics, and contexts. Processes covered include small groups, spectrograms, locograms, floor checks, step-in sociometry, sociograms, and circle of strengths. Each of these will be described and depicted with emphasis on employing them in trauma-informed and trauma-focused ways. The six trauma-informed prin-ciples outlined by SAMHSA will be highlighted as inherently embodied in experiential sociometry processes. These experiential group tools can be integrated into any group setting including group therapy, community organ-izing, education, supervision, training, and organizational leadership.

Experiential Sociometry as Trauma-Informed Group Processes

The clinical applications of sociometry include a variety of pen-to-paper activities that explore an individual's social atom or social network, or expe-riential action structures that explore the series of attractions, repulsions, similarities, and differences within the group (Hale, 1981, 2009). In the con-text of this discussion of group psychotherapy, clinical applications for groups

DOI: 10.4324/9781003277859-4

will be primarily emphasized – though sociometric tools are also used in individual settings, community work, and education (see Giacomucci, 2021a; Giacomucci & Skolnik, 2021).

There are numerous other commonly used experiential sociometric group processes that are employed in clinical settings including dyadic or triadic sharing, spectrograms, locograms, floor checks, step-in sociometry, and hands-on-shoulder sociometry (Dayton, 2005, 2014, 2015; Giacomucci, 2017, 2018a, 2019, 2021a; Giacomucci, Gera, Briggs, & Bass, 2018; Hale, 1981, 2009; Hudgins & Toscani, 2013). Each of these processes can be modified with content appropriate for any population or chosen topic. In terms of clinical uses of sociometry, these sociometric tools often stand on their own as multi-dimensional action-based group processes that provide the group with an avenue to discover and enrich their connections with each other. Sociometry can also be employed with an objective of recognizing shared identity between group members including membership to privileged or oppressed groups (Nieto, 2010). These same sociometric action structures frequently serve as a group warm-up exercise before conducting a psychodrama but can be used in the beginning, middle, or ending stages of a group. Each of these experiential sociometry structures can be used for group assessment, exploration, intervention, and evaluation. These sociometry structures can be used as psychoeducation and effectively cultivate all 11 of Yalom and Leszcz's therapeutic factors (2020).

Embodying Trauma-Informed Principles with Experiential Sociometry

Regardless of which sociometry tool is being utilized, it is useful for both the group and the facilitator if a clinical map is employed. To cultivate an experience of safety, vulnerability, containment, and warming-up, it can help to select criteria for prompts while adhering to the three clinical map for trauma (Chesner, 2020; Courtois & Ford, 2016; Herman, 1997; Giacomucci, 2018b; Hudgins & Toscani, 2013). Initial prompts would be simple and strengths based with the goal of facilitating connection. The next prompt(s) invite the group to share deeper with a focus on difficult emotions, defense mechanisms, trauma, loss, addiction, or mental illness. And to finish, making an offer of prompt(s) that facilitate or engage with meaning making, integration, future projection, and posttraumatic growth. Essentially, this clinical map starts with *positive* prompts, moves into *negative* prompts, and ends with *positive* prompts again (see Chapter 2 for more on the clinical map). This process reflects the process of slowly moving in and out of difficult emotional content – called pendulation and titration described by trauma experts (Courtois & Ford, 2016; Herman, 1997; Levine, 2010; Shapiro, 2018; van der Kolk, 2014). While providing containment, direction, and safety for the larger group process, this practice may also help clients internalize a sense of containment, self-efficacy, and safety related to their trauma (Giacomucci & Marquit, 2020).

The experiential group processes described in this chapter can be conceptualized as trauma-informed processes as they reflect the six principles outlined by SAMHSA (2014a) (see Figure 4.1).

Experiential sociometry is particularly useful in promoting connection within the group and enhancing interpersonal relationships. It cultivates peer support, safety, and trustworthiness while illuminating and making transparent the sociodynamics within a group. Participants are able to see clearly where they fit in within the group on various topics or preferences while reflecting on and articulating their experience. As the connection and group cohesion increases, so too does the felt sense of safety for each participant. Experiential sociometry provides multiple opportunities for choice, indicating preference, and elevating voices within the group while empowering participants with the power to influence the group process – sociometry

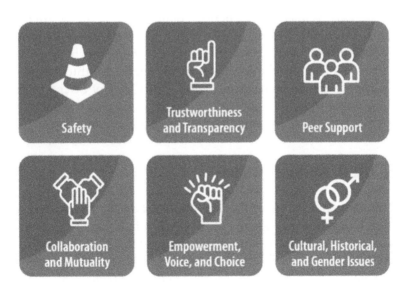

Figure 4.1 SAMHSA's six trauma-informed principles (republished with permission from Giacomucci, 2021b, p. 128).

is most frequently used as a warm-up to psychodrama during which the director tunes into the warm-up of the group and channels it into a psychodrama enactment. This process is inherently collaborative as the group-as-a-whole is seen as co-responsible for the group process (Fleury & Marra, 2022). A sense of mutuality and universality is inherently rooted in these exercises as they position participants as therapeutic agents for each other, honoring their capacity to promote healing, education, and support for one another. Experiential sociometry promotes a less hierarchical group structure in that instead of positioning the facilitator as the primary source of education or healing, the group-as-a-whole is elevated to this position. These action-based group processes are fundamentally anti-oppressive in the way that they disrupt traditional power dynamics in a group setting and promote co-creation (Giacomucci, 2021b).

Not only do they offer trauma-informed and action-based processes, but they can also be adapted for trauma-focused or trauma-informed content. For examples, a facilitator could ask spectrogram prompts related to gender issues, safety, or trustworthiness. A locogram or floor check can easily be employed using the six trauma-informed principles as the locogram/floor check options which allow the group to explore their relationship with them. This floor check is particularly useful for organizational workshops or meetings as it helps the organization-as-a-whole reflect on how they already incorporate these principles and where they have room to grow in this regard. Step-in sociometry can be used with clients, communities, staff, or students to explore their shared experiences related to the trauma-informed principles or aspects of identify/experience. Sociogram prompts can be generated to help a group explore how the principles are experienced within interpersonal relationships in the group or organization. The Circle of Strengths process can be modified to either concretize strengths to support trauma-informed work or to concretize the trauma-informed principles themselves.

Dyads, Triads, and Small Groups

Jacob Moreno often wrote of the importance of dyadic connection within groups and suggested that group cohesion was a function of the number of reciprocated mutual choices within the group (Hale, 2009; Moreno, 1934). Consequently, the use of dyadic sharing and breaking the larger group into smaller pairs can help facilitate interpersonal connection, mutual aid, and overall group cohesion (Giacomucci, 2021a). Using dyads, triads, or small breakout groups seems to be especially useful at the early stages of groups and when working with larger groups. Many clients do not feel comfortable sharing in front of large groups – using smaller groups allows for participants to feel safer as they are invited to share with one or two others. This process also mitigates the chances of one participant monopolizing the group discussion and preventing the more reluctant or introverted group members from actively engaging (Olesen, Campbell, & Gross, 2017). The process of a traditional talk-based group only permits one discussion to take place at a time but using dyads or small groups allows for multiple discussions to take place concurrently. The nature of small group discussions, especially dyads, invokes a role demand for each participant to respond, attend to, support, and share with their partner – thus engaging in mutual aid. The process of utilizing small group discussion frees up the facilitator to move around the room and listen to or check-in with each group. This allows the facilitator to take a less active role and indirectly reveals the facilitator's confidence, trust, and faith in each participant's ability to serve as a therapeutic agent for each other.

The method of choosing configurations of small groups or dyads can be modified depending on the facilitator's intention or the nature of the group. Partners or small groups can be assigned randomly, intentionally chosen by the facilitator, self-selected by participants, or chosen based on prompts. When inviting participants to self-select a partner or break into triads, participants are likely to choose the person(s) physically closest to them. Often, they are already sitting next to the group members that they feel most connected to so this may lead to already cohesive small groups and few new connections. Prompting participants to "partner with someone you don't know well" is a simple way to facilitate dyads ripe with new opportunities to connect.

In terms of the content of the discussion within the small groups, it helps to offer directed prompts related to the nature of the group or the therapeutic goals of the session guided by the aforementioned three stage clinical map. Generally, 3–5 prompts seem to be sufficient for small groups discussions in terms of adequately warming up the group without losing the interest of participants. Below are some examples of prompts following the aforementioned clinical map based on different topics for clinical groups.

Topic: Relationships

1) Share about one of your favorite relationships
2) Share about a person who has helped you in some way recently
3) Share about a relationship that you have difficulty or conflict in
4) Share how you would a difficult relationship to be different in the future

5) Share about one way you would like to change your behavior in relationships

Topic: Emotions

1) Share a memory that gives you a positive feeling
2) Share about the emotion that you have most difficulty with
3) Share about ways you could respond to difficult emotions different in the future

Topic: Mental Illness

1) Share about tools you have to cope with symptoms of mental illness
2) Share about one role model for living with mental illness (personal, societal, archetypal, historical, religious, or even a fantasy character)
3) Share about how your mental illness impacts you
4) Share about what you imagine your life would look like in the future without mental illness

Topic: Trauma

1) Share about one strength you have that can help you work through your trauma
2) Share about one step you have already taken toward healing from trauma
3) Share about one way your trauma has negatively impacted you
4) Share about one way you would like to grow from your trauma
5) Share about one step you plan to take in the future toward healing from trauma

Topic: Trauma-Informed Principles

1) Share about one principle you feel you embody well in your work
2) Share about one principle you feel your organization best embodies
3) Share about how you see the principles to be integrated and connected to each other
4) Share about one way you could grow in incorporating these principles in your work

Another method for facilitating dyadic connections within groups is to place cards, objects, or images in the center of the group space and ask participants to choose one based on a guiding prompt. Some prompts might include inviting participants to choose a card that can represent "your strength," "the next step on your journey of healing," "defense mechanism," "your spirituality," "your goal for today," or "your ideal self in the future." Once chosen, group members are instructed to share in dyads about their choice of cards and the symbolic representation. Sharing can be extended with new prompts and/or new partners to facilitate increased connection. This process can be done with any set of cards and used as a warm-up to any topic with various prompts.

The Therapeutic Spiral Model (TSM) utilizes this process of choosing cards to represent the role of the *observing ego* – sometimes called the *compassionate witness* or *caring observer* (Hudgins & Toscani, 2013; Lawrence, 2015). The observing ego is a concept, borrowed from Freud (1932), which in this context refers to the part of self that can accurately observe self and others without shame, blame, or judgment (Giacomucci, 2018b). In TSM groups, the cards are then placed on the walls of the group room to provide a conscious reminder of this role and its importance. The use of cards to concretize the observing ego, a strength, or any other positive role provides an anchor of safety for the group experience going forward (Giacomucci et al., 2018). The presence of the cards on the walls behind the group offers a sense of being contained as well as an already defined strengths-based role for the psychodrama director to utilize during the group if extra grounding is needed. TSM practitioners primarily use this process to concretize a psychodramatic role, but it is important to note here for the sociometric aspect of using cards or objects to cultivate dyadic sharing at the beginning of a group process. The experience of using small groups or dyads offers participants the opportunity to create new connections, deepen relationships, enhance their sense of belonging, warm-up to a topic, and increase overall group cohesion.

Spectrograms

The spectrogram is essentially a group-as-a-whole assessment tool that allows the facilitator to efficiently gather information about the group while providing participants with the chance to see where they fit in within the group and to connect with each other. A spectrogram is an action-based self-assessment along a spectrum within the room. Facilitation of a spectrogram is done by designating two different objects or two opposite walls of the room to represent the beginning and end of the spectrum. Generally, one side is designated as a 0/10 or 0% and the opposite side as a 10/10 or 100% while emphasizing that the imaginary line between the poles includes every possibility between 0 and 10 or 0% and 100%. Participants are invited to physically place themselves on the imaginary line based on where they believe they belong when considering the prompt(s).

The following video depicts the use of Spectrograms with a live group: http://www.phoenixtraumacenter.com/spectrograms/

Some examples of spectrogram prompts following the aforementioned clinical map are depicted below.

Topic: Connection and Loss

1) How many supportive relationships do you have in your life today?
2) How much loss have you experienced in your life?
3) How well do you think you handle grief?
4) How resilient do you judge yourself to be?

Topic: Addiction and Recovery

1) How many resources (supports, coping skills, tools, etc.) do you have to help in your recovery?
2) How motivated are you today for your recovery?
3) How much has addiction impacted your life?
4) How hopeful are you for your future in recovery?

Topic: Inpatient Treatment Experiences

1) How many days have you been in inpatient treatment?
2) How connected do you feel to the inpatient community of clients?
3) How difficult has it been for you to remain in treatment?
4) How much progress do you feel you have made since the day of your entered treatment?

Topic: Stress and Self-Care

1) How many tools for self-care do you have?
2) How often do you find yourself stressed out?
3) How much tolerance for stress do you judge yourself to have?
4) How many new strategies for coping with stress have you learned from the group?

Topic: Psychoeducation of Trauma

1) How curious are you to learn more about trauma?
2) How familiar are you with the common ways that trauma impacts people?
   a) how aware are you of how trauma has impacted you or your loved ones?

3) How knowledgeable are you in the different treatments and approaches to healing from trauma?

Topic: Trauma-Informed Principles

1) How well do you feel your organization implements trauma-informed principles?
2) How well do you feel like you embody trauma-informed principles in your own work?
3) How important do you think these six principles are for clients of the agency?

With each new prompt, it is helpful to change the axis of the spectrogram, using different areas in the room. This facilitates more physical movement and prevents participants from staying in the same physical place. Each prompt results in a new configuration of participants along the spectrogram. There are multiple ways to facilitate sharing. The simplest form of sharing is to have the group sharing in groups of 2–3 based on whoever is physically closest to them on the spectrogram. The use of dyadic sharing allows for everyone to share about why they are standing on the spectrogram at the point they are at without taking up too much time. Similarly, participants could be invited to share in clusters of larger groups about where they have chosen to stand on the spectrum. Another option is to ask for group members to share aloud to the group about their placement on the spectrogram. Other non-verbal ways to facilitate spectrogram sharing include with body posture, movement and gestures, or sound.

It is important to consider that the spectrogram is a self-assessment and how that may impact one's choices in the process (Giacomucci et al., 2018). There are spectrogram prompts where it would be advantageous to change the spectrum to a 1–10, or even a 5–10 spectrum. For example, when using the prompt "how resilient do you judge yourself to be?" with a group of trauma survivors, it may be empowering to limit the spectrogram to a 5–10 while indicating the belief that everyone in the room is at least of 5/10 in resilience whether they believe it or not. Most of the clients that we work with are struggling with trauma, loss, addiction, oppression, mental illness, or other forms of suffering and may have distorted judgments about themselves which will impact their self-assessment in the spectrogram process. When the facilitator notices this happening with a group member, it can be helpful to gently challenge the individual to reconsider or to reflect back to the group member where the facilitator would assess them to be on the spectrum. Another option would be to ask the group to share with the individual about where on the spectrogram they would assess that person to be based on the prompt – thus creating an opportunity for mutual aid.

A spectrogram prompt results in a distribution of group members along a continuum, sometimes with participants spread out, sometimes with clusters of participants in different places, and occasionally with isolates on the high or low end of the spectrum. When a prompt results in an obvious isolate on the spectrogram, it can be helpful to explore that person's experience at the group level. If they are an outlier on the higher end of a strengths-based prompt, they likely have important information that they could share to help the rest of the group. If they are an outlier on the lower end of a positive prompt, they might have questions about how to gain more understanding or competence related to the criteria. It can also be helpful to invite group members to raise their hands if they can remember a time in the past when they were at that point on the spectrogram and offer suggestions or identification with the person who is currently an outlier. A psychodramatist might also direct role reversals between group members on the spectrogram to have them explore what it is like to be at various spots. When participants have mobility limitations, the process can be modified by using an object to represent participants on the spectrogram or by having participants raise their hands to varying degrees (10/10 is as high as you can raise your hand; 0/10 is placing your hand on your lap) (Simmons, 2017). Spectrograms can also be easily modified for use during teletherapy or online teaching sessions by using the top and bottom of each participants video feed as the top and bottom of the spectrum. Participants are simply instructed to place their hand along the vertical spectrum of their camera window to indicate where on the spectrogram they are.

Spectrograms allow the facilitator to meet the group where they are at in terms of their warm-up to a specific topic or their understanding of the topic. They are especially useful in psychoeducational sessions, training workshops, classrooms, and supervision groups to assess the knowledge level of participants at the start of the session. This gives the facilitator the chance to change the content of the session to meet the learning needs of the group (Giacomucci, 2018a). Spectrograms are also useful for evaluation in that the same spectrogram prompt could be asked at the beginning and end of a session or program or pen-to-paper assessments can be modified into experiential spectrograms (Giacomucci, 2020).

What topics and prompts might be applicable as spectrograms in my own clinical groups or organizational meetings?

Locograms

The locogram is a sociometry tool that offers a quick visual group assessment or democratic group vote in an experiential format based on different options or categories. As suggested by the prefix of the term *loco-gram*, this process is an exploration of choices using places in the room. While the spectrogram orients itself upon a spectrum, the locogram is oriented based on designated locations in the room. One of the simplest ways to facilitate a locogram is using the four corners of the room to each represent a different choice and asking participants to physically indicate their preference by standing at the corresponding location (Giacomucci, 2020). Other styles of directing a locogram involve using objects or chairs to represent the various choices. Most locograms offer at least three options which usually includes an option for "other" – this invites other suggestions from the group. Locograms are useful for quick assessments or group choices in action. They can be used for many purposes including choosing a topic, discerning when to take a break, making a group decision, assessing group preference, uncovering similarities, and exploring a group's warm-up.

Here are some examples with the bullet points representing the different locations in the room (represented by the corners of the room or objects).

Purpose: Choosing a Topic in an Outpatient Group

- Anxiety
- Depression
- Trauma
- Other

Purpose: Discerning What the Group Is Warmed-Up for Next

- Discussion
- More sociometry
- Psychodrama
- Writing activity
- Other

Purpose: Outpatient Group Decision about Holiday Scheduling Conflict

- Schedule the session on the holiday
- Cancel the session on the holiday

- Meet a different day that week
- Meet twice as long the following session
- Other

Purpose: Uncovering Shared Experiences in School

- I hated school
- I loved school
- I had mixed feelings about school
- Other

Purpose: Exploring Religious/Spiritual Beliefs

- I am religious
- I have a belief in higher power
- I am uncertainty about spirituality
- I don't believe in God or a higher power
- Other

The locogram can be used for a quick group-as-a-whole assessment and group choice, or for an exploration of shared perspective, experience, or identity. When facilitating a locogram, it helps to limit or expand the number of options based on the size of the group. The facilitation of a locogram may or may not include sharing. If the goal is to make a quick group choice, then sharing is likely unnecessary. But if the goal is to facilitate connection and explore shared experience, then sharing is likely to be helpful.

A locogram can also be used in teletherapy groups and online teaching sessions. This could be done in a variety of ways including using a poll feature, instructing participants to write their choice/preference in the chat box, or assigning numbers to each locogram choice and instructing participants to indicate their choice/preference by showing the number of fingers that corresponds with their choice. If the technology platform utilized allows for breakout rooms, the facilitator can initiate breakout rooms which will allow for participants to talk about their shared preference/choice. This method of adapting the locogram for teletherapy or online sessions, is identical to how the floor check is modified for online groups. The floor check, a similar sociometry tool that evolved from the locogram, is outlined in the next section.

Floor Checks

The floor check is an experiential psychosocial process in the Relational Trauma Repair (RTR) model created by Tian Dayton (2014, 2015). It was inspired by the locogram process of using various places in the room for different options – the primary difference is that with the floor check the facilitator utilizes printed pieces of paper to label the options and offers a series of prompts each involving sharing. The floor check expands choice-making potential with increased options that transcend here-and-now prompts into past or future-oriented questions. The floor check expands the process with continual groupings and clustering which offer exponentially more chances for individual reflection, choice making, group connection, education, and healing. The floor check was developed, based on evolving research on trauma, grief, mental health, addiction, and posttraumatic growth, to meet the pressing needs within addiction treatment centers which were faced with shorter group times, larger group sizes, varying degrees of client vulnerability, and therapists with different levels of psychodrama training. When employing the floor check process, it is advantageous to construct prompts or floor check options with research-based content. This can be done by simply choosing floor check options that correspond to the recognized symptomology of a diagnosis or evidence-based research findings, theories, or practices (as described by Dayton, 2014, 2015). Thus, the floor check offers a psycho-educational and therapeutic healing avenue for addressing symptomology in an engaging and dynamic process involving intrapsychic and interpersonal explorations. The multiple, focused prompts in a floor check sociometrically align participants based on the content while providing a progression of spontaneous connection and healing.

With each prompt, participants physically place themselves at the paper that corresponds to their preference or response. A floor check prompt results in group members clustering in small groups based on shared experience for verbal sharing about their choice. The process, similar to the locogram, provides a group-as-a-whole assessment but also cultivates a deepening of sharing and connection between group members in small groups. Floor checks "put healing in the hands of the process itself rather than exclusively in the hands of the therapists" (2015, p. 10) while empowering participants to become therapeutic agents for each other and quickly activating the mutual aid within a group (Giacomucci, 2019, 2020; 2021a, 2021b).

Once a floor check is put into action and group members have physically indicated their choices, they are invited to share with whoever is standing with them. When participants are standing alone at a choice, the facilitator simply directs them to join others nearby for sharing about their choice. This process, creates sociometrically configured small groups, opening up opportunities for social-emotional learning and healing. Similar to the use of dyads or small groups, it allows the director to take a passive role in the process and move around the room listening or checking-in on each cluster of clients. Floor checks are versatile and can be used in any group context with nearly any topic.

> The following video depicts the use of Locogram and Floor Checks with a live group: http://www.phoenixtraumacenter.com/floor-check/.

Some useful examples are listed below (more detailed prompts available in Dayton, 2014) including prompts following the previously described clinical map:

Feeling Floor Check – anger; sadness; fear; guilt/shame; happiness; other

1) Which feeling best describes your experience today?
2) Which feeling most characterized your experience last week?
3) Which feeling do you most try to avoid?
4) Which feeling is hardest for you to tolerate in others?
5) Which feeling have you gotten better with?

Relationships Floor Check – family; friends; self; groups/communities; God/higher power; other

1) Which relationship do you feel most supported by today?
2) Which relationship has the most conflict in it for you?
3) Which relationship has improved the most since you started therapy?
4) Which relationship would you like/need to work on today?

Defense Mechanisms Floor Check – humor; denial or minimization; rationalization or intellectualization; acting out; passive aggression; dissociation; fight; flight; freeze; other

1) Which defense do you feel you are most aware of using in your life today?
2) Which defense do you feel you have used the most in this group?

3) Which defense is most difficult for you to tolerate when someone else uses it?
4) Which defense do you no longer uses as much as you used to?

Posttraumatic Stress Disorder Symptom Cluster Floor Check – avoidance; arousal and reactivity; re-experiencing and intrusions; negative mood and cognitions

1) Which would you like to learn more about?
2) Which best describes how trauma has impacted you?
3) Which describes symptoms you previously experienced but now have effective coping skills for?

Domains of Posttraumatic Growth Floor Check – personal strength; appreciation of life; relationships; spiritual/religious growth; new possibilities

1) Which domain do you feel you have grown in most?
2) Which domain do you feel you struggle with the most?
3) Which domain do you feel you could help someone in this group with?

Trauma-Informed Principles Floor Check – safety, trustworthiness and transparency; peer support; collaboration and mutuality; empowerment, voice, and choice; cultural, historic, and gender issues

1) Which principle do you feel is most central to your work?
2) Which principle do you feel you could be better at integrating in your work?
3) Which principle do you feel you have most grown in your ability to incorporate in the past year?

The floor check can be modified for any group topic or theme that can be sectioned down into categories or choices. Other useful examples include the stages of change, the stages of grief, the tasks of resilience in ambiguous loss, mental health diagnoses, treatment themes, and strengths. This process is also valuable in educational spaces and can be used as an experiential teaching tool promoting reflection and the integration of concepts into personal experience (Giacomucci & Skolnik, 2021). In social work education, it can be used with the social work core values, social work practice areas, or content from other theories (Giacomucci, 2019). The floor check is a holistic instrument that effectively warms people up physically, emotionally, socially, and to the chosen topic. It can be utilized alone as a group process or as a warm-up to another group process such as a psychodrama, art therapy piece, or writing process.

How might I use Floor Checks in my own clinical groups or organizational meetings?

Step-in Sociometry

The next sociometry process that we will explore is *step-in sociometry* – sometimes called *circle of similarities*. This experiential process is effective at quickly identifying shared experience or similarities in the group-as-a-whole (Archer, 2016). Buchanan (2016) notes that step-in sociometry is a newer addition to the sociometry toolbox in the 1970s from the New Games Movement (Fluegelman, 1976). Step-in sociometry is facilitated with the group stand in a circle. Prompts are offered with the instruction to step into the circle if you identify with the prompt. Prompts can be offered spontaneously, or the facilitator can ask participants to offer step-in prompts one at a time by going around the entire circle. It is helpful to encourage group members to make their statements broad and general rather than specific as it creates a more inclusive experience and prevents individuals from making statements so specific that they end up stepping in alone. If a prompt does result in one person alone in the circle, it is helpful to reframe the prompt in a more general way – for example, the prompt "I enjoy water color painting" could be generalized to "I enjoy creating art" which would result in more participants stepping in.

Either the facilitator offers prompts asking participants to physically step in if they identify, or group members take turns stepping in while making statements about themselves while others who identify also step in. Buchanan (2016) describes the latter as the *democratic approach* and the former as the *totalitarian approach* to step-in sociometry. This writer has discovered that the democratic approach is favorable in nearly all contexts. One exception where the totalitarian approach may be useful is when offering trauma-related prompts in a group where it could be harmful if the process goes too far into the trauma. The totalitarian approach would allow the facilitator to intentionally choose very broad trauma-related prompts that ensure the largest number of participants identify. In this context, the facilitator providing all of the prompts would contribute to group safety and containment. Another facilitation consideration is the facilitator's decision to participate in the process or not. The choice to participate or not, or participate in some rounds but not others, would come back to the facilitators style, the goals for the group, the group population, and the group context. In some groups and with some prompts, it may be advantageous for the facilitator to participate which allows the group to connect with them while in other groups and with other prompts, it may be best for the director not to participate (Buchanan, 2016; Giacomucci, 2017).

In facilitating this process, it is also important to inform participants that they can choose whether they want to self-disclose or not on any given criteria as there may be prompts offered that some participants are willing to self-disclose while others may not be ready to do so (Buchanan, 2016). When a group member offers a prompt and other participants step in, it allows the group to visually see others who have a shared experience. Step-in sociometry makes the invisible connections and similarities within the group visible and conscious – thus increasing overall group connection and cohesion (Giacomucci et al., 2018). Once participants have stepped in, concretizing their connection to the prompt, the facilitator invites them to quietly acknowledge others who have stepped in then step back into the larger circle. This process seems to be appealing to introverted clients and young adults who find it to be an opportunity for peer identification without much verbal sharing (Giacomucci, 2017). Alternative ways of facilitating include inviting participants who have stepped in to briefly share why they stepped in or to use sound or movement to express their connection to the prompt.

Step-in sociometry can be facilitated with multiple rounds, each with a larger theme, or as a single open-ended process without a theme. Both options have benefits. An open-ended step-in sociometry experience allows the group to choose any prompts which is likely to be revealing of the group's overall warm-up and allows the group to control the process (Archer, 2016). The method of using multiple rounds of step-in sociometry, each with themes, allows the facilitator to create a more directed and intentional group warm-up which may be most useful in clinical settings. When using multiple rounds of step-in sociometry, it is useful to follow the clinical map referenced previously.

The following video depicts the use of step-in sociometry with a live group: http://www.phoenixtraumacenter.com/step-in-sociometry/.

Below are some examples of different themes for step-in rounds.

Group: Inpatient Addiction Treatment

1) Step in and name something you like to do that is not related to your addiction
2) Step in and name a consequence of your addiction (medical, emotional, social, legal, etc.)
3) Step in and share a hope or goal for your future in recovery from addiction

Group: Immigrant Families

1) Step in and name something that is important to you about your family or culture
2) Step in and label something that has been difficult for you related to immigration
3) Step in and share a hope you have for you family going forward

Group: Grief and Loss Group for Parents

1) Step in and share one thing that has helped you in your grief and loss
2) Step in and share one difficult aspect related to your grief and loss
3) Step in and share one goal for yourself and your family going forward in the grief process

Group: Hospital-Based Cancer Support Group

1) Step in and share something about yourself beyond your medical condition
2) Step in and share one difficult aspect of your cancer diagnosis
3) Step in and name one goal for yourself going forward

Group: High School Group

1) Step in and share something about yourself
2) Step in and share one thing you find difficult about high school
3) Step in and share something you would like to accomplish by the end of high school

Group: New Social Work Graduate Students

1) Step in and share one thing that influenced your decision to get a graduate degree in social work
2) Step in and name one fear you have about the graduate program

3) Step in and name a professional role that you would like to have in the future

Group: Organizational Meeting on Trauma-Informed Care

1) Step in and share one way you feel our organization does a good job at providing trauma-informed care
2) Step in and name one way you feel we could improve as an organization in our provision of trauma-informed services
3) Step in and identify one goal for yourself about further integrating trauma-informed principles into your work

Step-in sociometry cultivates universality, curiosity, connection, and inclusion with the group experience and can be adapted for any topic or group setting (Buchanan, 2016; Giacomucci, 2020). Archer (2016) provides an in-depth exploration of various ways to adapt step-in sociometry with groups that consist of participants with physical limitations including group members who are visually impaired, wheelchair bound, or on crutches. In larger groups, or group spaces where creating a circle is not possible, the step-in sociometry process is often modified to utilize standing up or raising hands instead (Archer, 2016).

Similar to the previously described experiential sociometry processes, step-in sociometry can be used as a warm-up or as a group process on its own. Furthermore, the utilization of step-in sociometry for closure, processing and integration after a psychodrama enactment or other group process has been described (Giacomucci, 2017). This may be most useful in the context of large groups or when time is limited and a quick, efficient method for sharing is called for.

How could I use step-in sociometry to uncover shared experiences or preferences in my own clinical groups or organizational meetings?

Hands-on-Shoulder Sociograms

The sociogram was one of the first sociometry instruments that Moreno developed through his sociometric tests (Moreno, 1934; J. D. Moreno, 2014). A sociogram shows the number of times group members choose each other based on specific criteria. Using pen-to-paper sociometric tests, Moreno collected the written choices of participants and drew complex sociograms to depict the distribution of choices within the group. The hands-on-shoulder sociogram, sometimes called an action sociogram, moves this process from paper into the room as an experiential process. The action sociogram makes the unseen choices within a group conscious, revealing the invisible web of attractions, and repulsions within a group (Korshak & Shapiro, 2013). Hale (1981) refers to this as enhancing the sociometric consciousness of the group. While the previously described sociometry processes are all based in self-assessment, the sociogram is oriented on the assessment of others and the group's overall assessment of itself (Giacomucci, 2018a).

The experiential sociogram process prompts participants to put their hand on the shoulder of one other group member based on a specific prompt, simultaneously revealing the distribution of choices and preference within the group. This process uses physical touch, so it is important to check in with the group about their comfort level with physical touch and obtain their consent – especially when working with trauma survivors. Sometimes the aforementioned sociometry processes are used to explore comfort with physical touch such as a spectrogram, locogram, or step-in sociometry. If participants are not comfortable with others putting their hand on their shoulder, the process can be amended by having participants indicate their choices by touching their shoe to the shoe of another, standing next to another, pointing at their choices, or holding a scarf or string to indicate their choice (Hudgins & Toscani, 2013; Olsen, Campbell, & Gross, 2017; Simmons, 2017). While some may find the experience of physical touch as uncomfortable or intolerable, others may find it soothing and comforting (Giacomucci et al., 2018). Moreno wrote of the power of physical touch and highlighted the practice wisdom from the field of nursing in this area (McIntosh, 2010; Moreno, 1972).

The sociogram often helps participants become aware of their own tendencies around choosing, waiting to be chosen, and prioritizing their first choice. When one has difficulty with making a choice, they are encouraged to choose with their intuition or to trust their tele. Once each participant has indicated their choice by putting their hand on the shoulder of one person in the room, the facilitator may offer a brief interpretation of the sociometric constellation – for example noting prevalence of mutual choices, the equal distribution of choices, or the choices being highly concentrated with social stars and social isolates. The sociogram quickly depicts the distribution of criteria-specific social wealth within the group, thus highlighting the presence of tele and the sociodynamic effect. Then, participants are invited to share briefly with the person they chose about their reasoning for choosing them. This effectively increases interpersonal relationships within the group while enhancing overall group cohesion. Below are some examples of prompts tailored to different groups using the prescribed stages of the clinical map.

Group: Veterans Support Group

1) Place your hand on the shoulder of someone who you experienced take a significant step in their growth last month
2) Place your hand on the shoulder of someone who has said something related to your identity as a veteran which was meaningful to you
3) Place your hand on the shoulder of someone whose experience you would like to know more about
4) Place your hand on the shoulder of someone who you could see yourself connecting with outside of group

Group: Substance Use Relapse Prevention Group

1) Place your hand on the shoulder of someone who inspires you
2) Place your hand on the shoulder of someone who has said something that worries you
3) Place your hand on the shoulder of someone who you could call if you had a craving to use drugs
4) Place your hand on the shoulder of someone who you could call for relationship advice

Each of the given examples demonstrates the use of hands-on-shoulder sociogram criteria that is reality based and sociometric based. Another option is to offer prompts that are surplus reality and psychodramatically oriented. The difference between reality-based sociometric prompts and surplus reality-based psychodrama prompts is depicted below.

Sociometric Reality-Based Prompts

A. Place your hand on the shoulder of someone who you experience as courageous
B. Place your hand on the shoulder of someone who you look up to as a role model
C. Place your hand on the shoulder of someone who reminds you of yourself

D. Place your hand on the shoulder of someone who you would call for spiritual guidance
E. Place your hand on the shoulder of someone who you experience as motherly

Psychodramatic Surplus Reality-Based Prompts

A. Place your hand on the shoulder of someone who you would choose to play the role of your courage
B. Place your hand on the shoulder of someone who you would choose to play the role of one of your role models
C. Place your hand on the shoulder of someone who you would choose to play the role of yourself
D. Place your hand on the shoulder of someone who you would choose to play the role of God
E. Place your hand on the shoulder of someone who you would choose to play the role of your mother

Some find that psychodramatic prompts provide more distance and thus more safety for group members when choosing and being chosen. Psychodramatic prompts also have the benefit of getting participants warmed-up to choosing roles in a psychodrama. Many practitioners employ both sociometric and psychodramatic prompts in their use of sociograms in groups. Below are some examples of mixed prompts.

Group: Depression Support

1) Place your hand on the shoulder of someone who you would has helped you feel comfortable in the group
2) Place your hand on the shoulder of someone who you would choose to play the role of your resilience
3) Place your hand on the shoulder of someone who has helped you understand depression better
4) Place your hand on the shoulder of someone who you could call if your depression increased
5) Place your hand on the shoulder of someone who you would choose to play the role of yourself in the future no longer experiencing depression

Group: Healthy Relationships for Couples

1) Place your hand on the shoulder of someone whose sharing has helped you understand yourself better

2) Place your hand on the shoulder of someone who you would choose to play the role of your willingness to work on your relationship
3) Place your hand on the shoulder of someone whose love for their partner has inspired you
4) Place your hand on the shoulder of someone who you would choose to play the role of your honesty or vulnerability
5) Place your hand on the shoulder of someone who you would call if you needed support in the future

Group: Ongoing Agency Training on Trauma-Informed Care

1) Place your hand on the shoulder of someone who you feel best embodies the trauma-informed principle of "safety"
2) Place your hand on the shoulder of someone who you feel best embodies the trauma-informed principle of "addressing cultural, historic, and gender issues"
3) Place your hand on the shoulder of someone who you have seen significantly grow in their ability to implement trauma-informed services
4) Place your hand on the shoulder of someone who you would choose to play the role of "transparency"
5) Place your hand on the shoulder of someone who you feel is quick to offer peer support in your department

While these are examples of prompts that could be offered in groups, it is important for the facilitator to remain attentive to the group process and to offer new prompts when needed to create a more inclusive experience. For examples, if a facilitator notices that a participant repeatedly is unchosen, it would be important to spontaneously offer a new prompt that makes this person highly chosen. Group facilitators have a responsibility to be aware of the sociodynamic effect and to reverse its impact within the group to create an inclusive experience. While one may be unchosen in this group based on this criterion, they are almost certainly a social star when it comes to other criteria and in other groups. Korshak and Shapiro (2013) note that reversing the sharing in a sociogram is another method of reversing the sociodynamic effect. Rather than having participants *share their reason for choosing* another, the person chosen *shares their experience of being chosen* with the person choosing them. Zerka Moreno (2006) writes that the "essential reason for doing sociometric investigations is not just to make relationships visible and available for interpretation, but to reconstruct groups to maximize sociostasis and find some resolution to the problem of the unchosen and rejected" (p. 296).

At this point, it is important to note that of all of the experiential processes described in this chapter, the action sociogram has the most risk. Unless conducted attentively, spontaneously, and skillfully, the group may have a negative response to the hands-on-shoulder sociogram. This process is best utilized in higher functioning groups where participants are familiar with each other and have demonstrated a capacity for tolerating vulnerability and discomfort.

What topics and prompts might be applicable in hands-on-shoulder sociometry in my own clinical groups or organizational meetings?

Circle of Strengths

The circle of strengths is a safety structure that originates from the TSM (Hudgins & Toscani, 2013). It is an experiential process of concretizing the collective strengths of the group and strongly compliments trauma-informed care's strengths-based approach (Saleebey, 2012). Generally, this exercise begins with a large pile of scarves or other fabric in the center of the group room (though it can also be done with objects in the room or with pen/paper). As group members enter the room, the scarves spark their curiosity, playfulness, and creativity. One simple way of facilitating the circle of strengths is to have the group break up into dyads; if there are an odd number, the facilitator can join – this method of using dyads prevents anyone from being chosen last (Giacomucci et al., 2018). Participants are provided with psychoeducation on the importance of strengths and various types of strengths (intrapsychic, interpersonal, and transpersonal strengths). Participants are then asked to choose a scarf to represent a strength that they see in their partner and to present the strength to their partner one at a time while reminding their partner of examples of how they have demonstrated the strength. This provides a ritual for group members to practice healthy risks and vulnerability with each other based on positive criteria. The rest of the group witnesses the individual exchanges of strengths. As each strength is concretized (with scarves), they are placed on the floor of the group room, creating a large circle of strengths. This process can be repeated in new dyads or spontaneously between group members. The facilitator may choose to do one round in dyads, then a round where everyone identifies one of their own strengths, and finally a round where everyone concretizes a strength they experience in the group-as-a-whole.

The resulting circle of strengths on the floor serves as a conscious reminder of the individual and collective strengths within the group. They can be utilized by the facilitator later in the process if a group member becomes overwhelmed and might benefit from a reminder of their strengths. Symbolically, the circle is representative of the unity of the group and the ability of the collective group strengths to contain any participant's stories, experiences, trauma, or feelings. Logistically, the circle of strengths can serve as a stage for a future psychodrama in the group (Hudgins & Toscani, 2013).

The exercise was initially developed through the process of having group members choose scarves to symbolize their own personal strengths that they bring to the group. As TSM became utilized around the world, especially in Asia, this process evolved to become more culturally sensitive and new methods developed including having group members choose scarves to concretize the strengths they see in each other (Hudgins & Toscani, 2013). Novel methods for creating the circle of strengths continue to be developed including using short enactments of strengths, inviting group members to ask for reminders of specific strengths, and concretizing strengths of an organization or program. The experience of engaging in this process seems to significantly increase connections in the group, cultivate mutual aid, renegotiate one's sense of self, enhance group cohesion, and establish an "all in the same boat" mentality (Giacomucci, 2019, 2021a, 2021b; Giacomucci & Ehrhart, 2021 Shulman, 2010).

The following video depicts the use of Circle of Strengths with a live group: http://www.phoenixtraumacenter.com/circle-of-strengths/.

Some examples of statements from clients engaging in this process are provided below.

Interpersonal Recognitions of Strengths

- "I chose this for your courage because it is a strong and bold scarf. I have seen you demonstrate courage in the times you are vulnerable with us and in the stories you have shared about your childhood."
- "I chose this scarf to represent the compassion and kindness that I experience from you each time we are together. You always are friendly and are quick to offer support whenever anyone needs it – I know I can count on your support."

- "I picked this scarf to be your spirituality and the sense of purpose it gives you. It is clear that your spirituality is important to you and gives meaning to your life in the way you help others and maintain faith through uncertainty."

Acknowledging Personal Strengths

- "I chose this one to symbolize my resilience. Even though I have experienced hardship, I keep bouncing back and I survive no matter what."
- "This represents my relationship to my family. I believe family is the most important thing in life and they are always there to support me."
- "I chose this scarf for my ability to ground myself. I have learned breathing techniques and meditation which allow me to center myself internally even when things get chaotic."

Strengths in the Group-as-a-Whole

- "I chose this to represent our willingness to change. Everyone here demonstrates this strength each time you show up to group. Regardless of our failures or successes, we continue to be willing to change and grow."
- "I chose this colorful scarf to symbolize the diversity in this group. We all come from different walks of life and various backgrounds which gives us each a unique perspective that we bring to the group. I always learn new ways of looking at things because of you all."
- "I picked this scarf to represent the safety of this group. I usually don't trust people, but I know that this is a safe place and this group of people are worthy of my trust."

The circle of strengths process can be quite powerful for participants and has the potential of tapping into strong emotions for some. As group therapists and organizational leaders, we often are working with traumatized, oppressed, and disenfranchised populations. The process of taking the time to recognize strengths can be incredibly restorative, especially for those that have been marginalized within society, dehumanized in their interpersonal relationships, or stuck in self-loathing. This process could be employed as a warm-up for a psychodrama or as its own group process. The circle of strengths can also be facilitated in online groups by having participants choose objects in their own room to concretize the strengths of others and themselves. It can also be adapted for use in community groups, supervision groups, student groups, and organizational settings to increase confidence and cohesion in a meaningful and strengths-based process.

How could I employ the Circle of Strengths to build cohesion and connection in my own clinical groups or organizational meetings?

Conclusion

Experiential sociometry processes offer strengths-based and trauma-informed methods for engaging groups. These approaches intrinsically embody trauma-informed principles and can be used to further explore the six trauma-informed principles with clients, communities, students, and staff. Each of the aforementioned group processes can be adapted for use with any community and any topic making them valuable tools for group workers, psychodramatists, and leaders. While these exercises are often used as warm-ups for a psychodrama enactment, they can also be utilized on their own for group-as-a-whole assessment, engagement, intervention, and evaluation. These processes are also invaluable tools for organizational leaders as they offer avenues for active engagement, assessment, and intervention within organizational culture and the relational dynamics between staff.

References

Archer, M. (2016). Who, like me, loves to use the step-in circle? *The Journal of Psychodrama, Sociometry, and Group Psychotherapy, 64*(1), 79–82.

Buchanan, D. R. (2016). Practical applications of step-in sociometry: Increasing sociometric intelligence via self-disclosure and connection. *Journal of Psychodrama, Sociometry, and Group Psychotherapy, 64,* 71–78.

Chesner, A. (2020). Psychodrama and healing the traumatic wound. In A. Chesner, & S. Lykou (Eds.), *Trauma in the creative and embodied therapies: When words are not enough* (pp. 69–80). London: Routledge.

Courtois, C. A., & Ford, J. D. (2016). *Treatment of complex trauma: A sequenced, relationship-based approach.* New York: The Guildford Press.

Dayton, T. (2005). *The living stage: A step-by-step guide to psychodrama, sociometry, and experiential group therapy.* Deerfield, FL: Health Communications Inc.

Dayton, T. (2014). *Relational trauma repair (RTR) therapist's guide* (revised ed.). New York: Innerlook, Inc.

Dayton, T. (2015). *NeuroPsychodrama in the treatment of relational trauma: A strength-based, experiential model for healing PTSD.* Deerfield Beach, FL: Health Communications, Inc.

Fleury, H. J., & Marra, M. M. (2022). Theoretical and methodological foundations of socionomy. In H. J. Fleury, M. M. Marra, & O. H. Hadler (Eds.), *Psychodrama in Brazil* (pp. 17–29). Singapore: Springer.

Fluegelman, A. (1976). *The new games book.* San Francisco, CA: New Games Foundation.

Freud, S. (1932). *The dissection of the psychical personality. Standard edition* (Vol. 22, pp. 67–80). London: Hogarth Press.

Giacomucci, S. (2017). The sociodrama of life or death: Young adults and addiction treatment. *Journal of Psychodrama, Sociometry, and Group Psychotherapy, 65*(1), 137–143. https://doi.org/10.12926/0731-1273-65.1.137

Giacomucci, S. (2018a). Social work and sociometry: An integration of theory and clinical practice. *The Pennsylvania Social Worker, 39*(1), 14–16.

Giacomucci, S. (2018b). The trauma survivor's inner role atom: A clinical map for post-traumatic growth. *Journal of Psychodrama, Sociometry, and Group Psychotherapy, 66*(1), 115–129.

Giacomucci, S. (2019). *Social group work in action: A sociometry, psychodrama, and experiential trauma therapy curriculum.* Doctorate in Social Work (DSW) Dissertations, 124. Retrieved from https://repository.upenn.edu/cgi/viewcontent.cgi?article=1128&context=edissertations_sp2

Giacomucci, S. (2020). Addiction, traumatic loss, and guilt: A case study resolving grief through psychodrama and sociometric connections. *The Arts in Psychotherapy, 67*, 101627. https://doi.org/10.1016/j.aip.2019.101627

Giacomucci, S. (2021a). Experiential sociometry in group work: Mutual aid for the group-as-a-whole. *Social Work with Groups, 44*(3), 204–214.

Giacomucci, S. (2021b). *Social work, sociometry, and psychodrama: Experiential approaches for group therapists, community leaders, and social workers:* Springer Nature. https://doi.org/10.1007/978-981-33-6342-7

Giacomucci, S., & Ehrhart, L. (2021). Introduction to psychodrama psychotherapy: A trauma and addiction group vignette. *Group, 45*(1), 69–86.

Giacomucci, S., Gera, S., Briggs, D., & Bass, K. (2018). Experiential addiction treatment: Creating positive connection through sociometry and therapeutic spiral model safety structures. *Journal of Addiction and Addictive Disorders, 5*, 17. http://doi.org/10.24966/AAD-7276/100017

Giacomucci, S., & Marquit, J. (2020). The effectiveness of trauma-focused psychodrama in the treatment of PTSD in inpatient substance abuse treatment. *Frontiers in Psychology, 11,* 896. https://dx.doi.org/10.3389%2Ffpsyg.2020.00896

Giacomucci, S., & Skolnik, S. (2021). The experiential social work educator: Integrating sociometry into the classroom environment. *Journal of Teaching in Social Work, 41*(2), 192–202.

Hale, A. E. (1981). *Conducting clinical sociometric explorations: A manual for psychodramatists and sociometrists.* Roanoke, VA: Royal Publishing Company.

Hale, A. E. (2009). Moreno's sociometry: Exploring interpersonal connection. *Group, 33*(4), 347–358.

Herman, J. L. (1997). *Trauma and recovery: The aftermath of violence—From domestic abuse to political terror.* New York: Basic Books.

Hudgins, M. K., & Toscani, F. (2013). *Healing world trauma with the therapeutic spiral model: Stories from the frontlines.* London: Jessica Kingsley Publishers.

Korshak, S. J., & Shapiro, M. (2013). Choosing the unchosen: Counteracting the sociodynamic effect using complementary sharing. *The Journal of Psychodrama, Sociometry, and Group Psychotherapy, 61*(1), 7–15.

Lawrence, C. (2015). The caring observer: Creating self-compassion through psychodrama. *The Journal of Psychodrama, Sociometry, and Group Psychotherapy, 63*(1), 65–72.

Levine, P. A. (2010). *In an unspoken voice: How the body releases trauma and restores goodness.* Berkeley, CA. North Atlantic Books.

McIntosh, W. (2010). Walking with Moreno: A historical journey of psychodrama and nursing. *Australian and Aotearoa New Zealand Psychodrama Association Journal, 19,* 30.

Moreno, J. D. (2014). *Impromptu man: J.L. Moreno and the origins of psychodrama, encounter culture, and the social network.* New York: Bellevue Literary Press.

Moreno, J. L. (1934). *Who shall survive? A new approach to the problems of human interrelations.* Washington, DC: Nervous and Mental Disease Publishing Co.

Moreno, J. L. (1972). *Psychodrama volume 1 (4th edition).* New York: Beacon House.

Moreno, Z. T. (2006). The function of "tele" in human relations. In T. Horvatin, & E. Shreiber (Eds.), *The Quintessential Zerka: Writings by Zerka Toeman Moreno on Psychodrama, sociometry and group psychotherapy* (pp. 289–301). New York: Routledge.

Nieto, L. (2010). Look behind you: Using anti-oppression models to inform a protagonist's psychodrama. In E. Leveton (Ed.), *Healing collective trauma using sociodrama and drama therapy* (pp. 103–125). New York: Springer Publishing Company.

Olesen, J., Campbell, J., & Gross, M. (2017). Using action methods to counter social isolation and shame among gay men. *Journal of Gay & Lesbian Social Services, 29*(2), 91–108.

Saleebey, D. (2012). *The strengths perspective in social work practice (6th Edition)*. Boston, MA: Pearson Education.

Shulman, L. (2010). *Dynamics and skills of group counseling*. Belmont, CA: Cengage Learning.

Simmons, D. (2017). Implementing sociometry in a long-term care institutional setting for the elderly: Exploring social relationships and choices. *The Journal of Psychodrama, Sociometry, and Group Psychotherapy, 65*(1), 85–98.

Shapiro, F. (2018). *Eye-movement desensitization and reprocessing (EMDR) therapy (3rd edition)*. New York: Guilford Press.

Substance Abuse and Mental Health Services Administration. (2014a). *SAMHSA's concept of trauma and guidance for a trauma-informed approach*. HHS Publication No. (SMA) 14-4884. Rockville, MD: Substance Abuse and Mental Health Services Administration.

van der Kolk, B. A. (2014). *The body keeps the score: Brain, mind, and body in the healing of trauma*. New York: Viking Press.

Yalom, I. D., & Leszcz, M. (2020). *The theory and practice of group psychotherapy* (6th ed.). New York: Basic Books.

5
Safety in Group Therapy, Psychodrama, and Leadership

Chapter Summary

This chapter presents the first of SAMHSA's six trauma-informed principles – safety. The essential nature of safety will be underscored as it relates to working with trauma survivors. An experience of safety alone can be therapeutic for trauma survivors as trauma inherently robs one of a sense of safety. Strategies for cultivating safety will be offered including practical suggestions and examples from the author's clinical experience. Containment, consent, physical touch, group rules, clinical contracting, confidentiality, mutual respect, and boundaries will be covered. Attention will also be given to the varying contexts and levels of care that services are provided as it relates to safety before, during, and after the group process. The development of safety in group work and psychodrama work will be addressed. Maintaining safety for staff members is also important as it impacts the quality of their work and employees' ability to self-regulate. A clinical vignette on establishing safety after trauma is included to depict the power of psychodrama.

Trauma as a Threat to Safety

Trauma and safety are essentially opposites. Trauma is an experience that threatens one's sense of safety in their body, relationship, and the world. Many trauma survivors feel that they have lost their sense of safety and struggle to reconnect to a sense of safety long after the trauma is over. Some children grow up without safe caregivers and/or within structures that oppress,

DOI: 10.4324/9781003277859-5

marginalize, and dehumanize them in a way that they rarely or never feel safe in the world. Traumatic stress is characterized by ongoing sense of threat, arousal, reactivity, avoidance, intrusions, and negative changes in feelings and thoughts. Those struggling with posttraumatic stress disorder (PTSD) have lost a sense of safety in their body, in relationships, and in the world. There are multiple layers of safety that we must take into consideration when working with trauma survivors, some of these include physical safety, emotional/psychological safety, social safety, cultural safety, and moral safety (Bloom, 2013) (Table 5.1).

Table 5.1 Five types of safety to consider in organizations and groups

Five Layers of Safety				
Physical	Emotional/psychological	Social	Cultural	Moral

Incorporating the trauma-informed principle of safety means that we create spaces that promote physical safety, emotional/psychological safety, social safety, cultural safety, and moral safety for the clients we serve and for the staff employed at the agency.

Which of these five types of safety am I best at cultivating for my clients?

Which of these five types of safety could I most improve in my ability to cultivate for clients?

Safety is the most important aspect of trauma-focused work. No trauma processing can safely be done until the issue of safety has first been attended to. It is no coincidence then that safety is a core component of the three-stage clinical map that has been referenced throughout this book. For many trauma survivors, simply having an experience of safety is healing and a corrective experience. Providing a multi-dimensional experience of safety should be our priority when working with trauma survivors and especially in trauma-focused service offerings (Badenoch, 2018; Herman, 1992). Porges, Badenoch, and Phillips (2016) remind us that *safety is the treatment*. When considering the establishment and maintenance of safety, it is also essential that we consider safety as defined by those we serve. A provider's sense of safety may be different than a client's sense of what safety means or looks like. Safety is likely to be experienced differently from client to client and from community to community as well. There are usually greater risks to safety for folks who have marginalized identities or social memberships. This must be attended to. Many challenge the concept of "establishing safety" arguing that "safety" is relative and never absolute. Instead, some have suggested a goal of making spaces "safer." Furthermore, it is important to remember that safety is not a simple cognitive experience; it is an embodied experience involving one's senses, sensations, emotions, thoughts, and socio-cultural experience (Malchiodi, 2020).

Traumatization and Retraumatization by Service Providers

As noted previously, one of the underlying threads that lead to the development of SAMHSA's trauma-informed care content (2014a) was the painful realization that many service providers were (and continue to) traumatizing or retraumatizing the clients that they are tasked to serve. This happens explicitly, implicitly, unconsciously, and through negligence. No social service agency is entirely free from the potential of harming a client. It occurs through abuse of power, through the reenactment of discrimination or unconscious bias, a documentation mistake that leads to harming a patient, a forgotten task that negatively impacts a client's experience, and/or through violations of professional conducts of ethics. Unfortunately, these types of harms take place regularly in hospitals, prisons, policing, government, treatment centers, clinics, residential programs, universities, and community organizations.

The ongoing harms experienced by those accessing services are good reasons to elevate trauma-informed principles to the same level as ethical standards. As a trauma therapist, I consistently learn of ways that clients have been taken advantage of or directly abused by other therapists, programs, or social service agencies. The sad truth is that many clients are in trauma therapy in part to address trauma that they experienced from professionals. In my experience, these past experiences of traumatization at the hands of other professionals make it particularly hard for the client to ask for help and re-establish enough safety within our therapeutic relationship to begin processing the trauma. Even more tragically perhaps is that there are countless individuals who have been traumatized by professionals or providers and as a result are unwilling to seek services again. Instead of reaching out for help or accepting help, they suffer from both their trauma but also the sense of betrayal in being neglected and betrayed by those who were meant to help them.

The fourth "R" of trauma-informed care is devoted entirely to "Resisting Retraumatization." This could be conceptualized as similar to the ancient medical motto "first, do no harm." This may seem like a simple task but becomes ever more complex when we consider the often unconscious reenactments that come with trauma work – as well as the potential for retraumatization through a provider's neglect, oversight, or decisions influenced by unconscious bias. So many trauma survivors are seeking services due to abuse, violence, gaslighting, neglect, abandonment, and discrimination; thus, we need to avoid reenacting the same harms that led to their initial traumas. Ensuring safety and preventing retraumatization with trauma survivors includes consistently revisiting consent, permission, willingness, and choice – which will be revisited in Chapter 9. Forcing clients to engage in trauma-focused therapy is potentially retraumatizing in itself and should be avoided.

Trauma-Informed Leaders Prioritize Safety in the Workplace

There is an old saying that "hurt people hurt people." Perhaps many instances of service providers causing harm to clients reflect this old saying. After all, professions are humans and trauma survivors too. Various studies have pointed to the high prevalence of childhood adversity and trauma experienced by those of us that choose the social services fields (Bryce et al., 2021; Esaki & Larkin, 2013; Keesler, 2018; Steen, Senreich, & Straussner, 2021). Many of us explicitly choose this field as a direct result of our previous experiences of adversity and it improves our ability to be compassionate, understanding, and empathetic with clients. The overwhelming majority of educators, social workers, direct service providers, and child welfare professionals have histories of childhood trauma. Keeping this in mind, it would be important for organizations to consider that their staff are inevitably going to be largely comprised of trauma survivors. Sandra Bloom, a pioneer in trauma-informed care, sums it up well:

> Not only are our systems of care frequently unsafe for the clients but they may be unsafe for our staff and administrators as well – sometimes physically unsafe, but even more commonly psychologically, socially, and morally safe. Recovery begins with safety…
>
> (2011, p. 25)

The degree of safety felt by organizational staff is going to impact their ability to provide high quality services, their work efficiency, their job satisfaction, the work atmosphere/culture, and the overall sense of cohesion within the organization. Various studies on psychological safety in workplaces highlight how it increases learning, performance, and even lowers workplace mortalities

(Edmondson, 2018). Professionals who feel safe and supported will simply do a better job than professionals who feel unsafe and threatened (Handran, 2015). Google's five-year study, *Project Aristotle*, on work team productivity found psychological safety to be, by far, the most important dynamic in successful teams (Duhigg, 2016). As organizational leaders, we must prioritize the safety for our staff while preventing harm to them. There is often a parallel process between the level of safety felt by an organization's staff and the corresponding level of safety felt by the organization's clients (see Chapter 11 for more on this) (Bloom, 2011). When staff feel unsafe their anxiety, hyperarousal, and stress is inevitably felt and transferred through their interactions with clients and patients. Bloom and Farragher (2013) articulate how this lack of safety in organizations can evolve into chronic stress and what they describe as *organizational hyperarousal.* To mitigate this, trauma-informed leaders prioritize safety of their staff in the workplace.

As noted earlier in this chapter, there are multiple layers of safety to consider – physical, emotional/psychological safety, social safety, cultural safety, and moral safety. At the same time, it is also important to consider what safety means and how it is defined by the staff themselves rather than organizational leadership defining safety alone. General considerations for physical safety will vary between agencies but often include working to mitigating harm and hazards related to the organization's building, campus, and neighborhood. There are, especially in higher levels of care for mental health treatment, inherent risks of physical or emotional harm from patients toward staff members. These risks should be addressed by leadership providing front-line staff with support, protection, and resources as needed. Leadership can demonstrate to their commitment to their staff's safety through swift, decisive, compassionate, and generous responses to issues of safety in the workplace. Policies, procedures, and organizational culture are to organizations what group norms and rules are to group work. They provide a framework and container for safety and a safe work environment. Organizational policies and cultures that promote self-reflection, self-awareness, and personal/professional growth appear to be most effective at establishing safety and wellness for workers.

Beyond physical and emotional safety, we must also consider social and moral safety for staff. Unethical organizational practices are a violation of moral safety. Ethical practice is trauma-informed practice. Moral, cultural, and social safety are promoted in organizations through nondiscrimination, equity, and anti-oppressive organizational practices. Leaders who honor the inherent dignity and worth of each employee, regardless of gender, race, ethnicity, religion, age, ability, title, and salary help to cultivate safe and empowering workplaces. In organizational contexts, safety in the supervisory relationship parallels the centrality of safety in the therapeutic relationship for psychotherapy contexts. In group work, the cohesion of the group-as-a-whole exerts a determining influence upon each of its members; similarly, in organizations (or departments) the cohesion of the staff significantly impacts each individual employee. The organization is fundamentally a group and, thus, group work skills, theories, and interventions can be effectively applied to organizational settings for similar outcomes. The same methods a group worker uses to promote safety within the group can be applied by organizational leaders to promote safety in the workplace.

Some simple ways of operationalizing this could include providing meaningful employee benefits, staff appreciation, wellness funds for workers, Employee Assistance Programs (EAPs), critical incident response teams within the organization, transparency from leadership to staff, discussions and actions related to equity and equality in the workplace, celebrating staff successes or milestones, beginning staff meetings with a few seconds of mindfulness practice, or providing other self-care services or reminders for staff. Resources and possibilities related to enhancing safety within the organization will differ significantly between agencies depending on context, funding, and the nature of services provided. It is important that leaders involve staff in decisions related to enhancing safety and connection in the workplace (this will be discussed further in future chapters). A worker who feels unsafe is simply unable to consistently help clients feel safe. Without the foundation of safety, providing services – especially trauma-focused treatment, becomes significantly more complicated, dangerous, and arduous. Staff who feel safe are better able to connect with clients and coworkers, self-regulate, make complicated decisions, generate or implement sophisticated ideas, and contribute to the overall wellness of an organization. In the context of hiring decisions, organizational leaders can borrow ideas from the group therapy client selection process to guide their interviewing and screening of new staff. Will the organization be a good fit for this new staff member? Will they be a good fit for the team? Will they feel safe as part of this team, and will others feel safe with them? Whenever possible, organizational leaders should consider their organization's cohesion, safety, and culture when making hiring decisions.

What are the things that help me feel safest in the workplace?

What are some simple things I can do, or suggest, to enhance safety for my co-workers or staff?

Assessment, Referral, and Screening

"Good group therapy begins with good client selection. Clients improperly assigned to a therapy group are unlikely to benefit from their therapy experience" (Yalom & Leszcz, 2020, p. 293). Assessment and intake processes for trauma services can be stressful for both the client and the group therapist (Courtois, 2010; Courtois & Ford, 2016). It is important that the intake process meets the client where they are at. Proper assessment, referral, and screening for clients' needs, appropriate level of care, and goodness-of-fit within a group are all important in promoting safety for the client, staff, and other clients or group members. While the nature of promoting safety will be similar across agency types, there are inherently differences in the nature of services provided across various agencies. The context of our agency setting and, in particular, the level of care of a treatment center plays a significant role in maintaining safety for individuals. For example, promoting safety in a prison setting will look a lot different than promoting safety in a hospital, in a shelter for victims of domestic violence, or in an outpatient treatment center. These differences further highlight the importance of considering what safety means for the individuals or communities accessing services in different agencies. Consideration of safety must also extend beyond the agency and into the rest of the client's life experience. A client might feel safe at the hospital, but there may be a lack of safety at their home or in that they simple might not have a place to sleep. In these cases, our ethical responsibility for ensuring safety extends beyond the walls of the agency and includes helping clients to access services from other agencies that can help them secure housing, protection, or promote changes within a family or relationship. When a client has needs that our agency or group can't meet, we should refer the client to another provider or agency. Of course, there are also limits to a provider's power in ensuring safety – this is particularly true for clients who live in unsafe communities or who experience structural violence based on the very nature of their identity. Although we may be limited in creating change in some cases, we can still work toward promoting safety and help a client access resources that might also promote safety in their lives.

In terms of mental health treatment, thorough assessment and careful discernment about the appropriate level of care is an essential component of safety. Incomplete and inaccurate assessment leading to placement or referral at an inappropriate level of care can lead to harm and a loss of safety. A client presenting with the criteria warranting hospitalization who is referred for outpatient treatment is at risk. Similarly, safety is at risk when a client presenting with symptoms of a specific medical or mental health condition (such as substance use disorder, schizophrenia, or an eating disorder) is admitted to a facility that doesn't treat those conditions. When facilities admit clients whose conditions are outside of their scope of competence it impacts the integrity of services provided. Group workers within those facilities end up with group participants that don't fully fit in with the rest of the group based on the differences in their experiences, goals, and severity of symptoms. Assessment and pre-group screening requires careful consideration, clinical competence, and ethical standards (Brabender & Macnair-Semands, 2022).

When developing an outpatient group, the screening process is particularly important for the same reason. Groups tend to function best when there are overlapping individual goals, shared experiences, similar problems, and when the severity of participants symptoms are within similar thresholds. This is vital when screening participants for trauma or psychodrama groups as each individual's window of tolerance must be considered as it impacts the group-as-a-whole's ability to safely engage in trauma work. For example, when most of a group is stable, resourced, and willing enough to begin trauma processing work, but there are one or two group members who are not – the less stable members could be overwhelmed and/or harmed by the intensity of work that the more resourced group members want to engage in. This writer has found the following to be important criteria to consider when screening new potential group members for trauma-focused and/or psychodrama groups:

- Willingness to engage in trauma work
- Psychiatric stability – suicidality, psychotic symptoms, medication management, etc.
- Emotional containment skills and ability to tolerate discomfort
- Behavioral containment skills ensuring they will not disrupt safety of the rest of the group
- Severity of drug/alcohol use (and/or other process addictions)
- Social support – family/friends, therapist, community support, other support services
- Expected length of time in treatment (this especially important for inpatient groups) and/or ability to continue therapy at next level of care
- Some congruence between the individual's presenting symptoms, issues, goals and the group-as-a-whole

These criteria are meant to be guidelines (many are echoed in trauma group therapy guidelines offered by Courtois & Ford, 2016). They will differ depending on the nature of a group, the level of care, and the target population. For example, the criteria related to willingness will be more complicated in court-mandated settings. The criteria related to psychiatric stability will become more complex for groups in inpatient psychiatric settings. Severity of drug and alcohol use will be more in focus for groups within substance use treatment settings. A group focused on social anxiety and isolation may approach the criteria of social support differently. The guideline related to behavioral containment may need to be approached differently for groups facilitated within the prison system. Furthermore, trauma-focused group tasks or goals will differ in different phases of trauma recovery. What may be helpful in one phase can be harmful in another phase (such as attempting phase 2 trauma processing work before establishing the phase 1 safety, resourcing, and skills building groundwork) (Goodman & Weiss, 2000; Herman, 1992). In the screening phase, a group leader will need to discern the appropriate and reasonable thresholds for inclusion in the group related to each of these criteria, as it relates to the specific nature of the group at hand, and as it pertains to the different phases of trauma recovery. Yalom and Leszcz (2020) suggest that "the majority of clinicians do not select for group therapy. Instead, they deselect" (p. 295). In the group development process, clinicians must have some clarity on what exactly are the exclusionary criteria that indicate an individual would not be appropriate for the group at hand.

Cultivating Safety with Group Rules and Norms

Another important structure that provides safety is the establishment and maintenance of rules and norms within a facility and within group work. Policies, rules, and norms provide containment, consistency, clarity, expectation, and safety. Norms and rules naturally differ from group to group and from agency to agency based on context, population, and level of care. Other authors have proposed group norms and rules related to groups in different treatment contexts and stages of trauma recovery (see Courtois & Ford, 2016; Herman & Kallivayalil, 2018; Mendelsohn et al., 2011; Yalom & Leszcz, 2020). Group norms and rules also help provide safety and containment within educational spaces. In the group therapy research, group leader interventions that promote structure, a safe emotional atmosphere, and manage interactions are closely linked to the group cohesion while reducing social mistrust and conflict in the group (Burlingame, McClendon, & Alonso, 2011).

Some simple group rules that promote safety for trauma survivors include commitments to confidentiality, mutual respect, and asking permission for physical touch. Other rules or norms might include agreements related to attendance, financial costs, and dual roles in the group (Courtois, 2010; Goodman & Weiss, 2000) Confidentiality helps participants feel that they can share difficult details of their life experience without worrying that those stories or details will be shared with others. A commitment to mutual respect between participants highlights a collective agreement to honor each persons' dignity, regardless of their trauma history. I begin each group asking participants to agree to respecting everyone in the group for who they are, how they identify, what communities they are or aren't apart of, and for what they've experienced. This also helps to provide safety for participants who may be unsure if they can be themselves based on previous disrespect and perhaps trauma related to marginalized aspects of identity. Having a rule around physical touch is also helpful in a trauma group as many survivors of relational trauma struggle with safety related to physical touch. Requiring participants to ask permission before offering a hug or supportive hand on the shoulder is useful for multiple reasons – it helps normalize consent, provides opportunities for participants to practice boundaries, and mitigates the potential triggers of unexpected physical touch between group members. Another helpful rule in trauma work is to require choice and consent in every step of the group process. As noted previously, forcing clients to engage in trauma therapy is potentially harmful. Clients should be encouraged and reminded that they have the power to choose to join a trauma-specific group or not and that within the group process they have the power of choice related to group activities.

In trauma-focused group services, group members often feel expected or compelled to tell their trauma stories. While there is a place for sharing the details of one's trauma stories, it is also important to consider how this involves a vicarious traumatization potential for the rest of the group (Goodman & Weiss, 2000). In my group norms I find it helpful to let clients know that we are not going to sit in a circle and simply tell war-stories about trauma, but instead we will have a balance of considering strengths to face trauma and growth after trauma in addition to the details and impacts of the trauma itself. This group norm helps affirm group members' choice in revealing details of their trauma while providing containment for the group initially. It seems that the risks of vicarious trauma to the rest of the group decrease as the group establishes safety, containment, cohesion, and collective strength.

Beyond group rules, there are also safety-enhancing features of group norms. It can be particularly helpful to begin each group session with a brief ritual of renaming group rules, group norms, and the group purpose. Having a ritual of beginning the group provides a sense of consistency, familiarity, and structure for participants. In my groups, I invite the more senior group members to articulate the group norms to new group members to give them a stronger sense of co-responsibility and co-ownership of the group. This also helps cultivate peer support and mitigate power dynamics between facilitator and participants while increasing the likelihood of buy-in from new group members. Another norm that I find helpful at the start of the group in enhancing safety is to engage with as much transparency as possible about the group process and the agenda for the session at hand. I intentionally try to articulate a brief outline of the group session to participants before we begin so that they have a sense of what to expect.

The facilitator provides an essential function of both (co)establishing and enforcing group rules and norms until the group naturally begins to take co-responsibility for group norms. Nevertheless, the group leader is ultimately responsible for the final enforcement of rules, particularly rules that keep the group-as-a-whole safe. Group leaders must be willing to redirect clients who disrupt the safety of the group. I like to remind clients that when their behavior negatively impacts the rest of the group that I have a professional obligation to step in to prevent harm – that my primary responsibility is to the group-as-a-whole. As leaders, if we do not step in and redirect clients who break the rules, it implicitly gives others permission to do the same and impacts participants sense of security with the group. After establishing and/or re-articulating group rules at the start of a session, I find it helpful to ask participants to demonstrate their commitment to the rules and norms by physically standing up (for groups where everyone is physically mobile). This allows participants to concretize and embody their commitment to each other while also getting everyone out of their chair, thus making a seamless transition into an action-based warm-up for psychodrama groups.

There are other layers of norms beyond those that are verbally agreed upon with group members that can be helpful to consider as they also promote safety for the group. One such dimension is related to the physical layout of the group room. There are many aspects of the furniture, artwork, and décor which can improve clients' sense of comfort in the group. The temperature, smell, and cleanliness of the group room certainly also have an impact on group members. I often joke with my clients that the ongoing and frequent tweaks to the room temperature are a parallel process for the group's ongoing process of regulating emotions. Noise is another consideration for group facilitators. It is important that, as much as possible, noise outside the group room is minimized while mitigating the potential of people outside of the group hearing what is being said within the group. This can usually be accomplished with a simple white noise machine.

In almost all group therapy processes it is best to have the chairs set up in a circle rather than in a lecture style which inherently highlights the power-dynamic between facilitator and participants. The structure of the circle provides every participant with an equal position in the room. That being said, it is also helpful for the facilitator to consider occupying the chair with its back to the door. Many trauma survivors feel unsafe or uncomfortable sitting with their back to the door. When the group is organized in a circle it is inevitable that someone's chair will position them with their back to the door. Furthermore, if the group room has windows or a transparent door, it is important that clients feel that their privacy and confidentiality is not impacted. I find it best to cover windows and transparent doors where others outside the group are likely to see into the group room, while leaving any nature-facing windows uncovered. I also place an additional "do not disturb" sign on the outside of the door to further avoid unnecessary disruptions from other clients or staff.

A further dimension of norms that promote group safety are the norms related to the agency's relationship to the group at hand – this is notably true for inpatient or residential groups. In higher levels of care, it can be quite normal for patients to be pulled out of services to meet with the doctor, for a nursing assessment, to take medications, for an individual counseling session, to complete an insurance review, to sign paperwork, or even to clean/organize their messy room. I've found that in a trauma-focused group, it is not clinically appropriate to have unnecessary disruptions based on the nature of the work. Initially, for my inpatient trauma groups, my co-facilitator and I had to strongly advocate establishing a new agency norm that nobody was permitted to disrupt the trauma group sessions unless it was an emergency. This new norm made a considerable difference in the functioning of the group once it was accepted by the larger agency. Similarly, asking group members to avoid unnecessarily leaving the group can help keep the established group container strong. I find that this often involves asking inpatient clients to use the restroom, take medications, and handle any other needs before group begins – to ask outpatient clients to do the same while also muting their cellphones and not using them during the group. Shulman (2015) articulates a two-client system in which the group worker must not only promote change in the group but also within the system(s) or agency that the group takes place within. The norms and rules outlined thus far are simplified in Figure 5.1.

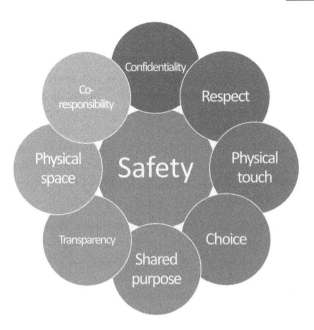

Figure 5.1 Norms and rules to establish safety in group therapy.

The norms and rules of a group will vary based on the nature of the group, its purpose, its members, and the context of where the group is held. Teletherapy groups will have different norms than in-person groups as additional considerations must be taken regarding the privacy and confidentiality, disruptions, internet connectivity, and technology (see Chapters 2 and 12 for ethical and clinical issues in trauma-informed group teletherapy). The suggestions above are meant to be guides for you as you create your own group norms and rules that establish and maintain safety for the groups you facilitate. Many of the group norms and rules that I use were not things that I originally thought of – instead they were suggestions from group members throughout the years that I have incorporated into the standard norms and rules of my ongoing groups. Trust the group to help articulate the norms and rules that it might need for safety and a helpful group process. The establishment and maintenance of group rules and norms is a collaborative process where the group holds co-responsibility.

Safety through Connection in Group Work

Safety is often a prerequisite for social engagement (Porges, 2011). Though, at the same time, one of the most important providers of safety is the group.

As human beings, we regulate our emotions and our sense of safety largely through relationships. The group provides a multitude of relational potentialities for cultivating safety. Gabor Mate and others have even suggested that safety is not so much about the lack of threat, but more so about the presence of human connection and attunement. The group provides a holding environment for each member through the matrix of relationships between each group member (Giacomucci, 2021b). The cohesion of the group offers a safe container within which trauma can be explored and transformed. Many experiences of trauma occur within social, group, or communal contexts. When one is harmed by the group, it makes sense then that healing would come in a group setting too.

Trauma so frequently leaves one feeling mistrust, shame, and isolation. Group work offers correction through authenticity, normalizing experiences, emotional support, and a sense of shared experience. The nature of trauma, especially relational trauma, and the symptoms of PTSD push survivors into isolation where they often feel alone, broken, worthless, helpless, and hopeless. Participants in a group of other trauma survivors quickly come to realize that they are not alone and that others are also struggling with similar symptoms, thoughts, feelings, and memories (Courtois, 2010). The connection between group members instills an "all-in-the-same-boat" awareness which becomes a foundation for safety, mutual aid, healing, and movement toward group and individual goals. The instillation of hope and a sense of universality are crucial therapeutic factors in effective groups (Yalom & Leszcz, 2020). As the group connects and develops a sense of cohesion, the mutual aid dynamics increase to the point where each group member is empowered as a therapeutic agent for each other. Each group member becomes an agent of safety for one another. Safety in the group process is nurtured through the other trauma-informed principles embodied in between group members – trustworthiness, transparency, peer support, collaboration, mutuality, empowerment, voice, choice, and addressing cultural, historic, and gender issues.

The group worker is tasked with transforming a bunch of individual trauma survivors into a cohesive group. This is done through prioritizing safety and leveraging relationships between group members as well as the relationship between participants and the leader. In the earlier phases of a group, it is more common for participants to be less connected to each other and more connected to the leader. As the group progresses, it is essential that the facilitator position individuals in ways that they can engage in safe connection with each other. At the same time, the facilitator inherently becomes a role model for the rest of the group on how to engage and interact with safety, appropriateness, and authenticity. Many trauma survivors find safety first in their relationship with the group leader before they are able to access safety with others in the group. Albeit there are, of course, other group members who will struggle to feel safe with the facilitator as a person in authority and power but will more quickly feel safe with their peers. In either case, the group leader has a responsibility to help participants feel safe while demonstrating and teaching others how to do the same. There are many tools available to leaders in this regard – some clients feel safe based on a group leader's age, gender, role, race, or credentials. Other clients find safety through a facilitator's demonstration of skill, competence, authenticity, empathy, passion, commitment, integrity, trustworthiness, knowledge, or wisdom. When appropriate, group leaders might make personal disclosures about their own past experiences which can also enhance participants' sense of safety. Many trauma specialists recommend a co-leadership model for trauma groups when possible (Courtois, 2010; Hudgins & Toscani, 2013). Group leaders need to be very self-aware as participants, especially hyperaroused clients, are picking up on our non-verbal gestures, our voice tone, the language we use, and especially how we interact with others in the group. In many ways, more safety can be communicated non-verbally and in action than simply through the words we articulate to the group.

What more can I do as a group leader to help my groups feel safer?

Developing Safety through Roles in Psychodrama

There are multiple unique opportunities within psychodrama groups to instill safety, especially through the use of sociometry warm-ups and the instillation of strengths-based roles (Giacomucci & Stone, 2019; Giacomucci & Ehrhart, 2021). One of the simplest ways to build safety in groups is to employ dyads, triads, or small groups within the process (Giacomucci, 2021a, 2021b). This was something I learned from clients in my ongoing inpatient trauma group. They repeatedly commented (both verbally and in written satisfaction surveys) that it was hard to talk about trauma at the group level with 10–15 people in the group that they didn't know well yet, but much easier to share with one or two other peers about their experiences. Taking their feedback into account, I began to use dyads or triads in every group session when new group members were beginning. I simply split the group into smaller groups and offer a series of structured prompts based on the topic of the group and following the clinical map. For example, in a trauma and loss group, I offer the following prompts one at a time:

1) Who is one person that you feel supported by in your recovery process?
2) What is one loss you've experienced that you feel ready to talk about, keeping in mind this can be any type of loss (death, ambiguous loss, loss of a part of self, loss of safety, hope, trust, faith, etc.)?
3) What are some of the unhelpful ways you have used to manage your grief and what are some other ways you can navigate grief going forward?
4) What is one way you have grown or developed a personal strength because of loss you've experienced?

The pacing of the questions, following the clinical map, helps establish safety and a structure for difficult topics to be discussed with containment and cushioned by positive criteria (Giacomucci, 2017, 2020). This provides everyone with a chance to connect on a more intimate level with others in the group. It also positions participants as therapeutic agents for each other and helps group members feel safe with each other. Any of the other experiential sociometry processes from Chapter 4 can also be utilized to help cultivate safety in groups.

In some psychodramas, "safety" becomes a role in itself offering messages to the protagonist and the group to help with regulation and soothing. Other strengths-based roles can also help promote safety in the psychodrama process as strengths are building blocks of safety (Giacomucci, 2021b). These roles might include any of the following – courage, willingness, empowerment, trust, empathy, wisdom, resilience, support, role models, archetypal figures, superheroes, protectors, nurturing roles, religious or spiritual figures, and/or God(s). Beginning a psychodrama scene with strengths-based roles helps the group to warm-up to the process while considering the trauma-based topic or issue from the perspective of multiple strengths. The strengths within the scene become symbolic, physical, and verbal markers of safety, especially if the psychodrama moves into more difficult content. Though the primary function of the strengths-based roles is to provide support within the role dynamics of the psychodrama scene, the humans playing the roles also provide implicit interpersonal support to the protagonist by joining them on stage.

Am I utilizing enough strengths-based roles to keep the group (and each group member) safe?

The double is another role or intervention that can promote safety within a psychodrama enactment. Enrolling a client into the double role for the full length of the psychodrama helps provide the protagonist with an attuned and empathetic support throughout the process. The Therapeutic Spiral Model has further developed the containing double and the body double as modified doubles for working with trauma. The Containing double works by skillfully providing containment or expression depending on what the protagonist needs for balance (Giacomucci, 2018). On the other hand, the body double offers consistent body awareness through physical mirroring as well as verbal and non-verbal reminders to return to body consciousness (Hudgins, 2019) (more on this in Chapter 3). In clinical practice, both of these doubles are often combined into one role. Doubling can also be used as an intervention rather than as an entire role. In this case, single sentence doubling statements are offered to the protagonist from the director or other group members who also have the potential of enhancing safety throughout the psychodrama process.

Chesner (2020) highlights other important considerations for healing trauma with psychodrama, including maintaining attunement to the group and each individual, centralizing the group contract, using appropriate pacing in the psychodrama, following a session structure (she suggests check-in, warm-up, action, sharing, and closure as a five-phase structure for psychodrama groups), working in bite-sized pieces, having a clear and specific focus for each enactment, and using doubling and strength-based roles. Other sources of safety in the psychodrama process include the therapeutic relationship between the protagonist and the director as well as the matrix of relationships between group members. The action-based nature of the process makes it easy for the director to instruct other group members on how and when to support the protagonist or other struggling audience members. As noted previously, relationships are one of the most effective methods for emotional regulation and building safety. These relationships can be leveraged within the psychodrama to enhance safety for the protagonist in very direct ways. Similarly, the director can enroll other safe relationships into the scene, even when that person is not physically present in the group. Furthermore, the director can use their own relationship with the protagonist to infuse additional connection and safety during the course of the session. The following example demonstrates a simple strengths-based psychodrama enactment that emphasizes safety.

> Lucy articulates her struggle feeling safe after multiple experiences of trauma throughout her life. She describes her sense of hyperarousal and dysregulation impacting her ability to be in relationships and do the things

she used to do in life before her trauma. After she and her topic are chosen by the group for the psychodrama, the director begins the contracting and initial interview of the psychodrama. Lucy articulates wanting to feel safe in her body and in the world again. After reminding Lucy that she has full control over the process, the director suggests that the psychodrama begin with an inner supportive voice role (or a double) to help Lucy with safety. The double offer statements such as "I can take a breath and relax my body" and "the trauma is over, and I am safe now". After a few minutes of connecting with her double, Lucy is noticeably more relaxed, though still anticipating what is next. The director works with Lucy to identify strengths and supportive figures that help Lucy feel safe. She identifies supportive peers, "boundaries" and a "protective guardian angel". All are enrolled into the scene. Group members are enrolled as themselves based on their connection to Lucy. They share supportive and encouraging messages with her throughout the psychodrama. In the exchange with boundaries, Lucy reminds herself of the importance of saying 'no' and maintaining boundaries with others in her life. She affirms her sense of choice in the world and her ability to keep herself safe. The psychodramatic dialogue with her guardian angel focused on protection and a sense of being guarded throughout her life. When she reversed roles with her guardian angel to speak to herself, she emphasized how her guardian angel had always been with her protecting her, safeguarding her, and guiding her – "even in your darkest moments of trauma when you felt alone and like you were going to die, I was there protecting you." The director guides Lucy, in the role of the guardian angel, to notice the sense of certainty, safety, and protection in her body and exaggerate her posture of protecting Lucy. As her guardian angel in a protective stance, Lucy begins confidently reminding herself of the various trauma's she has experienced and how she was protected, how she survived, and how she bounced back from the adversity each time. In a final statement before reversing roles back, she tells Lucy to remember that she is protected and safe today, even in the moments that she might feel unsafe. After returning to the role of herself, the auxiliary role player takes on the guardian angel role, assuming the same protective stance, and repeats the messages to Lucy. She gradually begins to weep while listening to the messages of safety from her guardian angel. As the guardian angel reminds her of the past traumas and how she survived, Lucy's double offers grounding statements such as "I am here in the safety of the group; the trauma is over," "I am protected and can protect myself today," and "I can notice the sense of safety in my body". Lucy's psychodrama moves towards integration through a continued discussion with the roles of her guardian angel and boundaries about moving forward in her life and facing whatever difficulties lie ahead for her.

Through this psychodrama scene, Lucy is able to experience an embodied sense of protecting herself and being protected. The support from her peers and the group helped cultivate the safety needed to continue with the psychodrama and explore other roles. The exchange and role reversal with the guardian angel provided Lucy with an opportunity to travel through her traumatic memory networks while in the role of a protective figure and to reconfigure these memories from the perspective and feeling of protection. The constant doubling statements help Lucy maintain a balanced experience of emotional and cognitive processing while also promoting dual awareness of the past trauma and present-day sense of safety and protection. The traumatic experiences did not need to be enacted, instead they were activated through strength-based roles. Lucy's psychodrama did not include any antagonist, trauma-based roles, or reenacting any trauma scenes. Instead, it was entirely focused on experiencing support, safety, and protection.

Though psychodrama has been used in unsafe ways in the past, it is regularly practiced in trauma-informed ways that enhance safety and promote incredible healing. One of the misleading ideas that fueled harmful practices within psychodrama and most other therapy approaches is the mistaken belief that abreactive catharsis in itself is curative or helpful (Giacomucci, 2019). This idea prompted many to use group therapy and psychodrama interventions or roles to provoke intense expressions of emotion that caused harm to participants. As noted in Chapter 2, psychodrama's primary objective is not simply catharsis of abreaction, but to follow it up with catharsis of integration (Giacomucci, 2021b). The larger group therapy research supports this finding in that emotional catharsis only promotes change when followed by cognitive learning (Lieberman, Yalom, & Miles, 1973). The use of strengths-based roles and doubling within psychodrama offer avenues for this type of cognitive learning along with catharsis in a titrated way. Psychodrama and drama therapies offer the therapist greater control in titrating and gradually moving into traumatic content then other verbal or exposure therapies (Sajnani & Johnson, 2014). Without strength-based roles, and the safety they provide, a trauma-focused psychodrama can quickly descend into overwhelming trauma content. However, the practice of installing positive roles provides a sense of containment, safety, titration, empowerment, support, and choice throughout the psychodrama process (Giacomucci & Marquit, 2020; Giacomucci, Marquit, & Miller Walsh, 2022). Safety is an embodied experience as such, psychodrama and other expressive arts therapies are uniquely situated to offer embodied healing (Malchiodi, 2020).

Conclusion

Safety is the number one priority in trauma-focused and trauma-informed work. Trauma and PTSD are characterized by threats to safety; therefore, trauma healing must begin with safety. Trauma-informed organization emphasize the multiple layers of safety through their policies and practices with staff, clients, and the communities they operate within. In mental health treatment, safety is emphasized through proper assessment, referral, and screening to ensure clients are receiving fitting services and the appropriate level of care within the treatment continuum. Within the context of group work, the group leader, group rules, and norms help to initially establish safety; however, the group becomes the primary source of maintaining and internalizing safety. Strengths-based approaches within group work and psychodrama offer foundations for establishing safety throughout the treatment process. Strength-based roles within trauma-focused role enactments provide additional containment, connection, safety, and cognitive learning necessary for ongoing change.

References

Badenoch, B. (2018). *The Heart of Trauma: Healing the Embodied Brain in the Context of Relationships*. New York: W.W. Norton & Company.

Bloom, S. L. (2011). *Trauma-informed system transformation: Recovery as a public health concern*. Philadelphia, PA: Trauma Task Force, Department of Behavioral Health.

Bloom, S. L. (2013). *Creating sanctuary: Toward the evolution of sane societies (Revised)*. New York: Routledge.

Bloom, S. L., & Farragher, B. (2013). *Restoring sanctuary: A new operating system for trauma-informed systems of care*. New York: Oxford University Press.

Brabender, V., & MacNair-Semands, R. (2022). *The ethics of group psychotherapy: Principles and practical strategies*. New York: Routledge.

Bryce, I., Pye, D., Beccaria, G., McIlveen, P., & Du Preez, J. (2021). A systematic literature review of the career choice of helping professionals who have experienced cumulative harm as a result of adverse childhood experiences. *Trauma, Violence, & Abuse*. https://doi.org/10.1177/15248380211016016

Burlingame, G. M., McClendon, D. T., & Alonso, J. (2011). Cohesion in group therapy. *Psychotherapy*, 48(1), 34.

Chesner, A. (2020). Psychodrama and healing the traumatic wound. In A. Chesner, & S. Lykou (Eds.), *Trauma in the creative and embodied therapies: When words are not enough* (pp. 69–80). London: Routledge.

Courtois, C. A. (2010). *Healing the incest wound* (2nd ed.). New York: W. W. Norton & Company.

Courtois, C. A., & Ford, J. D. (2016). *Treatment of complex trauma: A sequenced, relationship-based approach.* New York: The Guildford Press.

Duhigg, C. (2016). What Google learned from its quest to build the perfect team. *The New York Times Magazine.* Retrieved from https://www.nytimes.com/2016/02/28/magazine/what-google-learned-from-its-quest-to-build-the-perfect-team.html

Edmondson, A. C. (2018). *The fearless organization: Creating psychological safety in the workplace for learning, innovation, and growth.* Hoboken: John Wiley & Sons.

Esaki, N., & Larkin, H. (2013). Prevalence of adverse childhood experiences (ACEs) among child service providers. *Families in society, 94*(1), 31–37.

Giacomucci, S. (2017). The sociodrama of life or death: Young adults and addiction treatment. *Journal of Psychodrama, Sociometry, and Group Psychotherapy, 65*(1), 137–143. https://doi.org/10.12926/0731-1273-65.1.137

Giacomucci, S. (2018). Trauma survivor's inner role atom: A clinical map for post-traumatic growth. *The Journal of Psychodrama, Sociometry, and Group Psychotherapy, 66*(1), 115–129.

Giacomucci, S. (2019). Social group work in action: A sociometry, psychodrama, and experiential trauma group therapy curriculum. *Doctorate in Social Work (DSW) Dissertations,* 124. Retrieved from https://repository.upenn.edu/cgi/viewcontent.cgi?article=1128&context=edissertations_sp2

Giacomucci, S. (2020). Addiction, traumatic loss, and guilt: A case study resolving grief through psychodrama and sociometric connections. *The Arts in Psychotherapy, 67,* 101627. https://doi.org/10.1016/j.aip.2019.101627

Giacomucci, S. (2021a). Experiential sociometry in group work: Mutual aid for the group-as-a-whole. *Social Work with Groups, 44*(3), 204–214.

Giacomucci, S. (2021b). *Social work, sociometry, and psychodrama: Experiential approaches for group therapists, community leaders, and social workers.* Springer Nature. https://doi.org/10.1007/978-981-33-6342-7

Giacomucci, S., & Ehrhart, L. (2021). Introduction to psychodrama psychotherapy: A trauma and addiction group vignette. *Group, 45*(1), 69–86.

Giacomucci, S., & Marquit, J. (2020). The effectiveness of trauma-focused psychodrama in the treatment of PTSD in inpatient substance abuse treatment. *Frontiers in Psychology, 11,* 896. https://doi.org/10.3389%2Ffpsyg.2020.00896

Giacomucci, S., Marquit, J., & Miller Walsh, K. (2022). A controlled pilot study on the effects of a therapeutic spiral model trauma-focused psychodrama workshop on post-traumatic stress, spontaneity and post-traumatic growth. *Zeitschrift für Psychodrama und Soziometrie, 21*(1), 171–188.

Giacomucci, S., & Stone, A. M. (2019). Being in two places at once: Renegotiating traumatic experience through the surplus reality of psychodrama. *Social Work with Groups, 42*(3), 184–196. https://doi.org/10.1080/01609513.2018.1533913

Goodman, M., & Weiss, D. (2000). Initiating, screening, and maintaining psychotherapy groups for traumatized patients. In R. H. Klein, & V. L. Schermer (Eds.), *Group psychotherapy for psychological trauma* (pp. 47–63). New York: The Guilford Press.

Handran, J. (2015). Trauma-informed systems of care: The role of organizational culture in the development of burnout, secondary traumatic stress, and compassion satisfaction. *Journal of Social Welfare and Human Rights, 3*(2), 1–22.

Herman, J. L. (1992). *Trauma and recovery: The aftermath of violence—From domestic abuse to political terror.* New York: Basic Books.

Herman, J. L., & Kallivayalil, D. (2018). *Group trauma treatment in early recovery.* New York: Guilford Press.

Hudgins, K. (2019). Psychodrama revisited: Through the lens of the internal role map of the therapeutic spiral model to promote post-traumatic growth. *Zeitschrift für Psychodrama und Soziometrie, 18*(1), 59–74.

Hudgins, M. K., & Toscani, F. (2013). *Healing world trauma with the therapeutic spiral model: Stories from the frontlines.* London: Jessica Kingsley Publishers.

Keesler, J. M. (2018). Adverse childhood experiences among direct support professionals. *Intellectual and Developmental Disabilities, 56*(2), 119–132.

Lieberman, M. A., Yalom, I. D., & Miles, M. (1973). *Encounter groups: First facts.* New York: Basic Books.

Malchiodi, C. A. (2020). *Trauma and expressive arts therapy: Brain, body, and imagination in the healing process.* New York: Guilford Press.

Mendelsohn, M., Herman, J. L., Schatzow, E., Coco, M., Kallivayalil, D., & Levitan, J. (2011). *The trauma recovery group: A guide for practitioners.* New York: Guilford Press.

Porges, S. W. (2011). *The polyvagal theory: Neurophysiological foundations of emotions, attachment, communication, and self-regulation.* New York: W. W. Norton & Company.

Porges, S. W., Badenoch, B., & Phillips, M. (2016). *Feeling and expressing compassion [webinar].* Retrieved from https://bestpracticesintherapy.com/silver-month-long-july/

Sajnani, N., & Johnson, D. R. (2014). *Trauma-informed drama therapy: Transforming clinics, classrooms, and communities.* Springfield: Charles C Thomas Publisher.

Shulman, L. (2015). *The skills of helping individuals, families, groups, and communities* (8th ed.). Boston, MA: Cengage Learning.

Steen, J. T., Senreich, E., & Straussner, S. L. A. (2021). Adverse childhood experiences among licensed social workers. *Families in Society, 102*(2), 182–193.

Substance Abuse and Mental Health Services Administration. (2014a). *SAMHSA's concept of trauma and guidance for a trauma-informed approach.* HHS Publication No. (SMA) 14-4884. Rockville, MD: Substance Abuse and Mental Health Services Administration.

Yalom, I. D., & Leszcz, M. (2020). *The theory and practice of group psychotherapy* (6th ed.). New York: Basic Books.

6
Trustworthiness and Transparency in Group Therapy, Psychodrama, and Leadership

Chapter Summary

Trauma survivors have often suffered due to systems of oppression, people in power abusing their authority, betrayal in relationships, or harm caused by those closest to them. This underscores the importance of trustworthiness and transparency as trauma-informed principles in group therapy, psychodrama, and leadership. Providers and facilitators embodying these qualities offer participants corrective emotional experiences and the potential to trust again. This principle also applies to the facilitator approaching the client and community with a sense of trust. Treating clients as experts in their own experience while placing trust and faith in them effectively promotes empowerment, safety, and healing. Additionally, the clinician needs to be able to trust themself and to be transparent with themself, even when uncomfortable. Trustworthiness and transparency are of particular importance to organizational leaders, supervisors, and trainers as they reflect ethical principles for best practice. Both principles are significant in the psychodrama process, and at the same time, psychodrama can assist clients in redeveloping trust for others, themselves, their body, and their intuition.

Traumatic Disruption of Trust

Trauma and posttraumatic stress disorder (PTSD) rupture trust in self, others, and the world. Judith Herman, in her groundbreaking text – *Trauma and Recovery* (1992), describes trust as a foundational belief in the continuity

DOI: 10.4324/9781003277859-6

of life, a sense of safety in the world, and a formative core element sustaining one throughout their lifespan. Trust is the basis of all relationships and faith. In moments of terror and trauma, humans naturally cry out to those that they trust the most (often caregivers or God). When this cry for help and comfort is unanswered, a trauma survivors' basic sense of trust and faith in the world and others is destroyed (Herman, 1992). "When trust is lost, traumatized people feel that they belong more to the dead than to the living" (Herman, 1992, p. 52). A loss of trust in the world, trust in relationships, and trust in one's self and senses are core to the experience of trauma and PTSD.

Relational trauma has a particularly damaging effect on one's ability to trust others in the future. Harm and betrayal by others, especially those who are supposed to protect or nurture, can have a detrimental impact on one's ability to trust. This seems to manifest most often in romantic relationships and with figures of authority. Trauma can lead to the loss of a fundamental trust in the goodness of others and the world around us. The resulting PTSD symptoms tend to cultivate an inner battle between the survivor and their body in that they lose a sense of trust in their body's ability to protect and guide them. This loss of trust often occurs synonymously with the loss of safety. PTSD symptoms are the past resurfacing in the present moment – past images, emotions, beliefs, or sensations.

A trauma survivor often feels like their trauma is happening again here-and-now when the memory is reactivated. This leads to a mistrust of one's sensory information – being unable to always differentiate between what is real sensory experience in the here-and-now compared to the intrusive PTSD sensory information emerging again. The pain and suffering associated with trauma and PTSD often lead survivors to find ways of numbing their pain with drugs, alcohol, or other behaviors. Unfortunately, these behaviors, though they may temporarily numb the pain, frequently balloon into addictions or lead to additional problems. As many as half of all adults with PTSD also meet criteria for a substance use disorder (McCauley, Killeen, Gros, Brady, & Back, 2012). The concurrent experience of PTSD and substance use only further complicates one's ability to trust themselves and their experience again.

Considering the traumatic erosion of trust, it makes sense then that the trauma-informed principles would explicitly emphasize the importance of trustworthiness. Harris and Fallot remind us that "trust and safety, rather than being assumed from the beginning, must be earned and demonstrated over time" (2001, p. 20). Trust is foundational to the healing process and must be cultivated early on in groups, psychodrama, and organizations.

Trusting in Clients and Community

Trust goes both ways. It is a reciprocal and relational experience. Developing trust in the therapeutic relationship with our clients means that we must also extend a sense of trust from ourselves to them. A research study on trust in the doctor-patient relationship discovered a reciprocal relationship between the doctor and the patient's trust of each other (Petrocchi et al., 2019). This study suggests that the more we explicitly trust in our patients, the more their trust in us will increase. Trusting our clients means that we treat them as a collaborator and as the expert in their experience. It means we believe our clients unless presented with data that suggests that they are being dishonest. We give them the benefit of the doubt. Carl Rogers highlighted the importance of trust in psychotherapy suggesting that the therapist should specifically trust in the unrealized potential of the client (1951). Rogers believed that the therapist's attitude toward the client played a significant role in the development of the therapeutic relationship and successful outcomes in psychotherapy. He advocated that therapists should approach clients with unconditional positive regard, empathy, and trust (Rogers, 1961). A study by Peschken and Johnson (1997) on trust in the therapist–client dyad found evidence to support Rogers' claims.

There are few things more disheartening for a client than having their own therapist think they are lying when they are in fact being honest and transparent. Our mistrust for clients and communities only promotes more mistrust in return from them. Of course, there are limits to always trusting our clients as there may be an element of safety to also consider which will be uniquely different from agency to agency and based on the population treated. Perhaps, however, we can maintain trust for our clients' ability to heal even in moments of dishonesty or when challenging them on a lie. Clients can feel trust when it is given by their therapist. There are implicit ways that we demonstrate it – through our non-verbal responses, our suggestions or questions, and the way we structure our groups. Creating opportunities for clients to engage in peer support is one way of demonstrating our trust in them. By positioning clients in ways to support, heal, and educate each other we are showing our trust in action (the principle of peer support will be expanded on in the next chapter). We also demonstrate trust when we believe in our clients' innate ability to find their own way, to heal themselves with the right support, to ask for help, to bounce back from tragedy, and to achieve their goals.

How do my clients know that I believe in and trust them?

How do I actively safeguard and cherish the trust that clients extend to me as a professional?

As I write this, I am reminded of two moments in my own personal growth journey as a teenager and young adult. In the first experience, I was meeting with a psychiatrist and shared with them about my experience of depression and anxiety in the context of my ongoing recovery journey. They inquired about my drug and alcohol use, and I explained that I had been abstinent from drugs and alcohol for well over a year at the time. The psychiatrist rolled her eyes and made a sarcastic comment in disbelief. Even after reassuring her that I was abstinent and involved in various recovery and personal growth communities, she still did not believe or trust me. This brought about a disheartening feeling for me that quickly evolved into resentment and a discontinuation of my work with this professional. Knowing that she did not believe or trust me made it difficult to trust her or to trust that her services would be attuned to me and my experience.

This second experience was much more hopeful. After seeing a therapist for weekly session for about two years, the therapist suggested that we might shift our meetings to bi-weekly instead of continuing weekly. As a young client (I was about 18 years old at the time), I experienced this suggestion as a huge extension of trust. I remember thinking to myself that the therapist must really trust me and think I am doing well to suggest we reduce our meeting frequency. This simple suggestion, and the embodiment of trust within it, fortified me in my early recovery journey and helped me to further believe in and trust myself.

These examples highlight the importance of trusting our clients as it helps them to internalize the trust and learn to trust themselves again after trauma. As a trauma professional, it is particularly important that we consider the value of trusting our clients who are likely to have experienced minimization, dismissal, denial, and gaslighting related to their experience of trauma in the past. It seems that the reciprocity of trust experienced in the context the therapeutic relationship and/or a cohesive group experience allow trauma survivors to being to trust themselves and others again.

Trustworthy and Transparent Organizations, Supervisors, and Educators

The principles of trust and transparency must extend beyond the therapeutic relationship into the entire agency. There are often parallel processes in the way that trustworthiness and transparency are implemented between the agency leaders and staff and between the staff and clientele (Bloom, 2011). Staff who feel trusted by their leaders, especially to complete difficult tasks or projects, are more likely to excel then staff who feel untrusted by their colleagues. Similar to how the trust of the therapist is internalized and helps clients trust themselves, so too is the trust of the supervisor internalized by staff. Again, trust is a reciprocal process, so it is important that both staff and leadership demonstrate trustworthiness in their work and relationships. Sandra Bloom (2011) confirms that the "erosion of trust in the workplace has become a major barrier to instituting trauma-informed care" (p. 25). Without trust, we lose much of our capacity for safety, peer support, collaboration, mutuality, empowerment, voice, choice, celebrations of identity, and community.

The fact that "trustworthiness" and "transparency" are paired together by SAMHSA (2014a) in this second trauma-informed principle is no mistake. Trustworthiness and transparency are twin concepts that fuel each other and are closely related to each other. Trustworthiness promotes further transparency in relationships. And at the same time, transparency cultivates additional trustworthiness between parties (see Figure 6.1). Research from the fields of business, public relations, and organizational development highlight this connection between transparency and trustworthiness (Rawlins, 2008). Additional studies have uncovered that organizational transparency directly increases trust from the public, customers, and staff (Auger, 2014; Norman, Avolio, & Luthans, 2010; Williams, 2005).

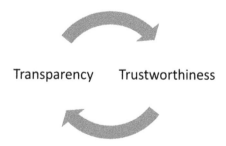

Transparency   Trustworthiness

Figure 6.1 Relationship between transparency and trustworthiness.

Staff are much more willing to follow a leader who they can trust to make decisions in the best nature of the agency's clients and employees. A meta-analysis on trust in supervisory relationships highlights that workers' trust in their supervisors appears primarily related to the supervisors' benevolence, competence, and integrity (Nienaber, Romeike, Searle, & Schewe, 2015) (see Figure 6.2). This means that as leaders, we can increase trust by demonstrating benevolence, competence, and integrity in our work, relationships, and actions.

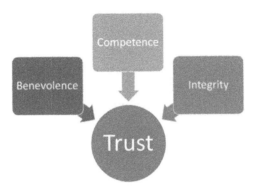

Figure 6.2 Trust in one's supervisor is fueled by a demonstration of benevolence, competence, and integrity.

The research literature points to the importance of ethical leadership in cultivating employees' sense of organizational trust while also promoting "extra-role service behavior" – which is where workers are willing to extend themselves beyond their defined role responsibilities to provide exceptional service (Kerse, 2021). Workers' trust in their leadership appears to promote self-efficacy, well-being, job satisfaction, work engagement, and even reduce work-related stress and exhaustion (Chughtai, Byrne, & Flood, 2015; Kelloway, Turner, Barling, & Loughlin, 2012; Liu, Siu, & Shi, 2009). Trust for leadership also tends to promote respect and admiration. Staff or clients who feel as though their leaders are untrustworthy are likely to develop resentment, fear, insecurity, and a loss of safety in the organization. A trauma-informed leader is trustworthy and transparent, demonstrating benevolence, competence, and integrity in their leadership.

Leaders who practice transparency are quick to develop trust from their staff, students, supervisees, clients, and communities. Being open and honest about decision making and other fueling factors of change helps others see the big picture which is sometimes only available to leaders. Many trauma survivors have experienced ongoing gaslighting, dishonesty, and abuse of power from others in authority. The practice of transparency, especially during organizational change, helps to promote trust and safety. When factors are left unknown, it can promote insecurity, fear, and projection; practicing transparency and openness helps to mitigate these. On the other hand, transparency is a principle to be demonstrated whenever possible – not just in difficult situations or change. Withholding important positive information such as gratitude, admiration, respect, and love from our clients or colleagues is also dishonest. A transparent leader or therapist is quick to also highlight the positive changes and goodness in their relationships. Undeniably, there are also limitations on leaders and therapists when it comes to transparency – some disclosures would simply be inappropriate, unethical, illegal, or a violation of client/student/employee confidentiality or privacy. This is a principle to be employed with careful discernment and care.

Transparency is not only about revealing details or decisions, but it is also includes transparency related to emotion and the use of self. While the use of self is a common relational intervention in psychotherapy contexts, it is less often considered as a helpful tool available to all leaders. Leaders, by the nature of their roles, are often idolized, feared, or resented. Perhaps due to the traumatic abuse of power and authority, many tend to have negative projections and transference toward people in power. Whether idolization or projection, both actively dehumanize people in power. The use of self and transparency are ways that leaders can engage human to human with their team and community. Sharing one's own inner conflict and emotions can help clients and staff see leaders as humans too. Leaders who are aware of their limits and emotions are much more effective than those who attempt to hide or deny their limitations and emotions. It seems that leaders who avoid personal disclosures, vulnerability, and humility are more likely to provoke negative projections from others.

How do the leaders that I admire demonstrate trustworthiness and transparency?

A recent example of this comes from my own leadership as director and owner of the Phoenix Center for Experiential Trauma Therapy, an outpatient psychotherapy center. We are a small practice with no outside funding and are entirely dependent on the income from our services to cover all operating costs. After much consultation, research, and consideration, I decided that we needed to increase our fee structure at the center and charge higher rates for our psychotherapy services. At the same time, we expanded our offerings of low-cost trauma therapy services provided through our graduate internship program and free community groups. There were multiple factors influencing this decision including the business growth, need for more support staff, increased expenses, realizing our rates were much lower than other similar centers, and the desire to also increase the pay for therapists/staff. After sharing these details and influences with the team, we created a new fee structure with tiered session fees varying based on the therapists' licensure, experience, and certifications. In creating the new fee structure, everyone's input and suggestions were considered, and it was modified based on the team's ideas and insights. We made it clear that the fee increases would be implemented with ethics, clinical consideration, flexibility and only for clients who could afford the increased cost - others would continue receiving services at the same cost previously agreed on.

In further discussions about how to best implement the fee increases with clients, it became apparent that many team members (and many therapists in general), were uncomfortable asking clients to increase their fee. Rather than being frustrated or dismissive, I opted to engage in a discussion with the team about my own insecurities related to raising fees at the center and increasing my own fees for consultation, training, and therapy sessions. I let the team know that I was with them in the discomfort and having the same types of conversations with my own clients, consultees, and community partners about increasing fees. This use of self and moment of transparency shifted the atmosphere in the team meeting and cultivated a greater sense of cohesion, unity, support, and vulnerability. I affirmed my belief that each team member is well worth their new fee based on their expertise, education, training, and skill. In reciprocity, one of the therapists offered me their feedback and affirmation that I am worth increasing my fee too! This is an example of a policy change that could have promoted mistrust, resentment, and projection towards leadership if it had been implemented without transparency and collaboration. It would have been easy for some to assume that I was greedily prioritizing profit over helping our clients and keeping services accessible. The transparency demonstrated throughout the process helped staff to better understand the invisible business complexities, contextualize our service costs with others, offer their own input as we co-created the policy change, and connect with authenticity and support.

Trustworthy and Transparent Leadership in Group Work and Psychodrama

Herman (1992) reminds us that the destructive potential of groups is equal to their therapeutic potential and that "the role of the group leader carries with it a risk of the irresponsible exercise of authority" (p. 217). A trauma-informed practitioner centralizes ethics in their work. Similar to organizational leadership, the trauma-informed group leader and psycho-dramatist must also demonstrate trustworthiness, transparency, and ethics. A group therapy leader needs to effectively gain the trust of their group members in order to guide them toward their collective goals. Perhaps this is even more poignant for psychodrama group leaders as we are not just leading groups but also working to get buy-in about the psychodramatic process. For psychodrama groups with participants unfamiliar with psychodrama, there is an additional layer of trust that must be developed. A simple, yet helpful, intervention related to transparency is to provide group members with a brief sense of what the plan for the group will be and what they can expect in the process. This act of transparency allows group members to warm up to the processes planned for the session while quelling initial uncertainties or fears about the unknown plan for the group.

One of the symptom clusters of PTSD is related to changes in arousal and reactivity. This effectively increases the sensitivity and vigilance of many trauma group members. Some research evidence suggests that one of the reasons clients may discontinue trauma therapy is related to an inability to trust the group (Chouliara et al., 2020). In the same study, trauma group participants who successfully completed the group process commented on the importance of developing a trusting bond with the group in order to feel safe and share openly. These findings demonstrate the significance of trust in both positive and negative group therapy outcomes. As group leaders, we are tasked with promoting trust between participants within the group (Klein & Schermer, 2000). This may be difficult at first and may require creativity, spontaneity, courage, and trust for the group. In the initial and beginning stages of the group process, one of the primary tasks of the group leader is to cultivate group cohesion, safety, and a sense of trust between group members (Yalom & Leszcz, 2020). The group therapy research confirms that mistrust in the group dissipates as group cohesion strengthens (Burlingame, McClendon, & Alonso, 2011). This experience of trust and connection becomes the foundation upon which the work in the middle stage of the group takes place (Courtois & Ford, 2016). Goldstein and Siegel, in their group psychotherapy chapter in *How People Change* (2017), articu-late that "trust facilitates learning as it harnesses neuroplasticity – the ways the brain changes in response to experience" (p. 283). This insight under-scores how trust is also important for learning and meaningful change at the neurobiological level.

Trauma survivors are often attentively assessing for safety and trustworthiness of the group leader. While trauma survivors are prone to projection and transference, many would agree that they are also more attuned to potential danger and often judging if the leader (and others) are safe. When working with trauma, I believe that ethics and integrity are especially important. Though we are human and make mistakes as group leaders, it is important that we work with our groups thoughtfully and carefully to avoid potential ruptures in trust. Inevitably we will blunder and unintentionally cause harm to some degree. In these moments we must demonstrate the ability to recognize our shortcomings, repair the harm caused, and get back in integrity with the group. Jon Allen, in the introduction of his book *Trusting in Psychotherapy* (2021), articulates this same concept – "To a great extent, trusting and trustworthiness are relationship specific, and they must be *created* anew in each relationship: developed, maintained, and repaired when disrupted. The creation is interpersonal" (p. xxviii).

This practice requires a unique blend of self-awareness, humility, and clinical skill. This ability is enhanced significantly through the therapist doing their own personal work and actively working to resolve their own issues which will reduce the frequency and intensity of unproductive countertransference. Yalom and Leszcz (2020) highlight that transparency and appropriate self-disclosures from group leaders can also help reduce transference from group members. The process of undertaking one's own personal work allows the group leader to better relate to clients and to develop and enhance various personal strengths that are helpful in group leadership – such as compassion, awareness, understanding, wisdom, courage, self-regulation, humility, confidence, resilience, and stability. This process also helps us as therapists better trust ourselves and be transparent with our selves – effectively applying these trauma-informed principles in relationship with ourselves. A group leader who hasn't developed trust and transparency in their relationship with themself is likely to struggle in their group leadership. Psychodrama training is unique in that it requires that the trainee take on the protagonist role on many occasions, doing their own psychodrama work while learning the process from the inside out. This is a real strength in psychodrama training as the training process integrates personal and professional selves through experiential learning. Clients working with a certified psychodramatist are working with someone who has completed not just 780 hours of professional training, but also hundreds of hours of personal growth work. Putting in these hours of personal growth helps to foster skilled professionals who are also more self-aware, compassionate, trustworthy, and humble humans and leaders.

Am I continuing to engage in my own personal growth work? How?

Trustworthiness and transparency are principles that I strive to employ in my work at all times. I am not perfect in this regard, but I am open and transparent with my clients, staff, and students whenever possible. Taking the time to explain clinical rationale, complicated processes, and behind the scenes business forces can really help with trust. For some, the experience of a trustworthy leader is a corrective emotional experience in itself. On multiple occasions I have had clients or students tell me that they were initially reluctant to work with me simply because I am a man. When I sense this with a client, I will explicitly check-in with them and see how it is to work with me as a male therapist by saying something to the effect of: "I want to recognize too that doing trauma work with me as a male therapist may be difficult as much of your trauma was from the men in your life. How is this going for you so far?" At the end of our work together, some of these clients and students reflected to me that most of their trauma (or other experiences of adversity) was caused by other men in power. They sometimes share that their experience with me was different as I endeavored to lead with integrity, humility, transparency, and trustworthiness. While their sharing with me stopped there, I like to think that our relationship may have had a lasting impact helping them to renegotiate their sense of hurt, betrayal, and mistrust for men. This is just one example of the transformative power of a trustworthy leader. As leaders, we are in positions to provide these types of powerful and meaningful corrective experiences for the clients, students, and trainees that we work with.

The experiential sociometry tools described in Chapter 4 are also quite useful in building trust and establishing a sense of transparency within the group process. Spectrograms, specifically, are useful in that they offer an experiential structure that makes some of the underlying group dynamics transparent in an unthreatening way. For example, in the beginning phases an LGBTQ trauma group, the following spectrograms could be employed to promote connection, trust, and transparency within the group:

1) How important is it to you to feel accepted by others for your gender and sexuality?
2) How comfortable are you sharing about your gender and sexuality in a group like this?
3) How accepted do you feel in your family related to your gender and sexual orientation?

4) How often do you feel anxious or fearful to be yourself in the workplace or in your neighborhood?
5) How willing are you to support and connect with others in the LGBTQ community?

This series of spectrogram prompts, following the clinical map, offers participants with a sense of transparency about where they fit in the group and how others in the group feel about important themes relevant to the group's focus. The spectrograms offer the group a chance to fulfill curiosities or uncertainties about other group members' experiences in a process of transparency. The transparency offered in spectrograms helps to build trust and safety as group members inevitably see that they are not alone in their experiences or wishes. Transparency and trustworthiness are essential to the process as "group psychotherapy is predicated on trust" (Brabender & Macnair-Semands, 2022, p. 26).

Trust in the Psychodrama Process

Beyond trusting one's self, trusting clients, and cultivating trust in organizations, we must also consider the significance of trusting the process. While this is a bit of a catchphrase in the therapy world, it certainly holds true once a practitioner has developed facilitation competencies and understands the process. This motto is also important for psychodrama directors to keep in mind. Though we are "directors" and take on a more active role in the psychodrama process, there is much wisdom in knowing when to trust the process and let the spontaneity unfold on its own. Perhaps the psychodrama slogan equivalent of "trust the process" is "follow the protagonist." This is classical psychodrama guideline for directors to allow their protagonists to lead the way and in doing so trust the process and the client. While I deem this as a generally good guideline to follow, I also believe that there are limits to always following the protagonist (or "trusting the process") – especially in trauma work where reenactments or retraumatization are more prone to occur. I might instead suggest the slogan of "follow-lead-follow the protagonist" (inspired from the follow-lead-follow approach outlined in Dyadic Developmental Psychotherapy by Hughes, Golding, & Hudson, 2019).

The experience of trusting the process in psychodrama largely involves trusting the spontaneity and trusting the tele in the group. When one believes in the model they are working from, it is much easier to trust the process and to trust one's self as the facilitator of the process. As described in Chapter 2, spontaneity is the manifestation of the warming-up process which leads to new creative action (Giacomucci, 2021b, 2021c). When the group has engaged in a wholesome warm-up process, we can trust that spontaneity will emerge within the group and the group-as-a-whole autonomous healing center will become activated (Giacomucci, 2019). The group will essentially heal itself. The tele in the group crystallizes through proper warm up and the establishment of cohesion and connection (Giacomucci, 2021a). The group develops a wholeness that promotes coordination toward the shared goal with each part doing its part to support the whole (Giacomucci et al., 2018). This group-as-a-whole phenomenon and the resulting self-healing seems to be largely related to tele – the unconscious two-way knowing and connecting between group members. Tele helps participants access a sort of intelligence within the group about what is needed next for completion. A director employing the essentials of the psychodrama process while maintaining safety can effectively trust the process, trust the tele in the group, and trust the spontaneity in the room to manifest the desired change.

One of the memorable things that I learned in my psychodrama training process was to embrace uncertainty as a director. I was taught that uncertainty creates space for spontaneity and new action or ideas and that we should create space for it rather than try to know all the answers all the time. My trainers taught me to acknowledge uncertainty when it arises in my directing and to literally take a step back creating space for the uncertainty. In my years of psychodrama directing, I have resorted to this intervention without fail. The act of pausing and taking a step back gives me new perspective while appearing to give the role players and protagonist more room to co-create the process. When a protagonist asks me what to do next, I sometimes will respond by telling them I don't know and suggest they ask one of the auxiliary roles that they've been interacting with or bring in a new role into the scene that would know where to go next. This intervention requires direct trust in the process, in the tele, and in spontaneity while empowering the group to engage as co-creators of the process. Similarly, in moments of the psychodrama where the process is working beautifully, I remind myself to step back (sometimes I'll even sit down in the audience) to non-verbally emphasize to the group that they are doing the work and they are the therapeutic agents for each other – not me.

Beyond the facilitators' trust in the psychodrama process, we can also explore issues of trust and mistrust explicitly through psychodrama processes and role-playing. One such example is through the use of a social atom and psychodramatic sculpting.

Through the process of drawing a family social atom (see Chapter 2) and exploring early family dynamics and relationships, Pete begins to realize how his adult trust issues may stem from his family of origin's culture of secrecy. He shares about being a child when he discovered that his mother was having an affair. His mother asked him to keep it a secret from his father which caused significant emotional conflict for Pete as a child. He begins to get in touch with his anger about this experience and how he didn't have a good role modeling of trust in relationships. The facilitator invites Pete to explore these feelings, dynamics, and relationships further by sculpting his social atom.

He chooses other group members to take on the roles of each person in on his social atom – his mother, his father, his siblings, and himself. The director instructs him to place the role player representing himself in the center of the stage and to symbolically portray the family relationships around himself using body posture and proximity to represent the relational dynamics and mistrust. He places his mother and father next to each other; his father facing his mother and reaching out to her, and his mother facing away from his father. He places his siblings close to himself and with open, trusting, postures in relationship to him. Pete explores the relationships further by offering a single doubling statement to each family member in the psychodramatic sculpture. The message from his father was one of longing for connection while the message from his mother was one of distraction and betrayal. The messages he ascribed to his siblings' roles were trusting, playful, and innocent. Through this process Pete begins to realize that his parents' relationship was characterized by betrayal and mistrust but his relationships with his siblings were trusting and intimate. The director asks Pete to step into the sculpture as himself and to hear the role players articulate the doubling statements recently provided. In doing so, he feels supported by his siblings but angered by his parents. The director invites him to articulate his feelings to each person in the psychodramatic family sculpture. He expresses his anger to his mother and his sadness for his father. He describes feeling like he had to carry his mother's burden as a child which wasn't fair. He shares about feeling unable to trust romantic partners throughout his life because of this. After his catharsis of anger and sadness, the director invites Pete to talk to his siblings in the sculpture and articulate what he did learn about trusting relationships from them. In this process, Pete uncovers new insights about trust in his family that he wasn't fully conscious of previously. In a final integrative dialogue, the director asks Pete to step into the mirror position and to speak to himself in the family sculpture about what he has learned about trust and how he will integrate it into his relationships going forward.

After the psychodramatic sculpture, the group shares with Pete about their learning and how they related to his experience in the family and with trust in relationships today. The group process helped Pete to examine his present-day trust issues in relationships and connect them to his childhood experiences. He was able to explore how his family's secrecy and betrayal have impacted his own relationships. The sculpting provided a simple scaffolding for working through the feelings associated with his childhood and integrating new insights about moving forward. This process offers a slower paced psychodramatic structure for exploring relationships in a way that is titrated and has less potential for overwhelming a protagonist or group than a full psychodrama. Sculpting is a great exercise for groups (or facilitators) new to psychodrama or when there isn't enough time for a longer experiential process. The social atom is a very useful warm up for psychodramatic sculpting but it can also be used in other contexts such as sculpting one's social relationships, strengths, social supports, core values, roles, or used in organizations to concretize and symbolically explore organizational structures. I often use psychodramatic sculpting with students or trainees to explore internal roles or even the four roles of the psychodrama director – analyst, sociometrist, therapist, and producer (Kellerman, 1992). This process helps participants reflect on their social relationships, inner experience, and/or role dynamics on a given topic.

Conclusion

Trauma is an antithesis to trust. It tends to destroy one's sense of trust in others, especially those in positions of power. Trauma even disrupts one's ability to trust self, senses, and memory. Trustworthiness and transparency are essential for healthy relationships of all kinds – including a working therapeutic relationship and relationships between leaders, supervisors, and staff. Trust is an interpersonal phenomenon that exists in a reciprocal state between both parties. As we increase our trust in others, they are likely to also increase their trust in us. Transparency plays an important role in promoting trust in organizations, in group therapy, and in psychotherapy in general. Trust in the process and in the group are both important for group therapists to demonstrate. Psychodrama offers various experiential avenues for exploring trust issues and cultivating deeper trust in action. Trust and transparency, as twin concepts, are essential for trauma-informed practice of group work, psychodrama, and leadership.

References

Allen, J. G. (2021). *Trusting in psychotherapy*. Washington D.C.: American Psychiatric Association Publishing.

Auger, G. A. (2014). Trust me, trust me not: An experimental analysis of the effect of transparency on organizations. *Journal of Public Relations Research*, 26(4), 325–343.

Bloom, S. L. (2011). *Trauma-informed system transformation: Recovery as a public health concern*. Philadelphia, PA: Trauma Task Force, Department of Behavioral Health.

Brabender, V., & MacNair-Semands, R. (2022). *The ethics of group psychotherapy: Principles and practical strategies*. New York: Routledge.

Burlingame, G. M., McClendon, D. T., & Alonso, J. (2011). Cohesion in group therapy. *Psychotherapy*, 48(1), 34.

Chouliara, Z., Karatzias, T., Gullone, A., Ferguson, S., Cosgrove, K., & Burke Draucker, C. (2020). Therapeutic change in group therapy for interpersonal trauma: A relational framework for research and clinical practice. *Journal of Interpersonal Violence*, 35(15–16), 2897–2916.

Chughtai, A., Byrne, M., & Flood, B. (2015). Linking ethical leadership to employee well-being: The role of trust in supervisor. *Journal of Business Ethics*, 128(3), 653–663.

Courtois, C. A., & Ford, J. D. (2016). *Treatment of complex trauma: A sequenced, relationship-based approach*. New York: The Guildford Press.

Giacomucci, S. (2019). Social group work in action: A sociometry, psychodrama, and experiential trauma group therapy curriculum. *Doctorate in Social Work (DSW) Dissertations*, 124. Retrieved from https://repository.upenn.edu/cgi/viewcontent.cgi?article=1128&context=edissertations_sp2

Giacomucci, S. (2021a). Experiential sociometry in group work: Mutual aid for the group-as-a-whole. *Social Work with Groups*, 44(3), 204–214.

Giacomucci, S. (2021b). *Social work, sociometry, and psychodrama: Experiential approaches for group therapists, community leaders, and social workers*: Springer Nature. https://doi.org/10.1007/978-981-33-6342-7

Giacomucci, S. (2021c). Traumatic stress and spontaneity: Trauma-focused and strengths-based psychodrama. In J. Maya, & J. Maraver (Eds.), *Psychodrama advances in psychotherapy and psychoeducational interventions* (pp. 1–44). New York: Nova Science Publishers.

Giacomucci, S., Gera, S., Briggs, D., & Bass, K. (2018). Experiential addiction treatment: Creating positive connection through sociometry and therapeutic spiral model safety structures. *Journal of Addiction and Addictive Disorders*, 5, 17. http://doi.org/10.24966/AAD-7276/100017

Goldstein, B., & Siegel, D. J. (2017). Feeling felt: Cocreating on the emergent experience of connection, safety, and awareness in individual and group psychotherapy. In M. F. Solomon & D. J. Siegel (Eds.), *How people change: relationships and neuroplasticity in psychotherapy* (pp. 273–289). New York: W. W. Norton & Company.

Harris, M., & Fallot, R. (2001). *Using trauma theory to design service systems. New Directions for Mental Health Services*. Hoboken: Jossey Bass.

Herman, J. L. (1992). *Trauma and recovery: The aftermath of violence—From domestic abuse to political terror*. New York: Basic Books.

Hughes, D. A., Golding, K. S., & Hudson, J. (2019). *Healing relational trauma with attachment-focused interventions: Dyadic developmental psychotherapy with children and families*. New York: W.W. Norton & Company.

Kellerman, P. F. (1992). *Focus on psychodrama: The therapeutic aspects of psychodrama*. London: Jessica Kingsley.

Kelloway, E. K., Turner, N., Barling, J., & Loughlin, C. (2012). Transformational leadership and employee psychological well-being: The mediating role of employee trust in leadership. *Work & Stress*, 26(1), 39–55.

Kerse, G. (2021). A leader indeed is a leader in deed: The relationship of ethical leadership, person–organization fit, organizational trust, and extra-role service behavior. *Journal of Management & Organization*, 27(3), 601–620.

Klein, R. H., & Schermer, V. L. (2000). *Group psychotherapy for psychological trauma*. New York: The Guilford Press.

Liu, J., Siu, O., & Shi, K. (2009). Transformational leadership and employee well-being: The mediating role of trust in the leader and self-efficacy. *Applied Psychology: An International Review*, 59: 454–479.

McCauley, J. L., Killeen, T., Gros, D. F., Brady, K. T., & Back, S. E. (2012). Posttraumatic stress disorder and co-occurring substance use disorders: Advances in assessment and treatment. *Clinical Psychology: Science and Practice*, 19(3), 283.

Nienaber, A. M., Romeike, P. D., Searle, R., & Schewe, G. (2015). A qualitative meta-analysis of trust in supervisor-subordinate relationships. *Journal of Managerial Psychology*, 30(5), 507–534.

Norman, S. M., Avolio, B. J., & Luthans, F. (2010). The impact of positivity and transparency on trust in leaders and their perceived effectiveness. *The Leadership Quarterly*, 21(3), 350–364.

Peschken, W., & Johnson, M. (1997). Therapist and client trust in the therapeutic relationship. *Psychotherapy Research, 7*(4), 439–447.

Petrocchi, S., Iannello, P., Lecciso, F., Levante, A., Antonietti, A., & Schulz, P. J. (2019). Interpersonal trust in doctor-patient relation: Evidence from dyadic analysis and association with quality of dyadic communication. *Social Science & Medicine, 235*, 112391.

Rawlins, B. R. (2008). Measuring the relationship between organizational transparency and employee trust. *Public Relations Journal, 2*(2), 1–21.

Rogers, C. R. (1951). *Client-centered therapy: Its current practice, implications, and theory.* Boston, MA: Houghton-Mifflin.

Rogers, C. R. (1961). *On becoming a person: A therapist's view of psychotherapy.* Boston, MA: Houghton-Mifflin.

Substance Abuse and Mental Health Services Administration. (2014a). *SAMHSA's concept of trauma and guidance for a trauma-informed approach.* HHS Publication No. (SMA) 14-4884. Rockville, MD: Substance Abuse and Mental Health Services Administration.

Williams, C. C. (2005). Trust diffusion: The effect of interpersonal trust on structure, function, and organizational transparency. *Business & Society, 44*(3), 357–368.

Yalom, I. D., & Leszcz, M. (2020). *The theory and practice of group psychotherapy* (6th ed.). New York: Basic Books.

7

Peer Support in Group Therapy, Psychodrama, and Leadership

Chapter Summary

The experience of trauma is inherently disconnecting and isolating, often causing symptoms that make relationships difficult. Relational trauma and complex trauma frequently result in a sense of mistrust, insecure attachment styles, and difficulty with intimate relationships. Group therapy and psychodrama offer exponential opportunities for peer support, renegotiating relational trauma, role training social skills, and experiencing healthy connection. The experience of supporting and being supported by one's peers provides a sense of hope, community, collaboration, and social confidence. Mutual aid uplifts all participants in a reciprocity that empowers. Psychodrama, similar to group work practice, centralizes the phenomenon of mutual aid and methods that promote it. While peer support is important for clients, it is equally significant in organizations, supervision, and education. Trauma-informed leaders promote peer support within their agencies while engaging in their own peer support.

Trauma as Inherently Disconnecting from Self and Others

Some have suggested that the presence or lack of presence of another attuned individual may be a primary mediator between a traumatic experience and posttraumatic stress disorder (PTSD) (Badenoch, 2018). The aloneness, that one experiences in trauma is particularly damaging. Trauma causes fragmentation and disruption in one's relationship to themselves, others, and the

DOI: 10.4324/9781003277859-7

world. Trauma within the relationship can leave a lasting impact on one's ability in relationships in the future to feel safe, to trust, to feel empowered, and to value self and others. When trauma is experienced in relationship, it can have a lasting impact on one's ability to develop and maintain secure attachments going forward. This is particularly true for attachment trauma and developmental trauma – adversity that takes place within the relationship between a child and their caregivers during critical developmental years. A child who grows up in the chaos of trauma without attuned and supportive caregivers is more likely to develop a mistrust for others, difficulty with self-regulation, low self-esteem, inhibited emotional and social intelligence, and limited relational skills. Trauma in one's early years without the benefit of other protective factors and opportunities for healing can prevent one from becoming all that they can become in life. At the same time, trauma is often a catalyst for posttraumatic growth and propels one into new potentials that did not exist prior to the adversity.

Negative belief systems often develop in the aftermath of trauma which can stay with an individual throughout their entire life. Beliefs related to unworthiness, unlovability, incompetence, stupidity, and helplessness are common for survivors of trauma. These beliefs may be introjections from the perpetrator or perhaps they are inferences from the mind of a victimized child that can't find any other way of making sense of the abuse they experienced other than to conclude that they deserved it. Regardless, these negative cognitions are prone to imprison an individual throughout the course of their life, disconnecting them from themselves, trapping them in a limiting narrative, and stunting the fulfillment of their individual potential in life.

Trauma promotes isolation. The internalized trauma essentially becomes a barrier disconnecting one from themself and from other human beings. It often promotes the chronic use of defense mechanisms such as projection, denial, and dissociation which significantly impact healthy relationship opportunities. Fight, flight, and freeze, the nervous system's innate (and quite helpful) defensive responses to threat, can also develop into chronic habits that prove relationally maladaptive long after the trauma is over (Porges, 2017).

Throughout the COVID-19 pandemic human beings have been more isolated than ever. Fear of getting the virus or spreading it to others has led to disconnection, separation, ambiguous loss, and dislocation from groups or communities for a large number of individuals within society. Peer support that was accessible prior to the pandemic has been significantly disrupted. Avenues for peer support have shifted into virtual platforms and programs which have proven to be a creative and modern adaptation to the limitations imposed on many due to pandemic restrictions. While virtual options for peer support are accessible and satisfactory to many, there are also many others who do not have access to internet or technology required, familiarity with computer programs needed to access connection online, or others who simply do not feel that engaging in peer support online fulfills their social needs in the same way as connection in person with others.

Trauma is disruptive to one's sense of usefulness to others. Though trauma can fuel enmeshment, over-giving, and co-dependency, it also has a determining effect on the survivor's sense of value and worth to others and the world. The feeling of being able to support and help others can dissipate as a result of victimization and adversity. In many ways relational trauma is the opposite of peer support in that the perpetration and harm create an imbalanced power differential. In the moment of trauma, there is a victim and a perpetrator rather than two equal peers. This trauma-informed principle of peer support is fitting then as it offers a remedy for this sense of worthlessness and disempowerment.

Reconnecting to Self through Group Therapy and Psychodrama

Group work and psychodrama are unique in their capacity to promote a reconnection and restructuring of the self. The self is largely developed through one's internalization of relationships, experiences, and social learning. Interpersonal neurobiologists highlight how the brain, mind, and self emerge through interpersonal experience (Cozolino, 2014; Shapiro & Applegate, 2018; Siegel, 2012). Various psychology theories propose that the self is composed of integrated parts of internalized representations, object relations, unconscious drives, and childhood experiences. Social work emphasizes how the self emerges and exists within a dynamic social environment. Psychodrama's theory of self is based on the development of roles from which the self emerges (Moreno, 1953). All of these theories of self overlap in that they underscore the essential nature of relationships and social experience in the development of the self. Group work offers exponential potentialities for self-shaping social experiences and relationships (Klein & Schermer, 2000). When a trauma survivor sees themselves mirrored, respected, and valued in the eyes of others in the group, a part of self is reawakened and reclaimed (Herman, 1992). A well-established and cohesive group has an influencing impact on each of its members. While the members each individually shape the group, the group also shapes the members. There is a reciprocity in the relationship between group member and the group. Participants give from themselves to the group and the group provides opportunities for reconnecting to self, renegotiating one's sense of self, and evolving and restructuring one's self. Through connection with others, we connect to ourselves.

How have my relationships and group experiences shaped who I am today?

Psychodrama takes this concept a bit further through role-playing. Psychodrama literally means "psyche in action" or "soul in action" (Giacomucci, 2019). A psychodrama enactment allows the protagonist to externalize parts of self in the group, renegotiate their intrapsychic relationships, and reintegrate the parts into a newly configured self. The experiential nature of psychodrama lends itself to other participants seeing themselves and parts of self within the protagonist and the other roles in the scene (Giacomucci, 2021b). The concept of "connecting with self" is deepened in psychodrama through roles (such as the double, future self, past self, and parts of self) while psychodrama interventions (doubling, mirror position, role reversal, role training, future projection, etc.) promote self-awareness, self-stabilization, and an expansion of self. Psychodrama allows a client to literally connect with themself and have a discussion with themself. Psychodrama's capacity to help an individual reconnect with self is depicted through the following vignette:

> Brian is chosen by the group to be the protagonist with his topic of becoming a better man and reconnecting with his goodness after years of addiction, trauma, and prison. He shares about years earlier in life when he felt a sense of hope, innocence, and integrity which he felt were quickly lost throughout his adult life. He comments on how he had to do things to survive in prison and become hardened and guarded in a way that he feels much shame, guilt, and disgust about. In the psychodrama enactment, Brian has a dialogue with his courage, his integrity, and his innocence as roles. His discussion with courage helped to clarify the importance of vulnerability and solidified his courage to change. The psychodramatic exchange with integrity allowed him to hone in on, and connect to, a sense of goodness and firmness within a set of personal values. "Brian, you may have done bad things to survive, but you can always reconnect with your integrity and values." Other group members took the opportunity to double for Brian in the role of integrity which further grounded him in the ways that others have experienced him as a man with integrity. One group member doubles, "Brian you demonstrate integrity in the way you help the group maintain safety." Another group member doubles, "Brian you are a good man and others around you know this to be true." In talking to his innocence, Brian expresses his sadness in feeling disconnected for years due to his addiction, trauma, and the ways

he has hurt others. Innocence affirmed that it exists deep within Brian and can reawaken through living with integrity in recovery. Finally, Brian engages in a dialogue with himself in the future. Reversing roles with himself in the future provides him with an embodied experience of being a man in long-term recovery, living with integrity, and helping others who have experienced similar things as he. As his future self, Brian was able to offer empathy to himself about the trauma he experienced and his powerlessness over his addiction – "you did what you had to do to get by Brian, now you can reconnect with all the goodness within you". He spoke directly to himself about his time in prison and validated that his actions in prison were self-defense and necessary to survive. In his discussion with himself, future Brian explains that "your recovery is a process or realigning with your values, regaining integrity with yourself, and helping others to do the same. He extended forgiveness to himself for his past and emphasized that he has the power to redefine himself, to be a better man, and to contribute goodness into the world going forward.

This psychodrama depicts the power of the method in helping individuals reconnect with a new sense of self in the aftermath of trauma, addiction, and adversity. The psychodrama process helped Brian to explore parts of himself and strengths that had become harder for him to connect with due to many years of trauma. Through the psychodramatic dialogues, he was able to express feelings of guilt, shame, and sadness while also reconnecting with a sense of hope, self-love, and self-worth. Doubling (and later sharing) from other group members helped Brian to see and hear how others in his group experienced him as a man with integrity and goodness, even though he had yet to see these things within himself. The final encounter with his future self facilitated reflection on where he is now compared to the potentialities of who he could become in the future. In the exchange between his current and future selves, he accessed self-forgiveness, self-love, and self-worth while also affirming a new commitment to this vision for himself going forward.

What insight or inspiration might my future self offer to me today about continuing forward towards my goals?

Group Work as Social Connection

Beyond connection to self, group work is fundamentally grounded in the importance of social connection. Group work provides social learning in the here-and-now. The group process helps participants to learn, practice, and refine their social skills with each other and the role modeling of the leader. Within the safety of the group, social experimentation is encouraged. Participants have a space to test out new social skills, develop new parts of self, and embody new ways of being and relating to others. The relational process of the group affords the possibility of reconfiguring attachment styles and relational templates through corrective emotional experiences with other participants. Yalom and Leszcz (2020) describe this as the corrective recapitulation of the primary family group in their list of therapeutic factors. Courtois and Ford (2016) articulate the unique benefits of group therapy for trauma survivors in that:

> Crucial features of psychological and interpersonal growth include individuation and differentiation not supported in the family of origin or in other victimizing context and relationships. These can be difficult or even impossible to evoke or rework in the same way in individual treatment.
>
> (p. 191)

Group work is a remedy for the isolation that often results in the aftermath of trauma and the experience of both PTSD and complex PTSD (Ford, Fallot, & Harris, 2009). Trauma survivors often can feel isolated in their experience and assume that they are alone. It can be hard to imagine that anyone else has could possibly understand or have experienced the same trauma. This is where group work excels beyond the limits of individual therapy. The group of clients comes together with a shared purpose, identity, or experience leading to the realization that they are not alone in their trauma or difficulties (Courtois, 2010). The group process effectively normalizes experiences of participants while providing new connection. As group cohesion is established, an "all-in-the-same-boat" phenomenon arises. Yalom and Leszcz (2020) describe this as a sense of universality. The solidarity of the group encourages peer support between its members. For some, the group might be the only social interaction in their life with others who have the same shared experience. There is a sense of social support that comes from the resulting empathy and normalization that often cannot be offered by a therapist – it can only be offered by peers with similar experience. For some trauma survivors, group participation may be a necessary precursor to individual therapy as they may need to learn to trust peers again before they can consider trusting another authority figure (Courtois & Ford, 2016). For other clients, individual therapy may be a necessary prerequisite to participation in a therapy group.

The experience of peer support proves helpful to both parties engaged in the process – the supporter and the supported. The supported receives help, care, empathy, insight, suggestions, information, and support while the supporter often leaves the interaction with a sense of pride, competence, value, empowerment, respect, and self-esteem. Yalom and Leszcz (2020) label this as altruism in their list of therapeutic factors in groups. They highlight how this process of give-and-take promotes role versatility in that participants are challenged to shift between providing help and receiving help (Holmes & Kivlighan, 2000, as cited in Yalom & Leszcz, 2020).

How has helping someone else helped me recently?

In the social work with groups tradition, we refer to this phenomenon as mutual aid (Giacomucci, 2021a). It is the cornerstone of social work with groups; the group worker's primary objective is to create the conditions for mutual aid and peer support within the group (Kurland & Salmon, 2005; Shulman, 2015). In this light, we can clearly see how this principle of peer support is also connected to other trauma-informed principles such as safety, trustworthiness, collaboration and mutuality, empowerment, and cultural, historic, and gender issues.

The collective strength of the group has a greater capacity to hold and integrate trauma and adversity than any of the individual participants alone; this collective resource becomes available to each participant through the group process (Herman, 1992). These same principles are also applicable within community frameworks. The centralization of peer support in community settings can be seen within religious communities, therapeutic communities, inpatient populations, recovery homes, 12-step fellowships, and other communities. Peer support is the mechanism by which healing is experienced and by which change ripples throughout the community.

Peer Support for Professionals, Employees, and Leaders

In the same way that peer support promotes healing in communities and groups, it also cultivates healing and resilience within organizations. At its core, an organization is also a group and a community. Social support within organizations can help reduce feelings of workload overwhelm and occupational stress which fuel negative impacts on attendance, well-being, organizational commitment, and employees' intention to stay with a company long term (Bowling et al., 2015; Whybrow, Jones, & Greenberg, 2015). The power of two colleagues supporting each other is sometimes even more powerful and significant than a supervisor helping a supervisee. Furthermore, there are likely to be certain topics, issues, and feelings that workers in any agency may experience that they are less comfortable sharing with a supervisor than with a peer. There is often an added layer of safety and mutuality within peer relationships that can be missing in supervisory relationships where there is a clear power differential. Peer support has shown promising positive impacts on confidence, self-esteem, resilience, well-being, job performance, and job satisfaction (Agarwal, Brooks, & Greenberg, 2020).

The research outcomes on peer support in the workplace have propelled many organizations to develop organizational peer support programs in their organizations to support their staff. These programs are staffed by other employees who have experienced emotional, relational, and occupational challenges who are positioned to help other staff struggling with similar problems. These types of programs are not a substitute for psychotherapy, but they certainly help staff feel that they are not alone while providing concrete support and suggestions for coping with or navigating the issues at hand. Sometimes staff may be more willing to speak with a peer than with a counselor. Peer support programs also provide employees with resources and referrals for continued support when needed.

Leaders in all organizations would benefit from an increased awareness of the importance and benefits of peer support in the workplace. Many staff members' relationships with their peers at work are a significant source of enjoyment, support, and learning in their lives. Perhaps many staff members' primary sense of fulfillment related to their job is entirely related to their relationship with their peers more so than the actual work responsibilities or organizational mission. In social work with groups, the primary duty of the group worker is to set into motion mechanisms that promote mutual aid – the capacity of each group member to support each other, educate each other, and contribute to the healing of each other. When we approach organizational leadership through this lens of group leadership, one of the primary duties of the leader is also to promote mutual aid and connection between staff. Not only does mutual aid between staff benefit the staff, but it also benefits the leadership, the organization, and the clients or communities served. Peer support can be cultivated in a variety of direct and indirect ways including supervision groups, peer supervision, training events, support groups, peer support programs, professional development initiatives, team meals, and team events. Peer support can also be indirectly cultivated through various smaller decisions that impact the sociometry of an organization such a hiring of staff in dyads or small groups, the positioning of offices or workspaces based on shared identities or interests, and the coordination of shifts based on interpersonal connection between staff. All of these examples promote connection, cohesion, and peer support between workers.

In my own organizational leadership, I found it important to create opportunities for peer support between therapists and interns on my team. I've noticed that individuals can easily feel isolated when they don't have others on the team who share the same identities, professional orientations, and/or level of experience. As my team grew, I have made hiring decisions partially influenced by this sociometric awareness. I often hire new therapist or interns in pairs so that they have a peer starting the same role with them at the same time. It not only is more efficient for me in onboarding and orienting, but it creates an opportunity for peer support in a way that wouldn't be possible otherwise. It appears that this is especially important for the graduate interns that we host as they inevitably become close to their peer who has the same placement timeline as them. With therapists on my team, I've found that these peer support dyads seem to emerge less related to hiring dates but more so related to one's theoretical orientation and amount of experience in the field. For example, the therapists on my team whose primary orientation is EMDR tend to naturally gravitate to the other EMDR therapists. Similarly, the IFS therapists organically pair with each other, the psychodrama practitioners gravitate together, the therapists of color naturally connect with each other, and the new graduates often form unique bonds. Being aware of this natural tendency to associate with peers who share similar experiences, identities, and professional orientations has helped me to develop organizational sociometry that promotes peer support and minimizes isolation.

Some of these same ideas were explored within organizational sociometry by Jacob Moreno (1953) who used sociometric tests and sociograms to uncover the sociodynamics impacting relationships between workers at his mental health hospital and other organizations. More recently, sociometrist Diana Jones offers an in depth look at leadership through sociometric and relational lenses (2022). In a study by Folette, Polusny, and Milbeck (1994), it was discovered that 95% of mental health professionals report engaging in peer support. Multiple research studies highlight the importance of peer support for professionals in the helping profession (Iliffe & Steed, 2000; Naturale, 2007). Peer support effectively helps to mitigate the impact of secondary traumatic stress while cultivating vicarious post-traumatic growth for professionals (Manning, de Terte, & Stephens, 2015; Sutton, Rowe, Hammerton, & Billings, 2022; Tehrani, 2010). The research literature compellingly articulates the benefits of peer support within organizations for helping professionals and specifically those working with trauma.

Peer support is also important for leaders to engage in with other leaders. When professionals are promoted into leadership roles, their work relationships shift with the role change. Many of their former peers may become supervisees and/or the relationships may shift in more subtle ways due to the changed power differential. Leaders can easily feel isolated and unsupported in their own agencies, especially when there are few or no other peers at the same professional rank as them. There are many nuances to in organizational leadership and unique work stressors for leaders that make peer support essential for them as well. In my own experience as a business owner, I occasionally feel isolated or feel that others in my organization might not fully understand the stressors that I experience which are specific to my role. Owning and leading a therapy center involves unique financial risks, legal liabilities, sacrifices, stressors, disappointments, and anxieties. One of my attempts to navigate this for myself was to invite a colleague who runs a similar business as mine to meet on a regular basis for unpaid peer consultation. Our informal meetings involve each of us taking 30 minutes to support the other in any topic or issue requested. While our discussions center around our professional roles, we inevitably also share of our personal lives. Our discussions have ranged from organizational, financial, educational, ethical, social, and emotional topics within the framework of peer support. Personally, I have found these meetings to be an invaluable resource and a unique opportunity to give and receive peer support with a colleague who owns and directs a center almost identical to my own. Through this mutual aid relationship, both participants are rejuvenated.

Who can I offer peer support to in my organization or professional circle?

Who is someone that I can seek out to receive peer support from in my organization or professional circle?

Psychodrama Centralizes the Power of Mutual Aid

One example of the power of psychodrama to promote peer support comes from my trauma-focused psychodrama group at Mirmont Treatment Center. The warm-up phase of the group employed the circle of strengths exercise (described earlier in Chapter 4) which helped establish safety, vulnerability, connection, and peer support early in the session. Through the presentation of strengths to each other, participants helped one another access strengths within the group and renegotiate their sense of self. The process of having one's peers concretize strengths and remind them of how they are demonstrated brought many group members to tears. Each client helped other clients to see their best qualities in a matrix of mutual aid.

A 30-year-old woman named Edie volunteered their topic of childhood molestation and their goal of unburdening themselves from it by sharing about it for the first time and building up the courage to tell their father about it. Other clients also volunteered topics so a sociometric protagonist selection was facilitated which resulted in the overwhelming majority of the group choosing her topic. By itself, the sociometric selection of the topic and protagonist helped Edie to see that she as not alone in this experience. Other group members who chose her topic based on their shared experience were also shocked to see that nearly three quarters of the entire group had also experienced childhood sexual trauma. This initial sociometric selection primed the group for peer support and mutual aid throughout the process.

As the psychodrama evolved, Edie chose peers to play the roles of 'courage,' 'positive inner voice,' and 'God' as the supportive roles necessary to work towards her goal. The role reciprocity and tele within the roles dynamics further deepened the experience for Edie and the role players who were emotionally connected to the topic based on their own childhood sexual trauma. At one point, the client playing the role of courage became overwhelmed stating that they had also been molested as a child and feared that they wouldn't be courageous enough to carry on. Two group members spontaneously emerged from the audience to fortify her in the role of courage while continuing the flow of messages from the role of courage to Edie. In her psychodramatic dialogue talking to God about her childhood trauma, Edie became overwhelmed with emotions. As the facilitator, I asked her if it would help to have more support from the group to which she agreed. When I prompted a few group members to join as supportive roles, nearly the entire group jumped into the scene offering peer support. When role reversed with God, Edie spoke to herself (a role now played by John who had been chosen as God) about forgiveness, healing, trust, strength, and truth. As she continued speaking as God, the John started to gradually become emotional – he stated that he had also been sexually abuse as a child and needed to hear the same messages from God for his own healing. Edie accessed a deeper level of healing due to this reciprocity within the role dynamics. On one hand, she was God speaking to herself, but on the other hand, she recognized that she was also speaking through the role to her peer (playing the role of Edie) who also needed support for himself. As the dialogue moved towards closure, Edie and John were instructed to role reverse back to their original roles and to replay the scene. Now, John, role-playing as God had the chance to offer support to Edie who found closure by handing her burden to God at the end of the interaction. She confidently told the group that she intends to request a family session with her counselor to disclose to her father about the abuse she experienced as a child. After the psychodrama enactment, the group shifted into the sharing phase where each client had a chance to share how they related to Edie and her psychodrama. The sharing from her peers reminded her again that she isn't alone in her experience while illuminating for Edie how her work had helped inspire and promote healing for other group members.

Edie's psychodrama depicts the trauma-informed principle of peer support embodied throughout each of the three phases of the group – warm up, action, and sharing. The sociometric warm up awakens peer support, the sociometric protagonist selection focuses the peer support on a specific topic/goal, the psychodrama enactment crystallizes the peer support on multiple levels (psychodramatically through roles but also socially through participants), and the sharing phase of the group helped Edie to hear how she had helped her peers through the work she had done in her psychodrama.

The psychodrama method emphasizes the importance of mutual aid and empowers every participant to contribute to the healing process (Giacomucci, 2021a, 2021b). Moreno's psychodrama and group therapy philosophy explicitly elevates each patient to become a therapeutic agent for the group (Giacomucci et al., 2018). In his *Open Letter to Group Psychotherapists*, Moreno exclaims that "one patient can be a therapeutic agent to the other, let us invent devices by which they can help each other, in contrast to the older idea that all the therapeutic power rests with the physician" (Moreno, 1947, p. 23). Moreno's original code of ethics even suggested that we should consider asking each participant to take the Hippocratic Oath, demonstrating this deep belief in each patient as a therapeutic agent (Moreno, 1957).

Experiential sociometry tools are especially potent in their ability to cultivate peer support within groups (Giacomucci, 2021a). Many of these experiential processes are outlined in detail within Chapter 4. The use of small groups, spectrograms, locograms, floor checks, step-in sociometry, hands-on-shoulder sociograms, and circle of strengths each help participants access mutual aid and peer support that is waiting to be tapped into within the group. Sociometry is uniquely connected to this trauma-informed principles of peer support as sociometry orients itself on uncovering and transforming the sociodynamics within groups and communities. Simply put, sociometry is an exploration and realization of the potentials of peer support within groups (Giacomucci & Ehrhart, 2021). Experiential sociometry processes not only illuminate these potentials for peer support but also manifest further peer support dynamics within the process.

While a psychodrama group may appear to consist of a single protagonist doing their personal work with the support of the group, if conducted properly it is really a group-as-a-whole process where the protagonist's work is representative of the rest of the group (Giacomucci & Stone, 2019). Essentially the protagonist becomes a mirror for other group members to see themselves and do their work symbolically through the scene and the roles. This is best supported through the group choosing a protagonist and a topic using a sociometric selection to ensure the psychodrama topic is reflective of the entire group and a sense of universality. The process builds upon the reciprocity within the roles and between participants while accessing mutual aid and peer support within the group in a profound way. Psychodrama group participants frequently comment on how it helped them in their own process to play auxiliary roles for someone else's psychodrama (Giacomucci & Marquit, 2020). The experiential aspect of psychodrama and other expressive arts therapies appear to further elicit unconscious and implicit trauma content through relational experiences and peer support (Malchiodi, 2020).

The experience of engaging in mutual aid is particularly transformative for patients struggling with a sense of worthlessness or the belief that they cannot offer value to others (Yalom & Leszcz, 2020). The mutual aid and peer support process is mutually beneficial and further feeds into other trauma-informed principles such as safety, trustworthiness, empowerment, collaboration, and mutuality. A group process centered on mutual aid and peer support, such as psychodrama, emphasizes the power within the group rather than the power of the group leader. As such it mitigates the potential of unhealthy power dynamics between the group facilitator and participants which could lead to retraumatization. Peer support as a trauma-informed principle is in particularly connected to the trauma-informed principle outlined in the next chapter – collaboration and mutuality.

Conclusion

Peer support offers a remedy for many of the negative impacts of trauma, especially the commonly resulting isolation, disconnection from self, and disempowerment. Centralizing peer support in group work and psychodrama elevates participants as therapeutic agents and helps everyone in the group to recognize their strengths, their agency, and their ability to help others while also helping themselves. Peer support is also important in organizations and educational settings as professionals are human too. We are prone to burn-out, isolation, and vicarious trauma which can be mitigated and transformed through the mutual aid process. As leaders, we need to create opportunities for peer support within our communities, within our service offerings, within our organization, and for ourselves.

References

Agarwal, B., Brooks, S. K., & Greenberg, N. (2020). The role of peer support in managing occupational stress: A qualitative study of the sustaining resilience at work intervention. *Workplace Health & Safety, 68*(2), 57–64.

Badenoch, B. (2018). *The heart of trauma: Healing the embodied brain in the context of relationships*. New York: W.W. Norton & Company.

Bowling, N. A., Alarcon, G. M., Bragg, C. B., & Hartman, M. J. (2015). A meta-analytic examination of the potential correlates and consequences of workload. *Work & Stress, 29*(2), 95–113.

Courtois, C. A. (2010). *Healing the incest wound* (2nd ed.). New York: W. W. Norton & Company.

Courtois, C. A., & Ford, J. D. (2016). *Treatment of complex trauma: A sequenced, relationship-based approach*. New York: The Guildford Press.

Cozolino, L. J. (2014). *The neuroscience of human relationships* (2nd ed.). New York: W.W. Norton & Company.

Folette, V. M., Polusny, M. M., & Milbeck, K. (1994). Mental health and law enforcement professionals: Trauma history, psychological symptoms, and impact of providing services to sexual abuse survivors. *Professional Psychology: Research and Practice, 25*(3), 275–282.

Ford, J. D., Fallot, R. D., & Harris, M. (2009). Group therapy. In C. A. Courtois, & J. D. Ford (Eds.), *Treating complex traumatic stress disorders: An evidence-based guide* (pp. 415–440). New York: The Guilford Press.

Giacomucci, S. (2019). *Social group work in action: A sociometry, psychodrama, and experiential trauma therapy curriculum*. Doctorate in Social Work (DSW) Dissertations. 124. https://repository.upenn.edu/cgi/viewcontent.cgi?article=1128&context=edissertations_sp2

Giacomucci, S. (2021a). Experiential sociometry in group work: Mutual aid for the group-as-a-whole. *Social Work with Groups, 44*(3), 204–214.

Giacomucci, S. (2021b). *Social work, sociometry, and psychodrama: Experiential approaches for group therapists, community leaders, and social workers.* Springer Nature. http://dx.doi.org/10.1007/978-981-33-6342-7

Giacomucci, S., & Ehrhart, L. (2021). Introduction to psychodrama psychotherapy: A trauma and addiction group vignette. *Group, 45*(1), 69–86.

Giacomucci, S., Gera, S., Briggs, D., & Bass, K. (2018). Experiential addiction treatment: Creating positive connection through sociometry and therapeutic spiral model safety structures. *Journal of Addiction and Addictive Disorders, 5*, 17. http://dx.doi.org/10.24966/AAD-7276/100017

Giacomucci, S., & Marquit, J. (2020). The effectiveness of trauma-focused psychodrama in the treatment of PTSD in inpatient substance abuse treatment. *Frontiers in Psychology, 11*, 896. https://dx.doi.org/10.3389%2Ffpsyg.2020.00896

Giacomucci, S., & Stone, A. M. (2019). Being in two places at once: Renegotiating traumatic experience through the surplus reality of psychodrama. *Social Work with Groups, 42*(3), 184–196. https://dx.doi.org/10.1080/01609513.2018.1533913

Herman, J. L. (1992). *Trauma and recovery: The aftermath of violence—From domestic abuse to political terror.* New York: Basic Books.

Holmes, S. E., & Kivlighan Jr., D. M. (2000). Comparison of therapeutic factors in group and individual treatment processes. *Journal of Counseling Psychology, 47*(4), 478.

Iliffe, G., & Steed, L. G. (2000). Exploring the counselor's experience of working with perpetrators and survivors of domestic violence. *Journal of Interpersonal Violence, 15*(4), 393–412. https://dx.doi.org/10.1177/088626000015004004

Jones, D. (2022). *Leadership levers: Releasing the power of relationships for exceptional participation, alignment, and team results.* New York: Routledge.

Klein, R. H., & Schermer, V. L. (2000). *Group psychotherapy for psychological trauma.* New York: The Guilford Press.

Kurland, R., & Salmon, R. (2005). Group work vs. casework in a group: Principles and implications for teaching and practice. *Social Work with Groups, 28*(3–4), 121–132.

Malchiodi, C. A. (2020). *Trauma and expressive arts therapy: Brain, body, and imagination in the healing process.* New York: Guilford Press.

Manning, S. F., de Terte, I., & Stephens, C. (2015). Vicarious posttraumatic growth: A systematic literature review. *International Journal of Wellbeing, 5*(2), 125–139.

Moreno, J. L. (1947). *Open letter to group psychotherapists.* Beacon, NY: Beacon House.

Moreno, J. L. (1953). *Who shall survive? Foundations of sociometry, group psychotherapy and sociodrama* (2nd ed.). Beacon, NY: Beacon House.

Moreno, J. L. (1957). Code of ethics of group psychotherapists. *Group Psychotherapy*, *10*, 143–144.

Naturale, A. (2007). Secondary traumatic stress in social workers responding to disasters: Reports from the field. *Clinical Social Work Journal*, *35*, 173–181. https://dx.doi.org/10.1007/s10615-007-0089-1

Porges, S. W. (2017). *The pocket guide to the Polyvagal theory: The transformative power of feeling safe.* New York: W.W. Norton & Company.

Shapiro, J. R., & Applegate, J. S. (2018). *Neurobiology for clinical social work: Theory and practice* (2nd ed.). New York: W.W. Norton & Company.

Shulman, L. (2015). *The skills of helping individuals, families, groups, and communities* (8th ed.). Boston, MA: Cengage Learning.

Siegel, D. J. (2012). *Developing mind: How relationships and the brain interact to shape who we are.* New York: Guilford Press.

Sutton, L., Rowe, S., Hammerton, G., & Billings, J. (2022). The contribution of organisational factors to vicarious trauma in mental health professionals: A systematic review and narrative synthesis. *European Journal of Psychotraumatology*, *13*(1), 2022278.

Tehrani, N. (2010). Compassion fatigue: Experiences in occupational health, human resources, counselling and police. *Occupational Medicine*, *60*(2), 133–138.

Whybrow, D., Jones, N., & Greenberg, N. (2015). Promoting organizational well-being: A comprehensive review of trauma risk management. *Occupational Medicine*, *65*(4), 331–336.

Yalom, I. D., & Leszcz, M. (2020). *The theory and practice of group psychotherapy* (6th ed.). New York: Basic Books.

8
Collaboration and Mutuality in Group Therapy, Psychodrama, and Leadership

Chapter Summary

Trauma leaves us with a sense of disconnection while threatening our sense of worthiness or innocence. In the moment of trauma, mutuality disintegrates, and the possibility of collaboration is lost. The victim-perpetrator reciprocity creates an unbalanced power dynamic often reenacted in post-traumatic stress. The resulting sense of unworthiness and self-hatred complicates one's search for belonging, self-love, and purpose. Group work and psychodrama offer avenues for participants to experience and engage in collaboration and mutuality while recovering self-worth and a feeling of belonging. Collaboration and belongingness are equally important in organizations as they help staff feel valued, a part of, and purpose driven. Trauma-informed leaders treat staff with dignity and respect while engaging in collaborative ways.

Trauma Is Characterized by an Absence of Collaboration and Mutuality

The experience of trauma is inherently void of mutuality or any spirit of collaboration. Trauma, especially relational or collective trauma, is characterized by unequal power dynamics and decision-making power which involuntary leads to harm and hurt. Collaboration and mutuality disintegrate in the moment of trauma between two parties. Instead of belonging or intimacy, there is a rupture of connection and a forced experience. In the trauma caused by oppression or marginalization, the marginalized group is dehumanized by

DOI: 10.4324/9781003277859-8

the oppressor. There is no room for authentic collaboration or mutuality in the midst of racism, sexism, gender violence, and discrimination. Trauma significantly impacts one's sense of worthiness and value, often having a determining impact on all aspects of one's life. In the critical moments of trauma, the overwhelmingly disproportionate imbalance of power appears to be internalized within an individual. Many trauma survivors report feeling as though they lose their innocence, self-worth, self-respect, and personal power in the aftermath of trauma. The shocking nature of the traumatic event is often too much for an individual to process or make sense of – especially in the case of childhood trauma. Perhaps the high rates of self-blame in childhood trauma survivors could be explained as the child's attempt to make sense of the unbelievable experience. How else could something this horrific happen or be done to me unless I deserved it? This internalization of unworthiness and powerlessness distorts one's sense of self and thus their decision-making throughout their life. The extraordinary imbalance of power in trauma can only be reversed through a healing process that centers collaboration and mutuality. Because we are so frequently wounded in relationship, our healing must also take place within the context of relationship.

Collaboration means that trauma survivors must be approached as active agents in their own healing process rather than simply as patients receiving a treatment. The dominant medical model in treatment centers has its benefits, but it also can become a barrier to implementing trauma-informed principles such as collaboration and mutuality. The provision of treatment without a collaborative relationship that elevates the client through mutuality risks reenacting unequal power dynamics that may resemble the hierarchical dynamic between perpetrator and victim. Collaboration in trauma-informed care means that we "do with" the client rather than "do for" or "do to" the client.

How can I offer further approach clients as active collaborators in my work with them?

Many social service programs, though initially developed with pure intentions, have evolved into bureaucratic agencies that tend to reenact oppressive power dynamics with clients though patriarchal decision-making and coercive practices. For example, treatment plans often become templated jargon based on diagnoses to satisfy insurance companies rather than a meaningful and collaborative goal setting process with a client. These norms in the treatment field seem to be furthered by burnout staff who often feel oppressed by the overwhelming demands from their employer and the systems that they operate within (insurance companies, legal system, licensing/compliance requirements, agency expectations/policies, etc.). Commenting on high rates of burnout and compassion fatigue in service providers, Douglas (2012) remarks that "delivering care without caring is simply wrong" (p. 419). Here we see a parallel process between the absence of collaboration and mutuality between staff and clients, as well as between staff and the larger system that impact their work. Policymakers are sometimes critiqued for developing policy or laws that are disconnected from the realities of those that the policy would impact. Leaders would benefit from collaborating with frontline workers and treating them with mutuality in the development of new policy. Doing so would enhance the capacity of providers to also implement the principles of collaboration and mutuality with their clients. Harris and Fallot (2001), in their seminal text on trauma-informed care, note that "the core of the service relationship in a trauma-informed system is open and genuine collaboration between provider and consumer at all phases of the service delivery" (p. 19).

Mutuality means that we connect with others helping them feel seen, heard, loved, valued, and empowered. A sense of belonging is crucial to this effect. This requires developing an atmosphere of acceptance and mutual respect in all aspects of the organization – with clients, community members, families, employees, and leaders. There sometimes can be a tendency to only consider these principles as applicable to victims of trauma, but they are also necessary for perpetrators of trauma (who are frequently past victims themselves). Furthermore, the concept of mutuality is primarily only examined through the lens of our perspective on others, but it is also applicable in how we view ourselves. As community members, professionals, and leaders, we must also learn to give ourselves the same respect that we strive to offer to others. We must recognize our own inherent worth, strengths, and goodness in order to better see the goodness in others. One will struggle to collaborate with others unless we come to believe that our own ideas are worth consideration. In this way, mutuality is a principle that upholds collaboration as its twin principle.

Do I fully recognize my own worth and strengths as a professional and as a human being?

How can help those that I work with further recognize their inherent worth and strengths?

Collaboration and mutuality are also principles that are fundamentally relational in nature. Both can only exist within the framework of a relationship. This is also true for other trauma-informed principles such as trustworthiness and peer support. The importance of relationships has been written about extensively and is core to group work, psychodrama, and leadership (Brown, 2018; Giacomucci, 2021b; Northouse, 2021; Sinek, 2014). Implementing these trauma-informed principles require the vehicle of a relationship between two parties. It is no surprise then that the therapeutic relationship in psychotherapy is often regarded as the most important aspect of treatment (Ardito & Rabellino, 2011; Horvath & Symonds, 1991; Lambert & Barley, 2001). The research literature actually describes this relationship as a "therapeutic alliance" which further articulates the role of collaboration and mutuality in the process. Through a collaborative and mutual partnership, the service provider and client engage together. A meaningful sharing of power and decision-making promotes co-creation. In this way, collaboration and mutuality are associated with the other trauma-informed principles. Collaboration and mutuality cultivate safety, trustworthiness, support, empowerment, voice, choice, and an honoring of differences or similarities in identities.

Mutuality as Respect for Identity and Culture

Mutuality is also connected to the final trauma-informed principle which urges us to consider the impact of cultural, historic and gender issues. Helping individuals to feel a sense of belonging and acceptance within our organizations requires that we embody a mutual respect for every individual regardless of their age, gender identity, sexual orientation, race, ethnicity, culture, religion, political beliefs, social class, language, education level, national origin, ability, etc. When an individual or group experiences discrimination (explicitly or implicitly) within agencies that are supposed to be helping them, it only adds another layer of retraumatization. Trauma-informed care implies that we create a culture within our organizations where staff, clients, and leaders are treated with respect regardless of their identities. The marginalization and privilege that certain identities tend to provide within the larger society must be actively addressed and renegotiated within a trauma-informed organization. Power dynamics based on identity (such as age, gender, race, and class) need to be rebalanced. Decision-making within the organization and within provision of services to clients must be shared equally between stakeholders and those involved.

Embodying mutuality and fairness in this context require that individuals, especially leaders, be willing to both utilize their privilege in responsible ways and take responsibility for healing from the ways they have been marginalized in the past. Leaders who have not worked through their own trauma are likely to cause harm to others, or at least, will be limited in reaching their potential as a leader. Similarly, those leaders who are unable to critically examine their own privilege while creatively leveraging it for good are also missing the mark on becoming the best leader they can be while risking being a part of reenacting oppression within their organization, relationships, and communities. This mutuality in relationship with all clients and staff must be more than performative. It must be an authentic and action-based rather than simply a public relations show. Belongingness for all will depend on the ability of leaders and staff to demonstrate mutuality in their day-to-day interactions with others regardless of their privilege or marginalized identities.

How do I actively cultivate mutuality and belonging in my work with folks with marginalized identities?

Finding a Place to Belong in Group

Trauma-informed groups promote a powerful sense of belonging for participants. Many trauma survivors struggle with a sense of belonging, which can be a resulting impact of their traumatic wounding. If we are wounded in groups, it makes sense then that we are healed by groups (Bloom, 1998). Judith Herman (1992) offers a powerful argument for groups as a remedy for trauma:

> The solidarity of a group provides the strongest protection against terror and despair, and the strongest antidote to traumatic experience. Trauma isolates; the group re-creates a sense of belonging. Trauma shames and stigmatizes; the group bears witness and affirms. Trauma degrades the victim; the group exalts her. Trauma dehumanizes the victim; the group restores her humanity.

(p. 214)

A sense of belonging comes from a warm, welcoming, cohesive, and purposeful group experience (Foy, Unger, & Wattenburg, 2005). Not every participant will feel as though they belong in every group, and perhaps that is okay (for example, a doctor is less likely to feel a sense of belonging in a support group for teachers). However, we must ensure that our groups promote a sense of belonging for those that it was designed to serve (Giacomucci, 2017). We must also ensure that we are not unknowingly developing groups with good intentions that participants have unwelcoming and rejecting experiences within. SAMHSA's six trauma-informed principles offer a solid framework and basis for initiating groups that provide a sense of belonging to participants. When issues of safety, transparency, trustworthiness, peer support, collaboration, mutuality, empowerment, voice, choice, and cultural/historical issues are addressed in groups, the group is likely to be one that is experienced by most as supportive, welcoming, and helpful. A sense of belonging is often included in discussions of diversity, equity, and inclusion. Belonging is elevated beyond simply being given a space and a voice, but to include that one's voice is heard and responded to by others (Fosslien & Duffy, 2019).

The principle of collaboration speaks to the shared vision, purpose, and goals within a group. Groups with an explicit purpose are more effective groups. In the spirit of transparency, the group purpose(s) should be explicit to all members and prospective members. A clear group purpose helps to prevent traumatic reenactment (Herman, 1992). As group leaders, we initiate a collaborative process with participants throughout the stages of group development to move together towards fulfillment of group goals and purposes. The group goals and purpose provide a direction, shared mission, and a sense of universality. Participant's individual goals may be slightly different and varied but it is essential that their individual goals also relate to the shared group goals. We all have been in groups where there is an individual with a wildly different agenda for the group than what the group is intended for – these situations often are unpleasant for everyone involved.

A shared group purpose (often relating to individuals' goals) helps to provide the group with the glue and direction necessary for the collective to work together and move in the same general direction as a group-as-a-whole (Shulman, 2015). Group cohesiveness is described by SAMHSA as being related to the sense of belonging that an individual feels within the group (1999). The experience of belonging is core to a cohesive group, which has been shown as important in the effectiveness of group therapy research (Burlingame, McClendon, & Alonso, 2011; Burlingame, McClendon, & Yang, 2018; Yalom & Leszcz, 2020). Yalom and Leszcz (2020) suggest that cohesiveness may be a precondition for change. A cohesive and collaborative group process promotes the presence of therapeutic factors – especially those of a social nature such as imparting information, altruism, development of socializing techniques, imitative behavior, and interpersonal learning.

In group work of any kind, a collaborative process helps to uphold the principle of mutuality. When participants are determined to work together towards a common goal, they are likely to help each other leverage their unique strengths in service of the group. There is often a sense of empowerment and peer support that emerges in this way in that many participants, especially trauma survivors, may struggle with recognizing their own worth or strengths – but are quick to see and recognize the value and strengths that others in the group demonstrate. As the group works together on its shared mission, the value, worth, and strengths of individual members become more evident to all. This process helps individuals to access and accept their strengths while developing a sense of purpose, self-respect, self-worth, and perhaps even self-love. The strengths, gifts, and contributions of each group member configures together in a way that supports the trajectory of the group towards its primary purpose. Mutual respect for each other's contributions often becomes evident. Collaboration and mutuality often exist in a reciprocal relationship with each other in cohesive groups. Courtois and Ford (2016) articulate the power of collaboration, mutuality, and peer support in group therapy, "Group therapy directly and experientially addresses interpersonal and relationship difficulties and gives a unique opportunity for 'give and take' and for *in vivo* interaction and feedback" (p. 191).

Trauma-Informed Leaders Promote Collaboration, Mutuality, and Belonging

Collaboration and mutuality are important principles for organizational leadership, educators, and supervisors. Organizations and classrooms where collaboration and mutuality are centralized are likely to be more cohesive, effective, successful, and enjoyable. By their very nature, an organization or classroom is a group of individuals who come together with a shared mission to collaborate towards agreed upon goals. Organizations where individuals struggle to collaborate with each other are ripe with conflict, mistrust, abuse of power, inefficiencies, and an overall experience of being ineffective in meeting goals. A study by Cockshaw, Shochet, and Obst (2013) even discovered a correlation between workers sense of belonging at their place of employment and depressive symptoms. When workers are disconnected, disengaged, and disrespected in their workplace, they are likely to feel disempowered and depressed. SAMHSA's trauma-informed principles promote collaboration and mutuality within organizational and educational settings. Trauma-informed workplaces "create a sense of belonging, connection, and safety through their attitudes, policies, and practices" (Gerbrandt, Grieser, & Enns, 2021). When staff and students feel a sense of mutuality and mutual respect from others in the organization, they are likely to reciprocate. Collaboration and mutuality in organizations promote a sense of belonging for staff and students in the same way these principles promote belonging in groups.

A study by Slattery and Goodman (2009) highlights the importance and effectiveness of peer support, mutuality, and a collaborative workplace as factors reducing secondary traumatic stress for domestic violence advocates. Furthermore, Hartmann's (2018) exploration of 94 different workplace teams summarizes the central role that mutuality plays in prompting high-quality connection, resilience, and performance within organizational teams. Staff who experience a sense of belonging and consistent respect from others in the workplace, especially from their leaders, seem to be more often committed to the organization's success. Similar to the experience of peer support, a workplace atmosphere of collaboration and mutuality appears to have a positive impact on workers' self-worth, self-esteem, confidence, well-being, job satisfaction, and job performance while also reducing social isolation. Mutuality within organizations means that there is a mutual respect and honoring of value between staff, regardless of their rank in the hierarchy of the organization. All are treated equal, and none are given special treatment or privileges simply based on their role. Mutuality in the workplace can help individuals combat self-doubt and a sense of personal disempowerment that they may feel based on their own personal life experiences.

Do I really treat everyone in my organization with equal respect, regardless of their title or role?

There are various ways that leaders can integrate the principles of collaboration and mutuality in their organizations and classrooms. Many of the practical suggestions offered in the previous chapter related to peer support will also inherently promote collaboration, mutuality, and a sense of belonging. Positioning team members or students in ways to support each other will naturally result in increased collaboration and mutuality. Another simple process includes creating projects, committees, task forces, or teams with shared leadership to create systems that inherently integrate collaborative leadership roles (co-chairs, co-leaders, co-facilitators, etc.). Collaboration works best when it is role modeled by the leadership within an organization and a team. Leaders can initiate collaboration through decision-making and empowering staff as active agents in policy-making or organizational initiatives. Democratic and collaborative leadership approaches to decision-making include frontline workers or students as active agents in change regardless of their status in the hierarchy of the organization. A collaborative leader is quick to ask staff for feedback, to listen to staff, and to create changes based on the ideas of team members.

Psychodrama as Catalyzer for Collaboration and Mutuality

Psychodrama practice significantly emphasizes collaboration and mutuality as core elements through its focus on co-creation and co-responsibility (Fleury & Marra, 2022). In psychodrama philosophy, each person is recognized for their strengths, their inherent worth, and even their "genius" or "godlikeness" (Moreno, 2019). Psychodrama's founder attempted to elevate all patients in a group to the same level as the group leader by emphasizing their therapeutic power (Giacomucci, 2021a, 2021b). His experimental work in communities, group therapy, sociometry, and psychodrama made clear that every individual has the ability to help others in the group (Giacomucci, 2019). As noted previously, he went as far as suggesting in his code of ethics (Moreno, 1962) that elements of the Hippocratic oath should also apply to patients in the group. If we are going to fully recognize patients as collaborators and healing agents, then we should extend aspects of the Hippocratic oath to them as well. "In group psychotherapy the Hippocratic Oath is extended to all patients... Like the therapist, every patient is entrusted to protect the welfare of the co-patients" (Moreno, 1962, p. 5). Moreno's code of ethics embodies the spirit of trauma-informed care, in particular the concepts of collaboration, mutuality, peer support, safety, and empowerment. The therapists' belief in each client as a therapeutic agent is likely to have a determining influence and empower participants to experience themselves in a similar way. This role expectation for participants promotes a sense of co-creation, control, and helps participants increase a sense of ownership over the group (Giacomucci et al., 2018). While the organization or therapist may have initiated the group, Shulman (2015) reminds us that the participants should have control in the process – after all it is their group.

This emphasis on collaboration and mutuality in the psychodrama process promotes a sense of value and worth for participants. Multiple studies on the effects of psychodrama with various populations demonstrate its effectiveness in increasing self-esteem and self-worth (Gorji, Mohammadi, Mansur, & Konesh, 2011; Mosavi & Haghayegh, 2019; Perry et al., 2016; Ron & Yanai, 2021). Furthermore, a study by Davelaar, Araujo, and Kipper (2008) discovered a positive relationship between spontaneity and both self-esteem and self-efficacy. The mutual aid process within psychodrama groups positions group members to leverage their strengths, experience, and relationship for the greater good of the co-created process. In doing so, all participants are likely to access a deepened feeling of self-worth. This process is depicted in the examples below.

Each of the sociometric processes covered in Chapter 4 offer facilitators with action-based tools that inherently promote collaboration, mutuality, and a sense of belonging in groups. One specific tool that does this well is step-in sociometry. This process quickly and efficiently helps group members to uncover similarities in identity, experience, and goals. Step-in sociometry can help shift a group from isolation and disconnection towards belongingness and collaboration (Giacomucci, 2017). Step-in sociometry organizes the group into a circle where everyone has an equal place which inherently promotes mutuality. An example of this comes from the beginning phases of a mental health support group where most group members struggled with anxiety and depression. Participants were still struggling with a sense of connection to each other and the group-as-a-whole, so the facilitator employs step-in sociometry with the following three prompts for each round:

1) Step in and share something that you like to do in your free time;
2) Step in and share one way thing that you struggle with related to your mental health; and
3) Step in and share one hope or goal you have related to attending this group.

This process quickly illuminates for group members that there are far more similarities and shared experiences in the group than anyone fully realized. While the symptoms of depression and anxiety proved barriers to effortless connection, the step-in sociometry structure provided a container for participants to articulate their interests, struggles, and goals while visually seeing everyone else in the group who shared the same interest, struggle, or goal. A sense of belongingness quickly emerges in sociometric exercises which fuels collaboration and instills mutuality between participants (Giacomucci & Ehrhart, 2021). These tools can be used as stand-alone group interventions or as warm-up processes for a psychodrama enactment or other activity.

The following vignette depicts the power of psychodrama as a catalyzer for collaboration and mutuality within groups.

> Kira is chosen as the protagonist of a psychodrama in an ongoing trauma group. The group chose her topic among others through a sociometric selection, indicating that an overwhelming majority of the group relate to her experience and her goal. Her topic is related to addressing her sense of unworthiness and negative beliefs about herself resulting from complex childhood trauma beginning at age eight. Her goal for the psychodrama is to increase a sense of self-love and self-esteem. As the psychodrama process is beginning, she appears hyperaroused and anxious. As the facilitator, I check-in with her to see if she is okay. She shares about feeling anxious, and in particular, feeling like she doesn't deserve to be the protagonist for the psychodrama. She expresses a sense of guilt in being the center of attention and asks that someone else be the protagonist. I affirm for her that she is in control of the process and that she can choose not to be the protagonist if that is right for her. She quickly moves out of the center of the room (off of the psychodrama stage) and returns to her individual chair in the group circle. Multiple group members begin to spontaneously offer support and encouragement for Kira. I remind her that the group chose her topic because they relate to it and that by being the protagonist, she is helping the rest of the group heal from their trauma too. I reflect to Kira that her topic and her goal were related to worthiness. I suggest that perhaps there is something important for her recovery in feeling worthy to set boundaries and step out of the protagonist role, or in allowing herself to feel worthy enough to be the protagonist for the group. The group continues to offer their support and affirm her worth. Just as quickly as she had stepped out of the center of the group, Kira jumped back into the center of the room indicating her willingness to be the protagonist if the group would support her.
>
> We begin to move into the psychodrama by enrolling strength-based roles. Kira struggles to identify strengths within herself so I ask the group to call out the strengths that they notice Kira demonstrate that may be helpful for the topic and goal at hand. Kira identifies love and determination as roles needed. She chooses two group members to play these roles and starts to create a scene in the center of the group room. Initially Kira struggled to connect with her strengths in the role play but other group members were quick to offer doubling statements for the strengths, conveying to Kira how they see her as loving and determined. Through a series of role reversals and doubling statements she connects with her strengths in a meaningful way. When a role player began to have their own emotions and struggled to articulate supportive messages for Kira, other group members spontaneously emerged from the audience to support the group member while continuing the barrage of strength-based messages from the positive roles. The collaborative spirit of the group surpassed each potential barrier that Kira, other participants, and the group-as-a-whole faced in the process. Remembering Kira's goal,

I suggested that worthiness may be an important role to have in the psychodrama. She invited a group member to play the role and a dialogue with worthiness developed. She explored her relationship with worthiness today and throughout the timeline of her life, indicating that she felt a disconnect with her and worthiness at age eight at the time her trauma began. As she begins to cry, the chorus of positive affirmations from her strengths picks up. I invite any group member who wants to support Kira to step into the circle and onto the stage. To Kira's surprise, the remaining ten group members all stand up and step-in, indicating their desire to support Kira. After checking-in with her about her preferences, I facilitate the supportive group members in standing behind Kira and putting a hand on her shoulder so she can feel the support. Her tense body visibly softens in this moment, and she finds relief in the support of her peers.

Affirmed by the support of the group and her strengths, Kira is better able to connect with the role of worthiness. When I ask her if she wants to go one step further in the psychodrama, she agrees. I facilitate her in choosing a group member to play the role of her at the age of eight when she began to experience her trauma and feel disconnected from worthiness. She unknowingly chooses a young woman in the group who happens to have experienced her own developmental trauma (this is what we would call 'tele' in psychodrama). I coach the new role player on taking on the role of eight-year-old Kira and expressing the feelings of confusion, fear, anger, and unworthiness. I instruct Kira to practice validating this part of herself, to offer support, nurturing, perspective, and an affirmation of worth. With the help of the group, Kira begins to talk to her younger self, offering love and support – "those things that happened were not your fault," "it wasn't fair that you had to go through that, but you found your way and are stronger because of it," and "you may feel like you are worthless, but you have so much value to others – especially those that you will help based on your experience of recovery." Emotional, but grounded, she validates her experience as a child while sharing in the rage and grief of the trauma. By this point, the group member playing the role of younger Kira has accessed her own emotions related to her own childhood trauma and the role reciprocity draws Kira into a deeper place of validating and nurturing herself. I direct Kira to talk to her younger self about worthiness and to help her see her value as a human. She reminds her younger self that it wasn't her fault and that her trauma doesn't have to define her. As she continues to offer statements of worth, the other role player becomes more regulated. I role reverse Kira into the role of herself at age eight and ask them to replay the scene of validation and nurturing, this time with Kira in the opposite role. Through this experience, Kira has an opportunity to verbalize the horror and shame she felt as a child in the safe and nurturing space of the group, her strengths, and her adult self. The role player repeats supportive messages to her and adds new messages related to her worth and value. Kira role reverses back into the role of herself as an adult and ends the scene with a commitment to herself about continue to work on valuing herself going forward.

> After de-roling, the group moves into the sharing phase of the psychodrama and participants share about their own connection to the topic. Each group member took turns celebrating Kira's progress while also sharing about their own difficulties with past trauma and worthiness. Kira is the last to share. She thanks the group for their support and comments on specific points in the process where she felt like she wanted to stop but continued on due to the feeling of the group believing in her, valuing her, and being willing to support her. She shares about feeling lighter after the psychodrama and articulates a greater sense of belonging within the group.

Kira's psychodrama example highlights the role of mutuality and collaboration in the psychodrama process. Peer support became the vehicle for renegotiating a sense of self, enhancing worthiness, and practicing self-love. The psychodrama scene was co-created by the group around the shared topic and goal. The power of the group's collaboration, determination, and love for each other propelled the process forward. The group cohesion and sociometric protagonist selection cultivated tele within the group which ensured that the process was a group-as-a-whole journey and not simply Kira's topic. Kira was a mirror for the group to see themselves, access their own strengths, offer nurturing to themselves in the past after trauma, and affirm their own worth. The role reciprocity enhanced the dynamics within the role-playing. The roles in Kira's psychodrama, played by others in the group, facilitate the group members in accessing their own emotions and parallel parts of self. The sense of mutuality extended beyond the topic and goal into the roles, feelings, and younger part of self. The psychodramatic enactment provides an avenue for co-creation and co-regulation within the group process – "psychodrama, improvisation, and enactment offer multisensory ways to establish co-regulation through role play, modeling, mirroring, and enactment" (Malchiodi, 2020, p. 174).

Conclusion

The principles of collaboration and mutuality promote a sense of belonging, self-respect, self-esteem, trust, safety, peer support, and empowerment. The mutuality experienced in groups and in therapy challenges feelings of unworthiness and negative cognitions resulting from trauma in the past. The group's collaborative process pulls participants in as equals and co-creators – utilizing their strengths in service of the group-as-a-whole. The imprint of the past victim-perpetrator imbalance of power is renegotiated through collaboration and mutuality. The group offers belsonging and a place for everyone. Psychodrama puts this into action through role-playing, emphasizing all participants as therapeutic agents. Trauma-informed group leaders and trauma-informed organizational leaders work to cultivate collaboration and mutuality between all. Everyone's role is seen as essential and important. Trauma-informed leaders help group members and staff to feel a sense of belonging.

References

Ardito, R. B., & Rabellino, D. (2011). Therapeutic alliance and outcome of psychotherapy: historical excursus, measurements, and prospects for research. *Frontiers in Psychology, 2*, 270.

Bloom, S. L. (1998). By the crowd they have been broken, by the crowd they shall be healed: The social transformation of trauma. *Posttraumatic Growth: Positive Changes in the Aftermath of Crisis.* In R. G. Tedeschi, C. L. Park, & L. G. Calhoun (Eds.), *Posttraumatic Growth* (pp. 179–213). New York: Routledge.

Brown, B. (2018). *Dare to lead: Brave work. Tough conversations. Whole hearts*: New York: Random House.

Burlingame, G. M., McClendon, D. T., & Alonso, J. (2011). Cohesion in group therapy. *Psychotherapy, 48*(1), 34.

Burlingame, G. M., McClendon, D. T., & Yang, C. (2018). Cohesion in group therapy: A meta-analysis. *Psychotherapy, 55*(4), 384.

Cockshaw, W. D., Shochet, I. M., & Obst, P. L. (2013). General belongingness, workplace belongingness, and depressive symptoms. *Journal of Community & Applied Social Psychology, 23*(3), 240–251.

Courtois, C. A., & Ford, J. D. (2016). *Treatment of complex trauma: A sequenced, relationship-based approach.* New York: The Guildford Press.

Davelaar, P. M., Araujo, F. S., & Kipper, D. A. (2008). The revised Spontaneity Assessment Inventory (SAI-R): Relationship to goal orientation, motivation, perceived self-efficacy, and self-esteem. *Arts in Psychotherapy, 35*(2), 117–128.

Douglas, K. (2012). When caring stops, staffing doesn't really matter. *Nursing Economics, 28*(6), 415–419.

Fleury, H. J., & Marra, M. M. (2022). Theoretical and methodological foundations of socionomy. In H. J. Fleury, M. M. Marra, & O. H. Hadler (Eds.), *Psychodrama in Brazil* (pp. 17–29). Singapore: Springer.

Fosslien, L., & Duffy, M. W. (2019). *No hard feelings: The secret power of embracing emotions at work*. New York: Penguin.

Foy, D. W., Unger, W. S., & Wattenberg, M. S. (2005). Module 4: An overview of evidence-based group approaches to trauma with adults. In B. Buchele, & H. Spitz (Eds.), *Group interventions for treatment of psychological trauma* (pp. 116–166). New York City: American Group Psychotherapy Association.

Gerbrandt, N., Grieser, R., & Enns, V. (2021). *A little book about trauma-informed workplaces*. Winnipeg: Achieve Publishing.

Giacomucci, S. (2017). The sociodrama of life or death: Young adults and addiction treatment. *Journal of Psychodrama, Sociometry, and Group Psychotherapy, 65*(1), 137–143. https://doi.org/10.12926/ 0731–1273-65.1.137

Giacomucci, S. (2019). Social group work in action: A sociometry, psychodrama, and experiential trauma group therapy curriculum. *Doctorate in Social Work (DSW) Dissertations*, 124. Retrieved from https://repository.upenn.edu/cgi/ viewcontent.cgi?article=1128&context=edissertations_sp2

Giacomucci, S. (2021a). Experiential sociometry in group work: Mutual aid for the group-as-a-whole. *Social work with Groups, 44*(3), 204–214.

Giacomucci, S. (2021b). *Social work, sociometry, and psychodrama: Experiential approaches for group therapists, community leaders, and social workers*. Springer Nature. https://doi.org/10.1007/978-981-33-6342-7

Giacomucci, S., & Ehrhart, L. (2021). Introduction to psychodrama psychotherapy: A trauma and addiction group vignette. *Group, 45*(1), 69–86.

Giacomucci, S., Gera, S., Briggs, D., & Bass, K. (2018). Experiential addiction treatment: Creating positive connection through sociometry and therapeutic spiral model safety structures. *Journal of Addiction and Addictive Disorders, 5*, 17. https://doi.org/10.24966/AAD-7276/100017

Gorji, Z., Mohammadi, A. Z., Mansur, L., & Konesh, A. K. (2011). The effect of psychodrama on self-esteem and forgiveness of female adolescents with divorced parents. *Journal of Family Research, 7*(7.1), 195–209.

Harris, M., & Fallot, R. (2001). Using trauma theory to design service systems. *New Directions for Mental Health Services*, 89. Jossey Bass.

Hartmann, S. (2018). The power of we: The effects of mutuality and team reflexivity on team resilience in the workplace. *Academy of Management Proceedings, 1*, 11708.

Herman, J. L. (1992). *Trauma and recovery: The aftermath of violence—From domestic abuse to political terror*. New York: Basic Books.

Horvath, A. O., & Symonds, B. D. (1991). Relation between working alliance and outcome in psychotherapy: A meta-analysis. *Journal of Counseling Psychology*, 38(2), 139.

Lambert, M. J., & Barley, D. E. (2001). Research summary on the therapeutic relationship and psychotherapy outcome. *Psychotherapy: Theory, Research, Practice, Training*, 38(4), 357.

Malchiodi, C. A. (2020). *Trauma and expressive arts therapy: Brain, body, and imagination in the healing process*. New York: Guilford Press.

Moreno, J. L. (1962). *Code of ethics for group psychotherapy and psychodrama: Relationship to the Hippocratic Oath*. Beacon, NY: Beacon House.

Moreno, J. L. (2019). *The autobiography of a genius* (E. Schreiber, S. Kelley, & S. Giacomucci, Eds.). United Kingdom: North West Psychodrama Association

Mosavi, H., & Haghayegh, S. A. (2019). Efficacy of psychodrama on social anxiety, self-esteem and psychological well-being of university students that met diagnosis of social anxiety disorder. *Knowledge & Research in Applied Psychology*, 20(3), 22–30.

Northouse, P. G. (2021). *Leadership: Theory and practice*. Los Angeles: SAGE publications.

Perry, R., Saby, K., Wenos, J., Hudgins, K., & Baller, S. (2016). Psychodrama intervention for female service members using the therapeutic spiral model. *The Journal of Psychodrama, Sociometry, and Group Psychotherapy*, 64(1), 11–23.

Ron, Y., & Yanai, L. (2021). Empowering through psychodrama: A qualitative study at domestic violence shelters. *Frontiers in Psychology*, 12, 1017.

Slattery, S. M., & Goodman, L. A. (2009). Secondary traumatic stress among domestic violence advocates: Workplace risk and protective factors. *Violence against Women*, 15(11), 1358–1379.

Shulman, L. (2015). *The skills of helping individuals, families, groups, and communities* (8th ed.). Boston, MA: Cengage Learning.

Sinek, S. (2014). *Leaders eat last: Why some teams pull together and others don't*. New York: Penguin.

Substance Abuse and Mental Health Services Administration. (1999). *Brief interventions and brief therapies for substance abuse*. Treatment Improvement Protocol (TIP) Series, No. 34. Rockville, MD: Substance Abuse and Mental Health Services Administration.

Yalom, I. D., & Leszcz, M. (2020). *The theory and practice of group psychotherapy* (6th ed.). New York: Basic Books.

9
Empowerment, Voice, and Choice in Group Therapy, Psychodrama, and Leadership

Chapter Summary

Trauma is characterized by unspeakable terror, helplessness, and powerlessness which are fundamentally disempowering. In most cases, the victim of a trauma has their voice, choice, and power taken from them. Group work and psychodrama are methods that offer a multitude of possibilities for empowerment, voice, and choice. The safety and support of the group provide a container for one to reconnect with their autonomy and personal power. The psychodramatic approach places a strong emphasis on empowerment and choice while also including an intervention called *doubling*, which helps a client give voice to the unspoken. Empowerment, voice, and choice are also important principles for organizational leaders to incorporate into the culture of their workplace. Trauma-informed leaders honor the preferences and perspectives of their staff while empowering others.

Trauma Is Inherently Disempowering

An overwhelming traumatic experience is inherently disempowering. Trauma rarely involves much choice or respect for one's voice. Instead, trauma survivors are subject to a sense of powerlessness, voicelessness, and domination by a perpetrator of the circumstances. Terror and helplessness ensue. The loss of control, disempowerment, and sense of being trapped at the time of the trauma often carry over into other areas of a survivor's life. Other mental health issues or substance use disorders may develop, which

DOI: 10.4324/9781003277859-9

recreate a similar sense of powerlessness and disempowerment (SAMHSA, 2014b). These issues compound into a more complex and layered experience of stuckness.

Trauma has the power to corrupt core belief systems, arouse intense emotions, provoke unbearable physiological sensations, and discombobulate the nervous system for years to come. Even decades after a traumatic event, many trauma survivors continue to feel as though their past experience persists to have power over them – including their thoughts, feelings, physical sensations, relationships, sense of self, and behavior in the world. A traumatic incident often disintegrates one's sense of personal power, mastery, confidence, and control (Klein & Schermer, 2000) – even the healthiest and most resilient individuals. By its very nature, trauma is overwhelming and disempowering. It usurps power from the victim. The loss of personal power corresponds to a loss of confidence, safety, trust in the world, voice, and choice.

Trauma and traumatic stress impact one's ability to speak up and have a voice. In the moment of trauma, a victim cries out for help and protection. The unanswered cry at the time of trauma results in another layer of the experience – abandonment. The authorities, allies, and/or caregivers who were expected to protect or intervene did not. Instead, the trauma survivor experiences an abandonment on top of the perpetration. Along with this comes a sense of one's voice not being heard in crucial moments and a distrust that others will listen in the future when needed. Some have compared this compounded sense of voicelessness as similar to learned helplessness, even generating a new term – *learned voicelessness* (Hardy, 2019). It is important to include that learned voicelessness is less of a reflection on one's ability to speak up, and more of a reflection on the repeated dismissal and abandonment of those who refuse to listen or respond. Furthermore, trauma has a neuropsychological impact on one's ability to access language and speech. Rauch and colleagues' groundbreaking research (1996) highlighted how the speech and language centers of the brain are significantly impacted and inhibited when someone remembers a traumatic memory (van der Kolk, 2014). The voicelessness resulting from trauma has roots in the neurobiology of the survivor, the socioemotional impact of the trauma, and the failure of other people or systems to prevent or intervene on the trauma.

How am I elevating the voice of my clients and avoiding re-enactments of abandonment?

Trauma rarely involves choice. Instead, it is often characterized by a lack of choice, by coercion, and domination. In most cases, a victim's sense of choice is revoked from them in the moment of trauma – replaced with helplessness and powerlessness. In some cases of trauma, a survivor blames themselves for prior choices that they made which they feel directly or indirectly caused the trauma. In other situations, one might experience trauma as a direct result of choices that they made, which can also lead to a complicated relationship to one's sense of autonomy or ability to make healthy decisions. Furthermore, some experiences of trauma involve circumstances where a victim's choices are limited to multiple adverse options – a lose–lose situation. Regardless, in the aftermath of trauma, one's relationship to choice is tainted. A sense of autonomy becomes shaky due to the overwhelming experience of coercion, force, or subjugation. Klein and Schermer (2000) even describe trauma as "a terrifying experience of helplessness and entrapped dependency" (p. 10). This initial loss of autonomy may be at the root of reenactments of dependence, enmeshment, and unequal power dynamics within relationships long after the trauma is over.

In what specific ways do I promote choice and autonomy in my work with trauma survivors?

Trauma's devastating impacts on one's sense of empowerment, choice, and voice make each of these principles essential to a trauma-informed approach. Survivors' power, voice, and choice have been so often diminished; therefore, our approaches must orient around restoring power, voice, and choice (SAMHSA, 2014a). This process of empowerment must also involve a differentiation between healthy personal power and an abuse of personal power (Bloom & Farragher, 2011). The experience of accessing one's personal power or coming to roles of authority after being powerless, disempowered, and marginalized can easily flip flop to the opposite extreme, causing another reenactment of abusive power. The empowerment process in trauma-informed work is a rebalancing of power dynamics and a restoration of mutuality, voice, and choice. Herman (1992) even suggests empowerment as the first and foremost principle of recovery.

Empowered by the Group

Group work offers an intervention uniquely effective in its capacity for empowerment, voice, and choice. "The core experiences of psychological trauma are disempowerment and disconnection from others. Recovery, therefore, is based upon the empowerment of the survivor and the creation of new connections" (Herman 1992, p. 133). The connection and support within groups and communities are ripe with opportunities for empowerment, voice, and choice. The group provides a safe place for experimentation with choice and voice while also offering role modeling from other participants who have experienced similar trauma (Courtois, 2010). The mutual aid process and peer support within groups initiates a collective sense of empowerment for the group-as-a-whole and for each member within the group (Yalom & Leszcz, 2020). This group-as-a-whole process and synchronicity promotes a mutual regulation between group members (Malchiodi, 2020). The group that accesses its collective power also initiates a parallel process of each individual harnessing their own personal power and empowerment. Therapeutic factors such as hope, universality, altruism, imitative behavior, interpersonal learning, and cohesiveness fuel the reciprocity of empowerment between members and the group-as-a-whole.

Stark and Flitcraft define empowerment as "the convergence of mutual support with individual autonomy" (1988, pp. 140–141, as cited by Herman, 1992). This conceptualization of empowerment is particularly poignant in the context of group work. The group provides mutual support while recognizing individual autonomy of each member. Here we find a unification of all of the trauma-informed principles (safety, trust, transparency, peer support, collaboration, mutuality, voice, choice, cultural, historic, and gender issues) fueling a sense of empowerment. The group process provides a trauma survivor with a sense of being a part of something larger than self which is inherently empowering. Klein and Schermer (2000) describe by suggesting that "together we constitute the healing matrix of compassion and empowerment from which, individually, we have become isolated" (p. 17). This group matrix cultivates a sense of collective power that allows participants to also reconnect to the power within themselves individually.

When have I been in a (formal or informal) group, classroom, or community that felt empowering?

What were the conditions that led to this sense of collective and individual empowerment?

Part of the empowerment process is a reconnection to autonomy and choice. Trauma impacts one's ability to choose; however, the group process offers multiple opportunities for participants to practice making choices and setting boundaries. Boundary setting is often and undervalued, yet extraordinarily important skill in trauma recovery. In my experience, nobody can maintain long term trauma recovery (or any other recovery for that matter) without developing the ability to say no, set boundaries, and maintain those boundaries. Boundary setting is the utilization of choice and voice. The group process initiates a laboratory of sorts for experimenting with boundaries and choice – often role modeled by the group leader and other participants. This trauma-informed principle of choice promotes a reconnection to autonomy for the trauma survivor. In the aftermath of trauma, many feel that they have lost their autonomy; the group process helps recover this vital sense of ownership over one's life and choices.

Group empowerment also helps to cultivate one's ability to speak up and have their voice heard. The group becomes a safe place for participants to practice speaking up for themselves and others. Often in a group process when an individual is quiet, other participants or the group leader will encourage them to give voice to their experience or perspective on the issues at hand. In this way, the group process creates space for and elevates unheard voices while offering participants frequent role modeling of social skills and communication strategies. The overwhelming nature of trauma and the resulting posttraumatic stress disorder symptoms often makes it feel unspeakable. The experience of abandonment in the moment of trauma adds an additional layer of mistrust, and perhaps learned voicelessness – that even if one does speak up, their voice will be dismissed. Group therapy reverses this through corrective experiences – "the group serves as a symbolic societal witness to each victim's experience, as it is retold and relived in the group process" (Johnson & Lubin, 2000, p. 142). The group itself becomes a container for participants to share their story and be heard and seen by others who understand. The sharing of one's narrative and traumatic experiences in the safety of the group gives others the courage to also share their experiences. This is depicted in the group example below:

> New members are joining an ongoing trauma group for the first time. They appear timid, guarded, fearful, and hypervigilant at the start of the group. After the establishment of group rules and norms the group process continues to unfold. A longer standing group member initiates a discussion about how the current events related to the war in Ukraine have been triggering past memories of war trauma. He mentions thinking that others won't understand, but that he feels the need to share anyways. To his surprise other group members nod their heads in agreement. One group member, who hadn't shared about her childhood at all yet, jumps in the discussion revealing that images in the news were activating powerful emotions related to growing up in Bosnia and

leaving during the war. Others begin to empathize and offer their own sharing of how other current events trigger their past traumas. A queer group member shares about how painful it is to watch the news due to new anti-LGTBQ laws enacted throughout the country. Another participant reveals that current events about racism and hate crimes bring them back memories and experiences when they experienced racism themselves. As individuals shared their experiences, new group members began to chime in too. The group-as-a-whole spontaneously discovered a shared commonality and created a space for each person's experience to be voiced and heard. The courage and vulnerability of some group members prompted courage and vulnerability for others to speak up. With the guidance of the group leader, the group worked together to develop strategies and skills for coping with their trauma and how current events were triggering it. In this way, the group centered the principles of empowerment and voice.

Fostering Empowerment through Trauma-Informed Leadership

Organizational leadership, like group leadership, is enhanced through a process of centralizing empowerment, voice, and choice. This is also true for educators, supervisors, and other leaders. Trauma-informed leaders empower others to access their own leadership within. They elevate unheard voices and work with others to access power within the group rather than only use power over others. Gerbrandt, Grieser, and Enns, in *A Little Book About Trauma-Informed Workplaces* (2021), suggest to leaders that "one way to think about providing choice is to shift from holding *power over* to sharing *power with* others. A *power with* approach grows out of relationships that are built on mutual respect and support" (p. 38). Here, again, we see a convergence of other trauma-informed principles. In order to practice *power with* others and empowerment, a leader must attend to relational and organization safety, trust, transparency, peer support, collaboration, mutuality, voice, choice, and address issues related to culture, history, and gender.

In spaces where I have power, how can I practice "power with" rather than "power over" others?

A meta-analysis on empowerment in organizations discovered that individual empowerment and team empowerment are closely related, and that psychological empowerment is positively correlated with employee outcomes, job satisfaction, commitment to the organization, and performance while being negatively correlated with staff strain and turnover (Seibert, Wang, & Courtright, 2011). Empowerment in organizations is often fueled by the provision of choice, autonomy, and decision-making power. Staff who feel empowered by their leaders are better able to adapt to the needs of their clients (Chebat & Kollias, 2000). Leaders can promote empowerment, voice, and choice through collaboration with staff, providing professional development opportunities, involving staff in decision-making, giving staff some autonomy in defining/re-defining their role, providing access to organizational information, giving staff ownership in the organization and its initiatives, employing self-led teams, and utilizing democratic decision-making processes (such as employing sociometry tools from Chapter 4 to explore organizational preferences).

In group work, leaders are more likely to approach the group as belonging to the members rather than to the leader. This same paradigm may be useful for organizational leaders and educators. The organization doesn't exist without its staff. Leaders can empower their staff by creating space for their voices to be heard and their perspectives and ideas to be honored. When possible, leaders can prioritize the preferences of workers and provide opportunities for advancement and funding for professional growth. Leaders should strive to empower their staff, supervisees, and students to be the best that they can be. At times this might even mean encouraging and supporting staff to change roles or organizations. A therapy group becomes a container for participants to elevate their voice, practice decision-making and communication skills, and access a sense of empowerment – in a similar way, so too can the organizational group. Leaders need to engage in ongoing communication with staff and value their feedback and ideas. Staff who feel heard, respected, invested in, and empowered are going to not only be better workers and provide better services to clients, but are likely to also experience personal growth in the process. As leaders, we must keep in mind that a large portion of our staff are likely to be trauma survivors. Centralizing trauma-informed principles, in particular voice, choice, and empowerment, will help our staff to be the best that they can be.

When staff are empowered, supported, and involved in decision-making they will simply be better able to provide higher quality services and experiences to clients. Leaders who integrate feedback from staff and embody trauma-informed principles are also offering staff with role modeling for ways they can integrate these same principles with their clients. A parallel process will emerge between leaders–staff and staff–clients when empowerment, voice, and choice are centralized (SAMHSA, 2014a). Harris and Fallot remind us that:

> The goal of the trauma-informed service system is to return a sense of control and autonomy to the consumer-survivor. A trauma-informed system holds to the underlying belief that if consumers learn to understand and ultimately to control their responses, then they will need less, if any, help from service providers. Like the proverb, 'Give a hungry man a fish, and you feed him today, Teach him to fish, and you feed him forever,' the provider's job becomes helping the consumer to master the skills necessary to cope in healthy and constructive ways."
>
> (2001, p. 16)

Of course, this same wisdom also applies to empowering staff to be self-sufficient, autonomous, and to work with a sense of self-efficacy. The organization should cultivate a core belief in the resilience, strength, and capacity of both the clients served and the staff employed (SAMHSA, 2014a). Leaders and staff are approached as facilitators of recovery rather than controllers of recovery (Brown, Baker, & Wilcox, 2012 as cited in SAMHSA, 2014a). Trauma-informed leaders and staff are quick to seek feedback from those they work with and make program changes based on suggestions from staff and clients. The ongoing work and evolution of a trauma-informed workplace is informed by the experience of all involved.

How do I elicit and incorporate feedback from clients, community members, co-workers, and staff to refine my work, program offerings, and organization?

Is my workplace empowering or disempowering?

Empowerment through Psychodrama

The psychodramatic approach and philosophy center empowerment as a core principle. The philosophical commitment to empowerment in psychodrama is outlined in Moreno's code of ethics (1962) and his belief in every participant as a therapeutic agent (Giacomucci, 2019, 2021a). Psychodrama empowers participants to reclaim control of their life through role-playing. The role-playing process allows participants to enact scenes that one might crave to experience for closure, to change the outcomes of past experiences, to practice for future situations, and to explore various aspects of self and reintegrate them in a new way (Giacomucci & Marquit, 2020). In psychodrama, the protagonist can experience things that would be impossible otherwise. The surplus reality of the process is inherently empowering as it makes the impossible possible (Giacomucci & Ehrhart, 2021). This provides potent potentialities for corrective emotional experiences, renegotiated internalized trauma, and activating experiential healing possibilities within the body and brain (Dayton, 2015; Giacomucci, 2018, 2021b; Giacomucci & Stone, 2019; Malchiodi, 2020).

Morenean philosophy articulates the presence of an autonomous healing center within – a self-directed and self-healing capacity deep within the self, only activated through action (Z. T. Moreno, 2012). Zerka Moreno even suggests that the primary goal of all therapies is to help remove barriers so that the client can access this autonomous healing center (Giacomucci, Karner, Nieto, & Schreiber, 2021). A recent study demonstrated increases in psychodrama participants' autonomy, self-compassion, and sense of authorship over their own life, while also indicating decreases in one's susceptibility to control (Kantas & Mavili, 2021). Another study with Syrian refugees found participation in a psychodrama group empowered participants to increase their quality of life while decreasing frequency of domestic violence experiences (Damra, 2022). These findings help support psychodrama as an effective modality in promoting empowerment for participants. In the context of trauma-informed principles of empowerment, voice, and choice, it is important to emphasize that this core philosophical concept also inherently emphasizes a client's right to *autonomy* and choice. This is further operationalized in psychodrama practice through the popular director's motto, "follow the protagonist." Kellermann (2000) reminds us that the client-centered nature of following the protagonist is particularly important in terms of centering the trauma-informed principles of empowerment. Others have suggested that following the protagonist in trauma-focused psychodrama may be problematic, or even unsafe, at times due to the potential of following the protagonist into a trauma reenactment (Hudgins & Toscani, 2013). I would suggest a balanced approach to trauma-informed psychodrama directing, guided by the motto of "follow-lead-follow the protagonist" – borrowed from Dyadic Developmental Psychotherapy's "follow-lead-follow" approach (Hughes, Golding, & Hudson, 2019). This paradigm centers the client as the expert in their experience while promoting empowerment, voice, and choice but also articulates the psychodrama director's responsibility to safely lead the process. Each and every psychodramatic enactment contains a multitude of choice points as the psychodrama is co-created spontaneously. Most of these choices are protagonist driven based on the protagonist's goal, experience, or preference.

These principles of empowerment, voice, and choice are also embodied in the experiential sociometry processes outlined in Chapter 4, which are often used as warm ups for a psychodrama enactment. These sociometry tools empower the group to give voice to their concerns, identify a central concern of the group, and identify the protagonist for the session through democratic choice. The collective group choices and preferences allow the director to follow the group-as-a-whole. One simple sociometry tool that depicts this is the use of a locogram. A facilitator could initiate discussion in the group around options for topics in the current or future session and designate each corner of the group room to represent one of the different group topics. Then, each group member is asked to stand in the area of the room corresponding to the topic that would help them the most in that group. Instead of the facilitator choosing the topic, locograms can be used to empower the group to choose its own topic. Similar to locograms, the floor check sociometry process can also be used to promote empowerment, voice, and choice within groups. One such example is a floor check with the following prompts, using the five domains of posttraumatic growth: Increased Personal Strength, Appreciation of Life, Relationships, Spiritual/Religious Growth, and New Possibilities in Life.

1) Which do you feel you experience the most of due to trauma?
2) Which do you most need to work on in order to grow from your trauma?
3) Which do you feel you have been working on and made some progress in?

Each prompt in this floor check process would generate a new clustering of participants at each domain of posttraumatic growth and provide them with a chance to share their experience, name their struggles, and articulate their areas of growth for the future. The floor check is particularly adept at providing choices for participants and honoring each individual's choice while providing them with opportunities to voice the reasoning for their choice. Floor checks are innately empowering as they position participants as therapeutic agents for each other and promote mutual aid within the group, empowering each person as an agent of change for the group (Giacomucci, 2020).

Psychodrama elevates the voice of the group and the protagonist in each phase of the group process – warm up, action, and sharing. In the warming-up phase, the group gives voice to the shared concerns and issues while sociometrically/democratically choosing a topic and protagonist. In the action phase of the psychodrama session, the protagonist not only gives voice to their concerns but also goes beyond words to enact and embody the topic and goal. Rather than simply talking about experiences in the past, internalized aspect of traumas, defense mechanisms, symptoms, or other issues, the psychodrama process brings these issues to life through action. The psychodrama role/intervention of doubling is uniquely designed to help the protagonist give voice to unspoken aspects of the experience. In the final phase of the group, sharing, each group member has an opportunity to give voice to their experience in the group and their past experiences as they relate to the topic and goals of the psychodrama. In this way, the three phases of the psychodrama move the group process from centering the voice of the group-as-a-whole, the voice of the protagonist (who's issue represents the group's issue), and the voice of each participant individually. Furthermore, the role training capacity in psychodrama provides participants with opportunities to develop their voice, practice social skills, and strengthen their ability to speak up for themselves and others.

When directing psychodramas, it is important for the facilitator to be aware of their own identity and how it may impact one's sense of safety, voice, choice, or empowerment in the process. As a white male professional, I find it particularly important to remind participants, especially protagonists who have been harmed by white men in power, that they have full power and control over the process. I let them know that they will have the autonomy to make choices throughout the psychodrama and that we will co-facilitate it together. I explicitly ask the protagonist to let me know if anything feels inaccurate, or if they feel like the process is too much, too little, or going in a direction different than they'd like to. The following example depicts a psychodrama session with an ongoing psychodrama group focused on empowerment.

> After multiple sessions together and the warming-up process, the group has established the safety and containment necessary to move deeper into trauma processing work together. Jenn is chosen as the protagonist with the topic of finding her voice in recovery and developing self-worth. As the psychodrama emerges, the protagonist, shares about their past experience of abusive relationships and how her struggles with worthiness and speaking up seem to stem from here. The protagonist chooses strength-based roles of safety and determination to help with her goal. In the psychodramatic dialogue with safety Jenn develops a stronger sense of how to keep herself safe and how to access safety when she feels overwhelmed. In the role reversal with safety, Jenn reminds herself that she can find safety in her support system and by taking deep breaths. Through her connection with safety and determination, Jenn accesses the motivation and boldness to bounce back and speak up for what she needs or wants. The constant messages from determination and safety help provide Jenn with the mix of grounding and courage that she needs to feel empowered. Next, the director asks Jenn if she has any role models for empowerment and speaking up – she chooses Daenerys Targaryen (of the television

series Game of Thrones) and invites a group member to play the role. In her psychodramatic dialogue with Daenerys Targaryen, she finds inspiration and guidance on how to stand up for herself. Feeling fortified by the group, Jenn indicates that she is ready to practice standing up for herself.

The director asks Jenn if she'd like to practice this with her abusive ex-boyfriend, with the internalized messages of unworthiness from the abuse, or to practice it in a more symbolic manor helping Daenerys fight off a villain. Jenn chooses the second option, indicating that she isn't going back to her ex-boyfriend, but that the negative messages from him continue to impact her. She chooses someone to play the role of these negative messages and externalizes them through the psychodramatic role play. In the process, she practices combatting these negative voices with the support of her strengths, Daenerys Targaryen, and the group. The director instructs the role player of the negative voices to keep articulating the negative voices until they feel convinced by Jenn to back off. This puts a stronger role demand and stronger role reciprocity on Jenn to advocate for herself. Jenn struggles at first but is supported by the group. The director invites group members to offer doubling statements for Jenn to the negative voice which helps her find her own voice. As she practices advocating for herself and using her voice, the role of the negative voices gets quieter, less verbal, and starts to naturally step away from Jenn. The group applauds Jenn's success. As she stands with Daenerys Targaryen, her posture and sense of empowerment has visibly shifted. In a closing scene, the director helps Jenn integrate new, positive cognitions from her supportive roles to replace the old negative cognitions related to her abuse.

In this example, the empowerment potential within psychodrama is clearly demonstrated. Jenn was able to access the support of the group, expand her inner strength, and utilize archetypal support from Daenerys Targaryen to effectively renegotiate her relationship with the negative cognitions associated with her past abuse. The doubling statements of the group helped Jenn to find her own voice. The practice of speaking back to the negative voices offered Jenn an opportunity for role training and developing a new sense of voice and empowerment. The director offered Jenn multiple choices throughout the process rather than being overly prescriptive or being too passive that she felt a lack of guidance. This is a good example of the "follow-lead-follow" approach to psychodrama directing described previously. The choices toward the end of the process are particularly important to examine.

In this case, I offered Jenn with multiple choices for the next role. Each choice related to her goal and topic but addressed it from a different angle – from the interpersonal (her abusive ex-boyfriend), the intrapsychic (the introjected messages from the abusive relationship), or the symbolic (a villain). These three options each involved varying levels of intensity and proximity to the trauma and to the perpetrator. If I had assessed clinically that any of these options would have been too overwhelming, dysregulating, or retraumatizing for Jenn or anyone else in the group, I would not have offered them. Offering symbolic roles is a way of initiating aesthetic distance and playfulness into the process which helps keep the group within their window of tolerance – this is also routinely used in drama therapy (Sajnani & Johnson, 2014). In phase one trauma groups, it is not advisable to use perpetrator roles. Working with perpetrators in psychodrama should be reserved for phase two groups once safety, strengths, cohesion, and coping skills have already been established. Another possibility in this scene could have been to include some structured and safe physical exertion as Jenn fought back the negative voice. The physical act of pushing this voice off the stage while standing up for herself may have proved to have been even more corrective and empowering as it may have helped activate her sympathetic nervous system in the process and provide the completion of survival responses that may be incomplete from the time of the trauma. This process, informed by Polyvagal theory (Porges, 2017) and Somatic Experiencing (Levine, 2010), would have had to be carefully done to ensure physical safety for all involved. Furthermore, in any scene that involves antagonist roles, trauma roles, or perpetrator roles, it is necessary to engage in a more involved de-roling process. Generally, de-roling involves the role players verbally stating to the protagonist, in front of the group, that they are no longer the role and restating their name. This often involves a symbolic process of physically shaking off, or whipping off, the role to help the participant de-role psychologically. Another advanced de-roling strategy is to instruct the role player to place their role into an empty chair and speak to the role, telling it how they are different from it. These de-roling processes help prevent ongoing projections or transferences between participants related to roles and helps prevent a role player from getting stuck in an antagonistic role that they may have played in the scene (for more on de-roling, see Giacomucci, 2021b).

Conclusion

Trauma disrupts a sense of voice, choice, and empowerment. These trauma-informed principles help trauma survivors to reclaim the power and autonomy lost in the aftermath of adversity. Trauma-informed group leaders and organizational leaders work to embody these principles in their leadership. In trauma-informed spaces, participants and staff's voices are elevated. Feedback from all involved is considered and preferences are honored whenever possible. Group work and psychodrama both provide trauma survivors with increased potentialities for voice, choice, and empowerment. Psychodrama's action-based process initiates an embodied experience of empowerment with role training focused on trauma recovery tasks. Doubling in psychodrama helps the protagonist and the group to reclaim their voice individually and collectively. Trauma-informed psychodrama directors employ a follow-lead-follow approach that effectively empowers the group and offers choices for action while still delivering structure and guidance of the psychodramatic process.

References

Bloom, S. L., & Farragher, B. (2011). *Destroying sanctuary: The crisis in human services delivery systems*. New York: Oxford University Press.

Brown, S. M., Baker, C. N., & Wilcox, P. (2012). Risking connection trauma training: A pathway toward trauma-informed care in child congregate care settings. *Psychological Trauma: Theory, Research, Practice, and Policy, 4*(5), 507–515.

Chebat, J. C., & Kollias, P. (2000). The impact of empowerment on customer contact employees' roles in service organizations. *Journal of Service Research, 3*(1), 66–81.

Courtois, C. A. (2010). *Healing the incest wound* (2nd ed.). New York: W. W. Norton & Company.

Damra, J. K. (2022). The effects of psychodrama intervention on intimate partner violence and quality of life: Trial of Syrian refugee abused women. *Journal of International Women's Studies, 23*(1), 33.

Dayton, T. (2015). *NeuroPsychodrama in the treatment of relational trauma: A strength-based, experiential model for healing PTSD*. Deerfield Beach, FL: Health Communications, Inc.

Gerbrandt, N., Grieser, R., & Enns, V. (2021). *A little book about trauma-informed workplaces*. Winnipeg, B: Achieve Publishing.

Giacomucci, S. (2018). The trauma survivor's inner role atom: A clinical map for post-traumatic growth. *Journal of Psychodrama, Sociometry, and Group Psychotherapy, 66*(1): 115–129.

Giacomucci, S. (2019). Social group work in action: A sociometry, psychodrama, and experiential trauma group therapy curriculum. *Doctorate in Social Work (DSW) Dissertations*, 124. Retrieved from https://repository.upenn.edu/cgi/viewcontent.cgi?article=1128&context=edissertations_sp2

Giacomucci, S. (2020). Addiction, traumatic loss, and guilt: A case study resolving grief through psychodrama and sociometric connections. *The Arts in Psychotherapy, 67*, 101627. https://doi.org/10.1016/j.aip.2019.101627

Giacomucci, S. (2021a). Experiential sociometry in group work: Mutual aid for the group-as-a-whole. *Social Work with Groups, 44*(3), 204–214.

Giacomucci, S. (2021b). *Social work, sociometry, and psychodrama: Experiential approaches for group therapists, community leaders, and social workers.* Springer Nature. https://doi.org/10.1007/978-981-33-6342-7

Giacomucci, S., & Ehrhart, L. (2021). Introduction to psychodrama psychotherapy: A trauma and addiction group vignette. *Group, 45*(1), 69–86.

Giacomucci, S., Karner, D., Nieto, L., & Schreiber, E. (2021). Sociatry, psychodrama, and social work: Moreno's mysticism and social justice tradition. *Social Work with Groups, 44*(3), 288–303. https://doi.org/10.1080/01609513.2021.1885826

Giacomucci, S., & Marquit, J. (2020). The effectiveness of trauma-focused psychodrama in the treatment of PTSD in inpatient substance abuse treatment. *Frontiers in Psychology, 11*, 896. https://doi.org/10.3389%2Ffpsyg.2020.00896

Giacomucci, S., & Stone, A. M. (2019). Being in two places at once: Renegotiating traumatic experience through the surplus reality of psychodrama. *Social Work with Groups, 42*(3), 184–196. https://doi.org/10.1080/01609513.2018.1533913

Hardy, K. V. (2019). The sociocultural trauma of poverty: Theoretical and clinical considerations in working with poor families. In M. McGoldrick, & K. V. Harty (Eds.), *Re-visioning family therapy: Addressing diversity in clinical practice* (pp. 57–72). New York: The Guilford Press.

Herman, J. L. (1992). *Trauma and recovery: The aftermath of violence—From domestic abuse to political terror.* New York: Basic Books.

Hudgins, M. K., & Toscani, F. (2013). *Healing world trauma with the therapeutic spiral model: Stories from the frontlines.* London: Jessica Kingsley Publishers.

Hughes, D. A., Golding, K. S., & Hudson, J. (2019). *Healing relational trauma with attachment-focused interventions: Dyadic developmental psychotherapy with children and families.* New York: WW Norton & Company.

Johnson, R. J., & Lubin, H. (2000). Group psychotherapy for the symptoms of post-traumatic stress disorder. In R. H. Klein, & V. L. Schermer (Eds.), *Group psychotherapy for psychological trauma* (pp. 141–169). New York: The Guilford Press.

Kantas, Ö., & Mavili, A. (2021). Self-determination theory as a suitable theoretical basis and measurement approach for psychodrama interventions. *Journal of the Psychodrama, Sociometry, and Group Psychotherapy, 68*(1), 7–32.

Kellerman, P. F. (2000). The therapeutic effects of psychodrama with traumatized people. In P. F. Kellermann, & K. Hudgins (Eds.), *Psychodrama with trauma survivors: Acting out your pain* (pp. 23–40). Philadelphia, PA: Jessica Kingsley Publishing.

Klein, R. H., & Schermer, V. L. (2000). *Group psychotherapy for psychological trauma.* New York: The Guilford Press.

Levine, P. A. (2010). *In an unspoken voice: How the body releases trauma and restores goodness.* Berkeley, CA: North Atlantic Books.

Malchiodi, C. A. (2020). *Trauma and expressive arts therapy: Brain, body, and imagination in the healing process:* New York: Guilford Press.

Moreno, J. L. (1962). *Code of ethics for group psychotherapy and psychodrama: Relationship to the Hippocratic Oath* (No. 31). Beacon, NY: Beacon House.

Moreno, Z. T. (2012). *To dream again: A memoir.* New York: Mental Health Resources.

Porges, S. W. (2017). *The pocket guide to the Polyvagal theory: The transformative power of feeling safe.* New York: W.W. Norton & Company

Rauch, S. L., van der Kolk, B. A., Fisler, R. E., et al. (1996). A symptom provocation study of posttraumatic stress disorder using positron emission tomography and script-driven imagery. *Archives of General Psychiatry, 53*(5), 380–387.

Sajnani, N., & Johnson, D. R. (2014). *Trauma-informed drama therapy: Transforming clinics, classrooms, and communities:* Springfield: Charles C Thomas Publisher.

Seibert, S. E., Wang, G., & Courtright, S. H. (2011). Antecedents and consequences of psychological and team empowerment in organizations: A meta-analytic review. *Journal of Applied Psychology, 96*(5), 981–1003. https://doi.org/10.1037/a0022676

Stark, E., & Flitcraft, A. (1988). Personal power and institutional victimization: Treating the dual trauma of woman battering. In F. Ochberg (Ed.), *Post-traumatic therapy and victims of violence* (pp. 115–151). New York: Brunner/Mazel.

Substance Abuse and Mental Health Services Administration. (2014a). *SAMHSA's concept of trauma and guidance for a trauma-informed approach.* HHS Publication No. (SMA) 14-4884. Rockville, MD: Substance Abuse and Mental Health Services Administration.

Substance Abuse and Mental Health Services Administration. (2014b). *Trauma-informed care in behavioral health services.* Treatment Improvement Protocol (TIP) Series 57. Rockville, MD: Substance Abuse and Mental Health Services Administration.

Van der Kolk, B. A. (2014). *The body keeps the score: Brain, mind, and body in the healing of trauma.* New York: Viking Press.

Yalom, I. D., & Leszcz, M. (2020). *The theory and practice of group psychotherapy* (6th ed.). New York: Basic Books.

10

Cultural, Historic, and Gender Issues in Group Therapy, Psychodrama, and Leadership

Chapter Summary

The importance of recognizing the influence of culture, history, and identity is highlighted through this final trauma-informed principle. When someone is treated unfairly due to their culture, history, or identity, it impacts not only their social mobility but also their psychological well-being. Collective trauma describes the experience of traumatization by an entire group of people, often based on discrimination or violence directed towards them due to their group identity. This chapter outlines the importance of group work and group leadership as they relate to social justice, anti-oppressive practices, and healing-centered engagement. Sociatry, psychodrama's social justice framework, will be discussed while demonstrating psychodrama's utility in promoting psychological healing and social change. Cultural and religious values will also be presented as strengths that can be accessed by participants to aid the healing process. Furthermore, the importance of considering the impacts of identity, culture, and history will be highlighted in organizational dynamics. Trauma-informed leaders actively prevent retraumatization and discrimination related to identity or social location, instead empowering and celebrating differences of identity in the agency. Multiple examples employing sociometry, sociodrama, and psychodrama around issues of culture and identity are included.

DOI: 10.4324/9781003277859-10

Traumatic Impacts of Oppression, Discrimination, and Collective Trauma

Trauma, for most, is contextualized in relationship to their gender, sexuality, race, ethnicity, religion, culture, citizenship status, or other aspects of identity. Culture plays an important role as it relates to one's relationship to trauma – perception, experience, vulnerability, protective factors, access to services, social dynamics, and recovery (Bryant-Davis, 2005, 2019). SAMHSA (2014b) articulates that "Culture is the lens through which reality is interpreted. Without an understanding of culture, it is difficult to gauge how individuals organize, interpret, and resolve their traumas" (p. 131). Many experiences of trauma are direct (or indirect) harm, perpetration, dehumanization, violence, or discrimination related to an individual, family, group, or community's identity. Experiences of discrimination, oppression, inequality, and hatred can have lasting adverse psychological and social impacts. Research on the impact of racism and other forms of oppression and discrimination continues to evolve, demonstrating a range of adverse psychological effects (Kirkinis et al., 2021; Pieterse, Todd, Neville, & Carter, 2012; Williams, Osman, Gran-Ruaz, & Lopez, 2021). Discrimination, race-related stressors, and racial trauma are strongly related to posttraumatic stress disorder (PTSD) diagnoses for Latinx and African American adults (Sibrava et al., 2019). Furthermore, trauma is often experienced through gender violence, religious discrimination, ablism, agism, classism, and other forms of xenophobia.

Trauma experienced by entire groups of people is described as *collective trauma*. Collective trauma includes a variety of different experiences, such as natural disasters, war, community violence, terrorism, genocide, poverty, famine, pandemics, and other forms of systemic oppression or discrimination (Hirschberger, 2018; Hübl & Avritt, 2020; Kellermann, 2007; Saul, 2014). Symptoms of collective trauma manifest in our collective bodies – groups, communities, organizations, and society (Hübl & Avritt, 2020). Hübl and Avritt (2020) explain that "collective traumas distort social narratives, rupture national identities, and hinder the development of institutions, communities, and cultures, just as personally experienced trauma has the power to disrupt the psychological development of a growing child" (p. 79). Furthermore, they suggest that the *collective trauma* responses in relation to *collective trauma* (including historical trauma and intergenerational traumas) could be described as *collective PTSD*. Some examples of collective posttraumatic stress are depicted in the research literature. For example, various studies have uncovered that in the aftermath of police violence or the police killings of unarmed black individuals there is a collective impact to the mental health, well-being, anxiety, stress, and even school performance for communities of color (Ang, 2020; Bor, Benkataramani,

Williams, & Tsai, 2018; Heard-Garris et al., 2018). Other studies, focusing on historical trauma and its intergenerational influences, suggest ongoing adverse psychological effects for Native Americans (Ehlers et al., 2013), second and third generations of Holocaust survivors (Scharf, 2007), and various other communities that have experienced collective and historic trauma (Mohatt, Thompson, Thai, & Tebes, 2014).

Oppression and discrimination based on one's identity can manifest in a variety of adverse symptoms including distress, hyperarousal, alienation, isolation, anxiety and worry about the future, fear of others, difficulty coping, loss of safety, negative cognitions, avoidance behaviors, intrusions and re-experiencing, dissociation, depression, anger, low self-esteem, shame, and posttraumatic stress (Bryant-Davis, 2019; Carter et al., 2013; Carter & Muchow, 2017; Williams, Printz, & DeLapp, 2018). Microaggressions, systemic inequality, biases, and stereotypes continue to impact individuals on an ongoing basis. The pervasive and ongoing nature of identity-based discrimination and oppression is similar to complex trauma. Marginalized groups experience the overwhelming majority of negative impacts from inequality and oppression, nevertheless, it is also important to acknowledge that privilege also can cause negative psychosocial impacts to individuals or groups that benefit from it.

Each individual has a multitude of identities and holds memberships in various social groups; these social memberships either provide privilege (agent ranks) or are subject to marginalization (target ranks) (Nieto et al., 2010). Nieto and colleagues draw from the "ADDRESSING" Model developed by Pamela Hays (2001, 2008) which outlines a multidimensional conceptualization of identity and intersectionality:

A. Age and Generational Influences
DD. Developmental and Acquired Disabilities
R. Religion and Spiritual Orientation
E. Ethnicity and Racial Identity
S. Social Class Culture
S. Sexual Orientation
I. Indigenous Heritage
N. National Origin
G. Gender

While SAMHSA's sixth trauma-informed principles only explicitly names cultural, historical, and gender issues, it is important that trauma-informed practitioners consider the multiplicity of identities and their determining influence on an individual's experiences of trauma, life, work, and treatment. It also appears that early publications on trauma-informed principles did not include this sixth principle – it was later added to the original list of five trauma-informed principles. This, by itself, is interesting in that without this final principle, SAMHSA appears to have concluded there was a missing piece to the puzzle of providing trauma-informed care.

Which of the ADDRESSING categories do I have privileged positions in? Which do I have marginalized positions in?

Show often do I work with clients who have marginalized positions in these layers of identity?

This final trauma-informed principle not only demands that we are aware of identity issues but that we are actively responding in ways that are helpful. Although it is not enough by itself, acknowledging identity is a good starting place – such as inquiring about gender pronouns, asking if anyone needs accommodations, and offering land acknowledgments to recognize the native people of the land. These practices help raise consciousness and inclusion but can be largely performative if they aren't also followed up with further action such as anti-oppressive and healing-centered policies and practices.

Healing-Centered Engagement

A new paradigm has been proposed in the past few years by Shawn Ginwright called healing-centered engagement (2018). Ginwright's approach builds off trauma-informed care philosophy while offering additional emphasis on the importance of culture and identity, strengths-based approaches, and conceptualizing trauma as a collective and systemic experience rather than an individual wound. Ginwright emphasizes that the term "trauma-informed" is deficit oriented and instead he proposes the term "healing-centered engagement" as a strengths-based way to describe the work. He writes that "the term trauma-informed care runs the risk of focusing on the treatment of pathology (trauma), rather than fostering the possibility (well-being)" (2018, n.p.).

Healing-centered engagement was created in the context of working with youth of color and emphasizes the collective nature of trauma. Ginwright critiques trauma-informed care philosophy for subscribing to medicalized perspectives of trauma and PTSD by framing it as an individual experience. He expands this conceptualization of trauma by defining it as a collective and systemic experience rooted in identity and culture. He argues that the environment is the root cause of trauma, and that trauma-informed care is too focused on individual treatment without offering guidance for addressing the causes of trauma in neighborhoods, families, schools, and larger society (Ginwright, 2018).

Ginwright's 2018 publication introducing healing-centered engagement proposes four key elements within its framework:

- Healing-centered engagement is explicitly political, rather than clinical
- Healing-centered engagement is culturally grounded and views healing as the restoration of identity
- Healing-centered engagement is asset driven and focuses well-being we want, rather than symptoms we want to suppress
- Healing-centered engagement supports adult providers with their own healing

These elements echo foundational trauma-informed care philosophy while also contributing new insight. Healing-centered engagement emphasizes the role of the environment in cultivating trauma or well-being and proposes systemic interventions instead of individual treatments. This approach points out that until we critically analyze the policies and systems that perpetuate trauma, individuals will continue to blame themselves and feel isolated within their personal experience of wounding. Ginwright highlights the importance of culture "as a way to ground young people in a solid sense of meaning, self-perception, and purpose" (2018, n.p.). He argues that healing is a collective experience achieved through the development of healthy identity and a sense of belonging within community. Ginwright's philosophy is strongly influenced by positive psychology and community psychology. The fourth element of healing-centered engagement elevates the importance of professional self-care as well as addressing burnout, vicarious trauma, and the primary trauma of the helping professional (more on this in Chapter 11).

Healing-centered engagement encompasses trauma-informed care while expanding it with emphasis on the sixth trauma-informed principle. It raises important questions and insights for trauma-informed practitioners, leaders, and group therapists to consider in their work – especially work with communities of color. The concept of healing-centered engagement is new but becoming widely accepted in many professional circles. At the time of writing this chapter, very few peer-reviewed publications have been published that focus on healing-centered engagement. As Ginwright's framework becomes more well known, I expect that it will prove to be an invaluable resource for practitioners and organizations.

In my own estimation, it seems that healing-centered engagement is re-emphasizing many of the components of trauma-informed care that are sometimes lost in the translation from theory/philosophy to practice (specifically the latter three key elements of healing-centered engagement listed above). Ginwright reminds us that working with trauma requires a systemic approach (or what social work calls "person in-environment") and demands a trauma-informed and healing-centered philosophy to guide not only treatment but also policy-making, community development, and organizational structures. In this context, I would also insert group work and psychodrama as inherently systemic approaches that can benefit from the infusion of healing-centered engagement.

Anti-Oppressive Group Leadership and Cultural Humility

Collective trauma and violence experienced due to one's social or group identity are often best addressed in group work. When harm is caused by groups, it makes sense too that healing takes place in group (Bloom, 1998). Groups have a unique potential to promote healing from discrimination, oppression, and collective trauma that is simply impossible to access in the same way through individual work. Group work offers individuals opportunities for solidarity and acceptance in groups which can help renegotiate the impacts of prior discrimination and oppression (Honig & Martinez-Taboada, 2022). The long history of the group work tradition can be traced back to social reform, democracy, social action, social responsibility, advocacy, and empowerment for oppressed communities (Lee, 1991; Singh & Salazar, 2010, 2011). At the same time, many of the most popular contemporary group therapy and group work approaches fail to adequately address issues of culture, diversity, and oppression (Burnes & Ross, 2010).

Every group member and every group leader have their own set of cultural beliefs, values, assumptions, biases, and experiences which will undoubtable impact their choices in the group process (Corey, Corey, & Corey, 2018). It is essential that group leaders consider frameworks for anti-oppressive group psychotherapy while working to address their own biases. Considering bias, diversity, oppression, and social justice is not just a clinical issue, but also an ethical imperative for group therapists (Brabender & Macnair-Semands, 2022). Timothy (2012) explicitly frames anti-oppressive psychotherapy as a form of trauma-informed practice and argues that we must expand our definition of trauma to include social and systemic marginalization. Similar to other health problems, the distribution and prevalence of trauma may mirror social inequalities and further contribute to those same inequalities in society (Poole & Greaves, 2012). An understanding and examination of intersectionality provides the therapist with a better sense of their own identity and its impact on the therapeutic alliance while also offering a deepened understanding of clients' lived experiences – "when therapists look at clients' identities as fluid and intersecting, their concepts of mental health supports expand to include both their intersectional experiences of trauma and their resiliency and resistance" (Timothy, 2012, p. 52). Without cultural humility and an anti-oppressive stance, practitioners are prone to inadvertently fall into traumatic reenactments related to issues of diversity, oppression, and marginalization. Burnes and Ross (2010) offer multiple recommendations for incorporating anti-oppressive methods into group work including the use of intake questions related to participants' ability to have discussions about oppression, considering diversity and intersectionality in the development of the group, using structured activities that center issues of privilege and oppression, processing issues of oppression in the here-and-now in the group.

How do I explicitly incorporate and address issues of identity, oppression, and discrimination in my groups?

Do I avoid discussions related to issues of identity when they emerge in the group?

Furthermore, in the discussion of group norms, it can be helpful to emphasize the importance of mutual respect and acceptance of differences between group members. At the start of my trauma groups, I ask participants to make a commitment to mutual respect – "respect everyone in the room for who they are, for how they identify, for their identities, for groups or communities that they are or aren't a part of, and to respect them for what they have experienced in their lives." The norms established by the leader and the group become a container for issues related to oppression and identity to be safely explored. It is also helpful to explicitly include reference to collective trauma, racial trauma, gender violence, poverty, and other forms of oppression as trauma when providing psychoeducation in trauma groups. This helps normalize these types of trauma and promote an inclusive group atmosphere. A group leader should also be ready to address microaggressions or other reenactments of marginalization such as inappropriate jokes, comments, assumptions, or actions between participants. While it can be tempting to address these infractions through a reciprocity of anger, shame, rejection, and dehumanization – we are likely to have more success using the previously outlined trauma-informed principles as guides to addressing these interpersonal conflicts when they emerge (safety, trust, transparency, peer support, mutuality, collaboration, empowerment, voice, choice, and a recognition of cultural, historic, and gender issues).

> One illustration of this comes from a mixed gender trauma group I was leading a few years ago. In the early phase of the group process, one of the male group members made an inappropriate sexual and homophobic joke. Instead of shaming him or yelling at him, I calmly, but directly highlight that his joke may be triggering or impacting others' sense of safety or trust – especially those who have experienced sexual trauma or discrimination based on sexual orientation. At this suggestion, he softened and looked around the group to see other participants facial expressions which appeared to confirm my response. Initially, he appeared ready to challenge my authority as group leader, but once he noticed his negative impact on his peers (disrupting safety, trust, collaboration, mutuality, and peer support), he shifted his stance and participated appropriately throughout the group. This intervention focused on the individual's impact upon others in the group instead of about a power dynamic between the leader and the individual. This moment then becomes an opening for the group to explore their own experiences of similar moments, both as a person initiating a hurtful joke and as a person targeted through someone else's microaggression or joke. Others are able to relate with the man who made the offensive comment so that he doesn't feel ostracized.

In most cases, the individual making a joke like this is doing it in unconscious an attempt to find connection through the creation of an in-group and out-group (Lichtenberg, Beusekom, & Gibbons, 2013). Keeping this in mind, connection becomes even more important in this moment. Group members are able to easily relate to those impacted by the offensive comment and share about past experience of being the target of inappropriate jokes based on other aspects of identity. The man who made the inappropriate joke gets to see and hear how others are impacted by jokes or comments of this nature which helps him develop a sense of empathy. This effectively promotes peer support, re-establishes trust and safety after the group rupture, empowers participants to elevate their voice, and promotes mutuality and collaboration within the group around a shared issue. However, if I had leveraged my authority and anger towards this group member to shame him or kick him out of the group, the group would have lost an opportunity for repair and identification. As noted in other chapters, these trauma-informed principles must apply to everyone, even those who are/were in perpetrator roles. It is much easier to ostracize, kick out, or cancel others than to engage in ongoing dialogue to promote connection, understanding, acceptance, and reconciliation. This requires considerable courage, tolerance, and self-awareness from the group leader, particularly when the microaggression relates to the identity of the professional.

Cultural humility and cultural responsiveness are other important frameworks for group leaders and trauma-informed practitioners. Many suggested that we abandon the goal of *cultural competence* and instead reorient with the goal of *cultural humility* and *cultural responsiveness* (Tervalon & Murray-Garcia, 1998). Cultural humility is defined as "an orientation to care that is based on self-reflexivity, appreciation of patients' lay expertise, openness to sharing power with patients, and to continue learning from one's patients" (Lekas, Pahl, & Lewis, 2020, p. 1). Cultural humility suggests a passive stance from the practitioner, whereas cultural responsiveness explicitly promotes action and appropriate responses to cultural differences. Interestingly, these definitions of cultural humility and cultural responsiveness are strikingly similar to definitions of trauma-informed care. Cultural humility and responsiveness, like the trauma-informed philosophy, is an ongoing commitment to continue learning, to emphasize ethics and transparency, to empower clients' voices and autonomy, and to engage with collaboration and mutuality. The term cultural competence is problematic in that it suggests that "mastery" of other cultures is possible and neglects to articulate the complexities of intersectionality (Lekas, Pahl, & Lewis, 2020). Alternatively, cultural humility and cultural responsiveness promote person-centered care, self-reflection on our own implicit biases, ownership of our own cultural and identities, and an ongoing practice of working to equalize power dynamics in relationships with clients (Agner, 2020; Botelho & Lima, 2020; Hook et al., 2013; Lekas, Pahl, & Lewis, 2020). Cultural competence is inherently focused on content while cultural humility and responsiveness are process-oriented (Lekas, Pahl, & Lewis, 2020); here we find another parallel to the process-oriented nature of trauma-informed care, group work, experiential methods such as psychodrama.

A group leader who fails to consider the influence of socio-cultural forces and aspects of identity within the group process is also failing to fully embody a trauma-informed approach (Giacomucci, 2021). Developing self-awareness of one's own biases and how one's social location impacts perspective is important. Cultural humility helps leaders and practitioners to treat the patient as the expert in their experience and their culture while prompting self-reflection. Social location and identity have a major impact on participants' experiences of each other and of the group leader. The group is a microcosm of society (Yalom & Lesczc, 2020), therefore issues of oppression and discrimination are inevitably going to emerge in groups. As group leaders, it is important that we can address these moments directly while avoiding retraumatization and reenactments of oppression, discrimination, or collective trauma. Without attending to issues of culture, the therapeutic factors in group therapy will be inhibited. In *Examining Social Identities and Diversity Issues in Group Therapy*, Ribeiro (2020) reminds us that:

> How the therapist successfully navigates social identities in the group can foster trust in members and create an opportunity to heal from oppressive experiences outside of the group. However, if left unexplored, socially marginalized or dominant identities can also cultivate destructive dynamics in the form of microaggressions that parallel larger sociopolitical events.
>
> (p. 15)

How do my own identities impact my perspectives and approaches to group work?

How might group participants experience me based on my gender, race, age, and other identities?

The various layers of identity (see ADDRESSING model outlined earlier), can also be a source of collective strength, wisdom, values, and direction rather than only a source of collective trauma. Group workers can foster a sense of celebration related to identity in both homogeneous and heterogeneous groups. The collective, cultural, and religious values associated with community identity are potent sources of goodness, unity, and healing. These values can become particularly important strengths for renegotiating collective trauma, recognizing similarities across different groups, and celebrating differences. Diversity in a group is an asset that provides novel insight and perspective. Group work provides a container for collective trauma to be addressed and collective strengths to be accessed.

Culture and Identity in Organizations

Trauma-informed organizational leadership, like group leadership, requires a commitment to anti-oppressive practices, cultural humility, and cultural responsiveness. This is important for all leaders including group leaders, organizational leaders, educators, trainers, and supervisors. Organizations, like groups, can become a vessel for collective trauma to be addressed and for collective strengths to be celebrated. Organizations can, and often do, become vehicles that reenact and uphold systems of oppression, marginalization, and collective trauma. Yalom and Leszcz (2020) suggest that the group is a microcosm of society; the same is also true for organizations. Discrimination, oppression, and racism exist within society, therefore when unchecked in organizations, they will also emerge in covert forms of structural violence and institutional racism. An organization that fails to incorporate trauma-informed principles and address cultural, historical, gender, and other issues of identity will inevitably recreate policies and practices that favor some while excluding others. Even in the best-intentioned organizations, this can happen unconsciously when these larger issues aren't consciously addressed.

This sixth trauma-informed principle, challenges organizations and leaders to consider social location and identity. Each of the ten agency domains outlined by SAMHSA (2014a) needs to be considered through the lens of this final trauma-informed principle (see Figure 10.1).

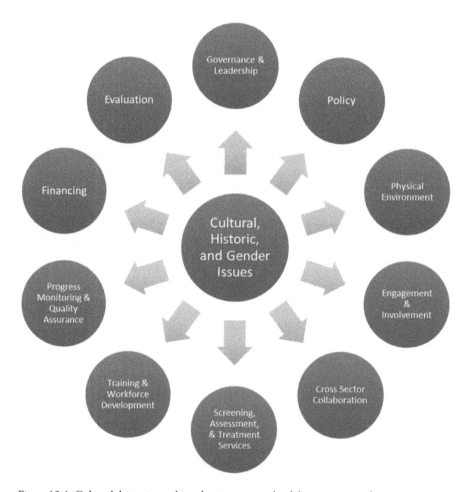

Figure 10.1 Cultural, historic, and gender issues in each of the ten agency domains.

While cultural, historic, and gender issues need to be considered in each of these 10 agency domains, policies and practices each of these 10 domains have the potential to privilege or marginalize staff and clients based on identity. Governance and leadership must attend to issues of identity and diversity while demonstrating culturally responsive policies, practices, pricing, and financing. Staff, clients, and community should be engaged and involved through culturally responsive means including physical environments, language, events, marketing, and staff that can attend to cultural values in diverse communities. Screening, assessment, and treatment services need to be responsive to individuals' cultural values. Cultural responsiveness of staff and leaders can be enhanced through cross sector collaboration, training, professional development, and regular progress monitoring and evaluation.

How does my organization consider and address issues of culture, gender, history, and identity into each of the 10 agency domains?

In which domain does my organization seem to best address issues of culture, gender, history, and identity?

Which domain does my organization seem to have the most room to grow in?

In the third trauma-informed principle of peer support, SAMHSA articulates that agencies should employ volunteers and staff who are trauma-survivors to promote peer support (2014a, 2014b). This must also include workers who have experienced collective trauma and identity-based trauma similar to those receiving services at the organization. Staff and leaders who better understand the lived experience of trauma and recovery, in this case collective trauma and recovery, will be better able to provide trauma-informed care for others experiencing trauma based on identity, gender, and culture. This expansive understanding of "who are trauma survivors" and "collective trauma survivors" mitigates the potential of *othering* which so frequently occurs in issues of identity, collective trauma, or inter-group conflict. At the same time, it can be tempting to discount leaders, CEOs, and others in positions of power in this regard. Many unconsciously project the role of *oppressor* or *perpetrator* onto people in power without evidence, perhaps due to unresolved trauma and the unjust history of people in power abusing their authority. The reality is that people in power are human and likely trauma survivors too – especially leaders in the social services fields. Everyone has a story and experiences of adversity which have shaped who they are and where they are today. This expansive focus of who are trauma survivors can help an organization and those who interact with it to do so with empathy, grace, understanding, inclusiveness, and responsiveness. In considering everyone in an agency may be a trauma survivor, this sixth trauma-informed principles must be considered as it helps to prevent potential retraumatization of staff based on reenactments of oppression, discrimination, or collective trauma. Far too many helping professionals have entered agencies whose goals are to support and empower others, only to reenact collective trauma, inequalities, and structural violence within the organization itself.

With the framework that clients, staff, and leaders are all trauma survivors, we can approach issues of identity, culture, gender, and history through the lens of trauma recovery rather than as simply issues of performative public relations, political correctness, and competitions for who is the most "woke," most progressive, or most radical. Addressing issues related to gender, race, and culture often become performative, superficial, or fear-based attempts by organizations to avoid being called out by others. The lens of trauma-informed care offers an action-based practice for actively addressing these issues which often feel complicated, elusive, philosophical, or like they are too large for a single professional or organization to address – especially while working within systems that continue to reenact the same collective harms. Nieto and colleagues (2010) remind us that awareness of social justice issues alone is not enough – true allyship is when awareness is combined with action.

There are numerous ways to take action around embodying this final trauma-informed principle, many of which have already been outlined. SAMHSA (2014b) endorses nine steps for cultural competency delineated by the Center for Mental Health Services (CMHS) (2003):

1) Recognize the importance of culture and respect diversity.
2) Maintain a current profile of the cultural composition of the community.
3) Recruit workers who are representative of the community or service area.
4) Provide ongoing cultural competence training to staff.
5) Ensure that services are accessible, appropriate, and equitable.
6) Recognize the role of help-seeking behaviors, traditions, and natural support networks.
7) Involve community leaders and organizations representing diverse cultural groups as "cultural brokers."
8) Ensure that services and information are culturally and linguistically responsive.
9) Assess and evaluate the program's level of cultural responsiveness.

Organizations can offer events, trainings, or direct services that focus on different aspects of identity such as gender-affirming care, racism, religion, accessibility, or historical trauma. The development of agency staff and hiring practices should also take into account this trauma-informed principle. Many clients and community members will inherently find safety and trust in working with staff who share identities or culture with them. This same safety and trust are likely to be developed from organizations who use language, marketing visuals, and promotional content that reflect diverse communities. This means that organizations would benefit from having staff whose identities mirror those of the clients and communities that they serve. This does not mean that every black client needs a black therapist, every trans client needs a trans therapist, every client with substance use disorder needs a therapist in recovery from substance use, and so on. While staff can certainly work with and be helpful for clients from different backgrounds and identities, there are also nuances of identity and cultural values that will be unknown to staff who don't share similar lived experiences and identities as their clients.

Do the identities of our agency's staff, at all levels of the organization, reflect the identities of the clients and communities that we serve?

In my experience providing trauma-informed trainings or assessments at various agencies, I find consistently that this final trauma-informed principle is most frequently the one that is lacking. In nearly every sociometric exploration of the six trauma-informed principles in groups and organizations, participants overwhelmingly indicate that this is the principle that they have the most room to grow in both as individuals and as organizations. A truly trauma-informed professional or organization takes into account this sixth trauma-informed principle and issues of identity and culture.

> One simple way that we have further integrated this principle into our organizational culture at the Phoenix Center is through regular discussions in our team meetings. Each week, we begin our Wednesday team meeting on Zoom with a breakout room discussion focused on a reflective prompt. This gives everyone a chance to connect with another team member, to critically reflect on their work, to learn from each other's experiences and perspectives, and to highlight areas of growth for the organization as a whole. One of our topic series for these breakout rooms was the ADDRESSING model, outlined at the start of this chapter. Each week we took one of the nine aspects of identity and focused our breakout room discussion on it. Participants were instructed to reflect on how each layer of identity impacted their experience as therapists, as

co-workers, and how it may impact their clients' experience. After each breakout room discussion, we returned together as a group to share some of the important insights and areas for growth that emerged from the dyads. The synthesis of collective insight, perspective, and feedback from the group provided individual staff and the organization with helpful avenues for continued growth every week. Together we discovered how age, gender, and sexuality might influence transference and countertransference, areas for increasing accessibility around disabilities, our biases related to religion and spirituality, the importance of talking about race and class, and the often invisible yet significant impact of issues faced by indigenous and undocumented communities. Together we explored how we as individuals hold privileged and marginalized positions in these nine areas. We considered from all angles how we might continue to grow as an organization that anyone, regardless of identity, could feel safe and welcomed in. This simple series of discussion resulted in changes to our marketing, our clinical and educational service offerings, our benefits offered to staff, our physical building layout, our intake questions, our hiring practices, and our evaluation processes. Furthermore, this process helped us as a team get to know each other better, celebrate the diversity of identities on our team, and reflect on how each individual could further embody the sixth trauma-informed principles in their work.

This is one simple example of how to approach conversations of identity, culture, gender, and history in an organization. Of course, doing this alone is not enough. Discussions of diversity and identity are helpful and important, but only meaningful when followed with purposeful action. Everyone, regardless of privilege is impacted by issues of gender, sexuality, race, ethnicity, class, national origin, indigeneity, age, disability, and religion/spirituality. We all have identities that are either privileged or marginalized in these nine categories, just like those of our clients. Organizational leaders and staff must commit to preventing retraumatization based on identity while developing practices and policies that are culturally responsive.

Addressing Impacts of Social Injustice with Psychodrama and Sociodrama

Jacob Moreno, psychodrama's founder, was a Jewish Romanian man who was a refugee in Vienna and later an immigrant to the United States. Moreno was also a trauma survivor – he writes of multiple experience of trauma or discrimination in his life including childhood sexual abuse, abandonment and disconnection from his father, discrimination based on his Jewish heritage, and later difficulties in the United States based on his ambiguous immigration status (Moreno, 2019). English was not his first, or even his second language. His layered experience of identities surely had an impact on his life experience and thus the development of his methods. When considering his experience as a refugee and an immigrant, it is not surprising that he spent significant time working with immigrants early in his career (especially related to the House of the Encounter) and that he worked in a refugee camp in Austria. Considering his multi-lingual experience, it makes sense that he developed methods that rely less on verbal communication and more so on body language and movement. His experiences of war and collective trauma in Europe likely fueled the development of his vision of Sociatry – healing for society. His experiences of discrimination as a Jewish man and immigrant are likely to have also influenced his decision to work with marginalized and oppressed communities most of his life. Similarly, Zerka Moreno was a Dutch Jewish immigrant to the United States. She met Dr. Moreno while seeking psychiatric treatment for her sister (see Figure 10.2). At age 40 she had an arm amputated due to cancer. Surely, her identities, experiences, and family history also had an impact on her thinking and practice. The rise of tyranny and fascism in Europe probably inspired their new ideas of group leadership which elevated every participant to equal status with the facilitator or leader. These are largely

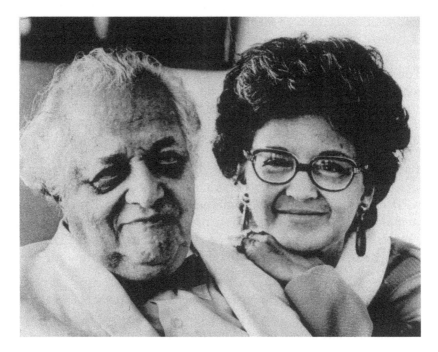

Figure 10.2 Jacob and Zerka Moreno in Amsterdam in 1971.

speculative conclusions, nevertheless, how could one's identity not impact the development of their ideas and approaches?

Moreno is primarily known for developing psychodrama and sociometry. However, his initial vision with of healing society and his initial implementation of "group therapy" would be more accurately described as community work by today's standards (Giacomucci et al., 2021). His work in Sing Sing prison, during which he coined the term "group therapy," involved a sociometry assessment of the identities of persons imprisoned at the time and a restructuring of the prison wing based on shared identities and preferences (Moreno & Whitin, 1932). Coincidentally, he was even using many of the nine aspects of identity outlined in the ADDRESSING Model by Pamela Hays (2001). Moreno's intention was to position the inmates in ways that they would become therapeutic agents and allies for each other based on their physical proximity to cellmates or neighboring inmates in the prison. His goal was to reduce the conflict and dysfunction within the prison community while promoting more harmonious relationships and social networks. Later, Moreno and his colleagues in Hudson Valley were some of the first in the social sciences to focus on racism and racial conflict within communities and organizations (Moreno, 1934, J. D. Moreno, 2014). He frequently promoted sociodrama (and sometimes ethnodrama) as methods of sociatry designed to promote healing related to inter-group conflict or collective issues in society and the culture. Moreno's early emphasis on culture, race, identity, and social justice has been carried on by other contemporary psychodramatists around the world. While many are using psychodrama and sociodrama to address issues of social injustice and identity (for example, see Galgóczi et al., 2021), this is also an area where the psychodrama community has much room to grow (particularly in the United States).

In transparency, I will also state that this embodying this sixth trauma-informed principle in my own psychodrama practice is an ongoing area of growth for me as a director and group leader. It is an area where I find that I make mistakes, have blind spots, act on my own biases, unintentionally reenact oppressive dynamics, and continue to learn and grow. At the same time, there are multiple examples from my clinical practice and training events that I will highlight and introduce in this section.

The sociometry processes outlined in Chapter 4 can be particularly useful for warming up a group to discussion and action related to identity or diversity. One simple example comes from a University of Pennsylvania guest lecture I provided in a course on racism and social work practice. I employed three spectrograms to assess the class while warming-up students to the topic and each other:

1) How comfortable do you feel talking about racism and white supremacy?
2) How prevalent do you think racism is in our society today?
3) How open are you to learning about racism and what you can do to combat it?

These three simple spectrograms positioned students along a spectrum and provided opportunities to connect with each other about shared experiences and beliefs. Each of the spectrograms initiated meaningful discussions while helping students see that they are not alone in their discomfort talking about racism as well as their desire to actively contribute to combating racism in the world today. The spectrograms also initiated discussion about performative allyship as many experienced stress and influence by the fact that their peers would see where they chose to place themselves on the spectrogram. After this sociometric warm up we were able to move into a sociodramatic role play exercise which included multiple short dyadic role plays related to addressing racism in everyday life. These short role plays offered a role training experience to practice responding to racist comments or microaggressions in personal and professional contexts while reflecting on one's own continued areas of growth in this regard (more detail on this in Giacomucci, 2021).

Sociodrama is sometimes a better option than psychodrama when working with collective issues as sociodrama orients on the group's collective experience rather than an individual's specific story (Giacomucci, 2017). This provides an enhanced sense of safety, distance, playfulness, and spontaneity that is often beneficial to groups when addressing uncomfortable and painful topics related to identity or social injustice.

> In the midst of the "MeToo Movement" in the United States, I was facilitating a workshop on sociodrama. The workshop participants, composed primarily of female therapists and graduate students, chose the topic of sexism, gender violence, rape culture, and sexual harassment for the sociodrama topic during the training. As a male facilitator, I determined it was necessary to acknowledge my position as a male in authority during the session while committing to facilitate the sociodrama with a sense of humility, following the lead of the group (follow-lead-follow). The group collectively co-created a scene of a mother prompting a difficult discussion with their teenage daughter about consent, sex, and sexual harassment. In the sociodrama, the daughter expressed her confusions with current events and national news related to prominent court cases during which men in positions of power seemed to be getting away with

sexual harassment or even rape without punishment or accountability. Feeling disempowered, both expressed their shared frustrations, fears, and hopes for a more equitable future. Group members offered doubling statements from each role to deepen their understanding and expression of the issues at hand. As the group articulated the important feelings and perspectives from each role, a sense of catharsis and new insight was achieved. The sociodrama still felt quite heavy as we organically were moving towards closure, so I suggested we incorporate an archetypal feminine role model to guide the teenager and mother in navigating these issues. The group chose Wonder Woman (the 2017 movie had recently been released at that time) who was enrolled into the scene to offer an enhanced sense of empowerment, safety, and powerful feminine energy. The sociodrama came to closure with Wonder Woman offering her guidance to the mother, the teen, and the group.

In this example, we can see the power of sociodrama in exploring collective issues within groups and society. Though sociodrama is often much less emotionally intense and involved as psychodrama, this specific sociodrama is testament to the fact that sociodrama scenes can be equally as intense and powerful as psychodrama scenes. Another sociodramatic example comes from a training workshop I presented on Moreno's developmental stages and relationships.

Mid-way through the half-day workshop, it became clear that multiple participants were very warmed-up to topics of race and the historical trauma of slavery as they had asked multiple questions related to these issues in the session thus far. The next piece of teaching that I had planned was to use two sociodramatic empty chairs to represent two people in relationship and explore Moreno's three developmental stages (doubling, the mirror, and role reversal) in the context of a relationship. Following the group's warm-up on the topic of slavery, we spontaneously changed the empty chair structure to explore the relationship between an enslaved black man and a white slave owner using the same framework of Moreno's developmental stages. Through a series of doubling statements, the group enriched an understanding of each person's experience of the relationship. The oppression and trauma experienced by the enslaved man was articulated and validated while the group also developed an increased sense of empathy for the white slave owner, also trapped in this system of oppression (albeit in a different way). The second developmental phase prescribed that we move onto the mirror position, during which participants took turns reflecting on the observations of the role reciprocity between the two roles. Finally, we moved onto the third phase of role reversal which provided participants with the opportunity to step into one of the role and reverse roles, becoming the other. In this process, the group moved towards closure through statements of recognition, validation, change, reconciliation, and equality. This process also highlighted the inherent dehumanization involved in the relationship between the two parties historically – there was not accurate attunement, doubling, mirroring, and role reversal between the two. If there had been, then it would have been impossible for whites to continue enslaving blacks. The sharing phase of the session involved a rich discussion on racism as it relates to doubling, mirroring, and role reversal and the continued impacts of historical trauma and slavery on racial tensions today.

In both of these sociodrama examples, we can see the symbolic enactments emerging from the group's warm up based on the groups' collective issue. The group is a microcosm of society so issues that are emerging the society are certain to show up in our groups, educational sessions, and organizations. Sociodrama offers a meaningful process for exploring these collective issues without requiring that a protagonist exhibit the vulnerability necessary for a psychodrama enactment (Giacomucci, 2019). Instead of focusing on an individual's concern and goal, sociodrama explicitly focuses on the collective issues in the group. While sociodrama is sometimes a better choice when working with collective issues, there are many times when psychodrama enactments are warranted.

> One of my first individual psychotherapy clients in my private practice was a young non-binary adolescent who had experienced multiple layers of trauma and loss, including discrimination and dehumanization based on their gender. This client had recently begun to ask others in their life to refer to them using they/them pronouns, though they had previously identified as a boy and used he/him pronouns. The client shared with me that they had a close relationship with their father who was accepting of their transition, but they were fearful of telling their mother. Using psychodrama, we employed an empty chair to represent their mother and to practice their upcoming discussion with their mother about their new gender identity and preferred pronouns. In this process, the client had the opportunity to practice varies ways of expressing and articulating themself to their mother while actively working through their fear and anxiety. Together we embodied and explored this discussion from multiple angles including the client's best case scenario, worst case scenario, and what they believed was most likely to occur. Through role reversals with their mother, they were able to get in touch with their mother's unconditional love for them and her own societal conditioning around gender. The client developed a sense of how their gender transition would impact their mother and how she may need time to process emotionally and to learn about pronouns. Having started the session feeling anxious and fearful of this future discussion with mom, they left the session feeling confident, prepared, and ready to offer their mother the patience, understanding, and information that she might need to better understand her child's gender identity and utilize non-binary pronouns.

This example depicts the use of psychodramatic role training in a one-to-one session. This process is useful for various reasons but primarily because it helps a client rehearse for future situations while expressing emotions and developing new insights that will contribute to the success of a future social interaction.

There are, of course, various other ways that psychodrama can be employed to explore issues of gender, culture, history, and identity. It is important that psychodramatists consider the cultural contexts of their work (Fleury & Marra, 2022). Nieto (2010) draws from Hays' ADDRESSING Model and urges psychodrama directors to develop awareness of their own identities and how they may influence the dynamics within their directing of protagonists based on the protagonist's identities. Nieto further highlights how other group members playing roles will also be influenced by their identities and the identities of the role they are playing, as well as the identities of the protagonist. For example, if we have a psychodrama protagonist who is an indigenous woman engaged in a psychodrama focused on healing from historical trauma who chooses a white woman to play the role of their courage – in this case, the nature of the white woman's spontaneity and performance in the role of courage may look different than if another indigenous woman where to play the role of courage. This is not to say that group members who do not share identities with the protagonist can't or shouldn't play supportive roles for them, but it does warrant that we carefully consider the sociodynamics and cultural dynamics that may emerge through the psychodrama for everyone involved. Cultural contexts must be considered by the psychodrama director as it relates to the contexts, issues, and participants within any psychodrama session (Giacomucci, 2021; Nieto, 2010; Remer, 2020).

Conclusion

Issues of culture, gender, history, and identity must be addressed and incorporated into trauma healing, group work, psychodrama, and organizations. Practitioners and leaders who neglect these issues are falling short of trauma-informed practice. So many of our clients and colleagues have experienced collective trauma related to experiences of dehumanization, discrimination, oppression, and structural violence due to their identities. Trauma-informed and trauma-focused approaches must take into account identity. Cultural values and diversity can be celebrated and employed as collective strengths in groups. Leaders must demonstrate cultural humility and cultural responsiveness in groups and organizations. Performative discussions about equality and justice are not enough; leaders must take action in implementing this sixth trauma-informed principle into each of the 10 agency domains outlined by SAMHSA. Anti-oppressive practices can be integrated into all settings to promote social justice for all. Psychodrama and sociodrama have a rich history in anti-oppressive work and collective trauma. Moreno's system of sociatry offers psychodramatists, group workers, and organizational leaders with experiential methods for intrapsychic and societal change.

References

Agner, J. (2020). Moving from cultural competence to cultural humility in occupational therapy: A paradigm shift. *The American Journal of Occupational Therapy*, 74(4), 1–7. https://doi.org/10.5014/ajot.2020.038067

Ang, D. (2020). Wider effects of police killings in minority neighborhoods. *Crime and Criminal Justice*. Retrieved from https://econofact.org/wider-effects-of-police-killings-in-minority-neighborhoods

Bloom, S. L. (1998). By the crowd they have been broken, by the crowd they shall be healed: The social transformation of trauma. Posttraumatic Growth: Positive Changes in the Aftermath of Crisis. In R. G. Tedeschi, C. L. Park, & L. G. Calhoun (Eds.), *Posttraumatic Growth* (pp. 179–213). New York: Routledge.

Bor, J., Venkataramani, A. S., Williams, D. R., & Tsai, A. C. (2018). Police killings and their spillover effects on the mental health of black Americans: A population-based, quasi-experimental study. *The Lancet*, 392(10144), 302–310.

Botelho, M. J., & Lima, C. A. (2020). From cultural competence to cultural respect: A critical review of six models. *Journal of Nursing Education*, 59(6), 311–318.

Brabender, V., & MacNair-Semands, R. (2022). *The ethics of group psychotherapy: Principles and practical strategies*. New York: Routledge.

Bryant-Davis, T. (2005). *Thriving in the wake of trauma: A multicultural guide*. Westport: Greenwood Publishing Group.

Bryant-Davis, T. (2019). The cultural context of trauma recovery: Considering the posttraumatic stress disorder practice guideline and intersectionality. *Psychotherapy*, 56(3), 400–408. https://doi.org/10.1037/pst0000241

Burnes, T. R., & Ross, K. L. (2010). Applying social justice to oppression and marginalization in group process: Interventions and strategies for group counselors. *The Journal for Specialists in Group Work*, 35(2), 169–176.

Carter, R. T., Mazzula, S., Victoria, R., Vazquez, R., Hall, S., Smith, S., ... & Williams, B. (2013). Initial development of the race-based traumatic stress symptom scale: Assessing the emotional impact of racism. *Psychological Trauma: Theory, Research, Practice, and Policy, 5*(1), 1.

Carter, R. T., & Muchow, C. (2017). Construct validity of the race-based traumatic stress symptom scale and tests of measurement equivalence. *Psychological Trauma: Theory, Research, Practice, and Policy, 9*(6), 688.

Center for Mental Health Services (2003). *Fact sheet (Rep. No. KEN 95-0011).* Rockville, MD: Substance Abuse and Mental Health Services Administration.

Corey, M. S., Corey, G., & Corey, C. (2018). *Groups: Process and practice* (10th ed.). Boston: Cengage Learning.

Ehlers, C. L., Gizer, I. R., Gilder, D. A., Ellingson, J. M., & Yehuda, R. (2013). Measuring historical trauma in an American Indian community sample: Contributions of substance dependence, affective disorder, conduct disorder, and PTSD. *Drug and Alcohol Dependence, 133*(1), 180–187.

Fleury, H. J., & Marra, M. M. (2022). Theoretical and methodological foundations of socionomy. In H. J. Fleury, M. M. Marra, & O. H. Hadler (Eds.), *Psychodrama in Brazil* (pp. 17–29). Singapore: Springer.

Galgóczi, K., Adderley, D., Blaskó, A., Belchior, M., Damjanov, J., Maciel, M., Teszáry, J., Werner, M., & Westberg, M. (Eds.) (2021). *Sociodrama: The Art and science of social change.* Budapest. L'Harmattan Könyvesbolt.

Giacomucci, S. (2017). The sociodrama of life or death: Young adults and addiction treatment. *Journal of Psychodrama, Sociometry, and Group Psychotherapy, 65*(1), 137–143. https://doi.org/10.12926/ 0731-1273-65.1.137

Giacomucci, S. (2019). Social group work in action: A sociometry, psychodrama, and experiential trauma group therapy curriculum. *Doctorate in Social Work (DSW) Dissertations,* 124. Retrieved from https://repository.upenn.edu/cgi/viewcontent.cgi?article=1128&context=edissertations_sp2

Giacomucci, S. (2021). *Social work, sociometry, and psychodrama: Experiential approaches for group therapists, community leaders, and social workers.* Springer Nature. https://doi.org/10.1007/978-981-33-6342-7

Giacomucci, S., Karner, D., Nieto, L., & Schreiber, E. (2021). Sociatry, psychodrama, and social work: Moreno's mysticism and social justice tradition. *Social Work with Groups, 44*(3), 288–303. https://doi.org/10.1080/01609513.2021.1885826

Ginwright, S. (2018). The future of healing: Shifting from trauma informed care to healing centered engagement. Medium. https://ginwright.medium.com/the-future-of-healing-shifting-from-trauma-informed-care-to-healing-centered-engagement-634f557ce69c

Hays, P. A. (2001). *Addressing cultural complexities in practice: A framework for clinicians and counselors*. Washington D.C.: American Psychological Association.

Hays, P. A. (2008). *Addressing cultural complexities in practice: Assessment, diagnosis, and therapy*. Washington D.C.: American Psychological Association.

Heard-Garris, N. J., Cale, M., Camaj, L., Hamati, M. C., & Dominguez, T. P. (2018). Transmitting trauma: A systematic review of vicarious racism and child health. *Social Science & Medicine, 199*, 230–240.

Hirschberger, G. (2018). Collective trauma and the social construction of meaning. *Frontiers in Psychology, 9*, 1441.

Honig, M., & Martinez-Taboada, C. (Eds.) (2022). *Cultural diversity, Groups and psychotherapy around the world*. Kreuzlingen: International Association of Group Psychotherapy & Group Processes.

Hook, J. N., Davis, D. E., Owen, J., Worthington Jr., E. L., & Utsey, S. O. (2013). Cultural humility: Measuring openness to culturally diverse clients. *Journal of Counseling Psychology, 60*(3), 353.

Hübl, T., & Avritt, J. J. (2020). *Healing collective trauma: A process for integrating our intergenerational and cultural wounds*. Boulder: Sounds True.

Kellerman, P. F. (2007). *Sociodrama and collective trauma*. London: Jessica Kingsley Publishers.

Kirkinis, K., Pieterse, A. L., Martin, C., Agiliga, A., & Brownell, A. (2021). Racism, racial discrimination, and trauma: A systematic review of the social science literature. *Ethnicity & Health, 26*(3), 392–412.

Lee, J. (1991). Forward. In M. Weil, K. Chau, & D. Sutherland (Eds.), *Theory and practice in social group work: Creative connections* (pp. 1–4). New York: Haworth Press.

Lekas, H. M., Pahl, K., & Fuller Lewis, C. (2020). Rethinking cultural competence: Shifting to cultural humility. *Health Services Insights, 13*, 1178632920970580.

Lichtenberg, P., Beusekom, J., & Gibbons, D. (2013). *Encountering bigotry: Befriending projecting people in everyday life*. New York: Routledge.

Mohatt, N. V., Thompson, A. B., Thai, N. D., & Tebes, J. K. (2014). Historical trauma as public narrative: A conceptual review of how history impacts present-day health. *Social Sciences & Medicine, 106*, 128–136.

Moreno, J. D. (2014). *Impromptu man: J.L. Moreno and the origins of psychodrama, encounter culture, and the social network*. New York: Bellevue Literary Press.

Moreno, J. L. (1934). *Who shall survive? A new approach to the problems of human interrelations*. Washington, DC: Nervous and Mental Disease Publishing Co.

Moreno, J. L. (2019). *The autobiography of a genius* (E. Schreiber, S. Kelley, & S. Giacomucci, Eds.). United Kingdom: North West Psychodrama Association.

Moreno, J. L., & Whitin, E. S. (1932). *Application of the group method to classification.* New York: National Committee on Prisons and Prison Labor.

Nieto, L. (2010). Look behind you: Using anti-oppression models to inform a protagonist's psychodrama. In E. Leveton (Ed.), *Healing collective trauma using sociodrama and drama therapy* (pp. 103–125). New York: Springer Publishing Company.

Nieto, L., Boyer, M. F., Goodwin, L., Johnson, G. R., Smith, L. C., & Hopkins, J. P. (2010). *Beyond inclusion, beyond empowerment: A developmental strategy to liberate everyone.* Olympia: Cuetzpalin Publishing.

Pieterse, A. L., Todd, N. R., Neville, H. A., & Carter, R. T. (2012). Perceived racism and mental health among Black American adults: A meta-analytic review. *Journal of Counseling Psychology, 59*(1), 1.

Poole, N., & Greaves, L. (Eds.). (2012). *Becoming trauma informed.* Toronto, ON: Centre for Addiction and Mental Health.

Remer, R. (2020). Culture-related psychodramatic techniques: Experiences with Asian cultures. *Journal of Psychodrama, Sociometry, and Group Psychotherapy, 67*(1), 25–40.

Ribeiro, M. D. (Ed.). (2020). *Examining social identities and diversity issues in group therapy: Knocking at the boundaries.* New York: Routledge.

Saul, J. (2014). *Collective trauma, collective healing: Promoting resilience in the aftermath of disaster.* New York: Routledge.

Scharf, M. (2007). Long-term effects of trauma: Psychosocial functioning of the second and third generation of Holocaust survivors. *Development and Psychopathology, 19*(2), 603–622.

Sibrava, N. J., Bjornsson, A. S., Pérez Benítez, A. C. I., Moitra, E., Weisberg, R. B., & Keller, M. B. (2019). Posttraumatic stress disorder in African American and Latinx adults: Clinical course and the role of racial and ethnic discrimination. *American Psychologist, 74*(1), 101.

Singh, A. A., & Salazar, C. F. (2010). The roots of social justice in group work. *Journal for Specialists in Group Work, 35*(2): 97–104.

Singh, A. A., & Salazar, C. F. (Eds.) (2011). *Social justice in group work: Practical interventions for change.* New York: Routledge.

Substance Abuse and Mental Health Services Administration. (2014a). *SAMHSA's concept of trauma and guidance for a trauma-informed approach.* HHS Publication No. (SMA) 14-4884. Rockville, MD: Substance Abuse and Mental Health Services Administration.

Substance Abuse and Mental Health Services Administration. (2014b). *Trauma-informed care in behavioral health services*. Treatment Improvement Protocol (TIP) Series 57. Rockville, MD: Substance Abuse and Mental Health Services Administration.

Tervalon, M., & Murray-Garcia, J. (1998). Cultural humility versus cultural competence: A critical distinction in defining physician training outcomes in multicultural education. *Journal of Health Care for the Poor and Underserved*, 9(2), 117–125.

Timothy, R. (2012). Anti-oppression psychotherapy as trauma-informed practice. In L. Greaves, & N. Poole (Eds.), *Becoming trauma-informed* (pp. 47–56). Toronto: Centre for Addiction and Mental Health.

Williams, M. T., Osman, M., Gran-Ruaz, S., & Lopez, J. (2021). Intersection of racism and PTSD: Assessment and treatment of racial stress and trauma. *Current Treatment Options in Psychiatry*, 8, 1–19.

Williams, M. T., Printz, D., & DeLapp, R. C. (2018). Assessing racial trauma with the Trauma Symptoms of Discrimination Scale. *Psychology of Violence*, 8(6), 735.

Yalom, I. D., & Leszcz, M. (2020). *The theory and practice of group psychotherapy* (6th ed.). New York: Basic Books.

11

Trauma-Informed Organizations: From Vicarious Trauma to Vicarious Posttraumatic Growth

Chapter Summary

Trauma-informed principles must also be applied in professional relationships, organizational culture, education, supervision, and leadership. This chapter orients on the incorporation of these principles in these areas with emphasis on addressing traumatic countertransference, vicarious trauma, compassion fatigue, and burnout. The phenomenon of vicarious posttraumatic growth will be introduced as another possibility for how trauma work regularly impacts professionals. SAMHSA's guidance for developing trauma-informed organizations will be outlined. Content from the Sanctuary Model is presented along with the idea that organizations are complex living systems impacted by trauma and loss in similar ways as individual trauma survivors. Experiential sociometric and psychodramatic processes can be employed within organizational meetings, supervision, or trainings to promote vicarious posttraumatic growth and peer support while mitigating the impacts of vicarious trauma. Examples from the author's experience will be provided throughout to depict concepts in action using sociometry and psychodrama techniques described throughout the book.

Vicarious Traumatization, Secondary Traumatic Stress, Compassion Fatigue, and Burnout

Vicarious traumatization (VT), secondary traumatic stress (STS), compassion fatigue (CF), and burnout are work hazards that impacts all social service industries, especially those professionals working directly with trauma

DOI: 10.4324/9781003277859-11

survivors and providing trauma-focused services. These negative impacts of the work can have a detrimental impact on the quality of services provided, the health of workers, and the success of an organization over time. If left unchecked, these work hazards can run amok and causing conflict, increasing organizational liability, disrupting relationships, impacting safety, decreasing staff morale, and usurping the staff and clients of inspiration and hope. Trauma-informed organizations need to consider the risks and presence of vicarious trauma, CF, and burnout within their staff while taking action to foster wellness and self-care. We could argue even that organizations have an ethical responsibility to consider staff's well-being through these lenses (Kanno & Giddings, 2017)

Vicarious trauma and secondary trauma are terms often used interchangeably but they actually were developed with a distinct differentiation. The concept of vicarious trauma was developed by Pearlman and Saakvitne (1995) to label the adverse changes that workers sometimes experience in their belief systems, cognitions, and worldview. For example, a divorce attorney may come to believe that healthy marriages are rare; an EMT in an area impacted by the opioid epidemic may come to believe that recovery from addiction is impossible, or a therapist in an inpatient psychiatric unit may develop a belief that trying to help others is pointless as they frequently return to the hospital suicidal. The term STS, however, was developed to describe the phenomenon of posttraumatic stress symptoms manifesting in professionals who were working with trauma survivors (Figley, 2013). Both vicarious and STS are experienced by a variety of professionals including healthcare workers, therapists, lawyers, law enforcement, case managers, advocates, activists, administrators, educators, students, supervisors, and leaders. Both of these conditions are also possible in everyday life from hearing disturbing details of the traumatic experiences of others, on the news, and in social media. Participants in group therapy also have some risk of experiencing vicarious trauma and STS through hearing the experiences of other group members. Perhaps the difference between VT and STS is less relevant since the 2013 publication of the DSM-5 which updated the posttraumatic stress disorder (PTSD) diagnostic criteria in two significant ways: (1) it includes recognition that one might develop PTSD through hearing repeated distressing stories or details of the trauma of others through their work or relationships and (2) it added a fourth symptom cluster of PTSD that focuses on negative changes to a trauma survivors moods and belief systems. These changes probably further contributed to the confusion between VT and STS as the latter was more focus on the original three PTSD symptom clusters (arousal/reactivity, numbing/avoidance, and intrusions/re-experiencing) while VT articulates how the fourth symptom cluster (negative changes in mood and cognitions) relates to professionals and vicarious trauma. To further complicate these concepts, Figley (2002, 2013) also used the terms STS and CF synonymously, believing that CF was a more user-friendly and less stigmatizing way of describing this phenomenon. In summary, there is not always agreement in the literature about clearly defining and differentiating vicarious trauma, secondary trauma, CF, and burnout (Kanno & Giddings, 2017).

Similar to vicarious trauma and secondary trauma, we also must define and differentiate the terms CF and burnout. CF was initially proposed as a concept by Carla Joinson (1992) to label nurses loss of their ability to nurture others. Figley and others adopted the term and integrated it into their work on STS and burnout, further leading to the confusion in these terms (Mathieu, 2021). CF is the process by which the worker takes on the suffering of their clients and develops adverse emotional and psychological impacts which impact their ability to continue as a healthy helper. CF is characterized by a sense of numbness, indifference, desensitization, and loss of morale in the work. Burnout, on the other hand, is a state of exhaustion resulting from overworking without proper self-care. It emerges as forgetfulness, irritability, anxiety, overwhelm, depression, and helplessness. Burnout is frequently, but not always related to vicarious trauma and STS. Burnout is less trauma related, though can certainly be fueled by trauma. Understanding and addressing these four negative impacts on workers and colleagues is essential for all trauma-informed organizations. The specific definitions of each are probably less important for practitioners than for academics or researchers. One study even found STS, VT, and burnout to be mainly measuring the same phenomenon (Devilly, Wright, & Varker, 2009). STS pioneer Beth Stamm touches upon this point in the first page of her seminal text in stating that "the great controversy about helping-induced trauma is not "can it happen?" but "what shall we call it?" (1995, p. 1, as cited in Mathieu, 2021).

The prevalence of STS and burnout is alarmingly high among therapists and other healthcare workers. A study of over 250 trauma therapists in the United Kingdom discovered that over 70% of participants were at high risk for STS (Sodeke-Gregson, Holttum, & Billings, 2013). Similarly, 70% of social workers reported at least one symptom of STS while 42% indicated that they suffer from STS (Adams et al., 2006; Bride, 2007). Shockingly, 34% of child welfare workers met criteria for PTSD based on STS (Bride, 2007). An alarming recent study discovered that 47.5% of frontline health care workers were suffering from STS during the COVID-19 outbreak in 2020 (Orru et al., 2021). Multiple studies highlight vicarious trauma as a predictor of staff turnover and negative outcomes for staff, organizations, and clients (Devilly, Wright, & Varker, 2009; Kim et al., 2018).

Like STS, burnout also is much more common and pervasive than one might expect. A systematic review of burnout in psychotherapists (including 8,808 participants total) resulted in a finding of over half reporting moderate–high levels of burnout (Simionato & Simpson, 2018). Similarly, a study of over 400 psychologists resulted in 49% reporting moderate–high levels of burnout (Simpson et al., 2019). Burnout has been demonstrated in various studies to impact professionals' physical and psychological well-being including sleep, medical issues, memory problems, mental health conditions, interpersonal difficulties, absenteeism and staff turnover, poor work performance, and misconduct (Simionato, Simpson, & Reid, 2019). "Hence, the ethical impact of burnout extends to our duty of care to clients and responsibilities to employer" (Simionato, Simpson, & Reid, 2019, p. 470).

In the discussion of vicarious trauma, STS, CF, and burnout, it is also important to highlight the potential that the organization and other systems have in fueling these experiences for staff. It can be tempting to frame these concepts as deficiencies on the part of the individual worker, but they are also manifestations of deficiencies in the system and organization within which services are provided. Bloom and Farragher (2013) write that "it is becoming increasingly clear that burnout is not a problem of individuals but of the environments within which people work" (p. 347). A 2007 NASW study showed that participants experience more stress from their workplace environment and working conditions than from the vicarious stress of working with trauma survivors (Dale, 2008, as cited in Handran, 2015). In my own experience as a therapist, supervisor, and educator, I have found this to ring true. In my work as a psychotherapist, it is hard to think of a client I've worked with who didn't spend considerable time in therapy talking about the stress of their workplace, work relationships, work expectation/pay, or conditions on the job. As a supervisor, I find that many supervisees at other agencies frequently seek emotional support in supervision related to workplace problems and unethical practices in the field. Similarly, as an educator, each year my students spend considerable time in class describing the work-related stresses and frustrations with their internship or field placement supervisors and sites. A study by Handran (2015) discovered higher rates of burnout and STS in social workers experiencing a lack of organizational support, lacking supervisory support, and limited training in trauma. These findings suggest that organizations can mitigate the potential hazards of burnout, CF, vicarious trauma, and STS by creating organizational structures that prioritize workers' well-being, peer support, supervision, and professional development. It isn't much of a stretch to conclude that an organization committed to trauma-informed care is also an organization that workers find more pleasurable and meaningful to work within.

Traumatic Countertransference

Countertransference is another phenomenon that can impact the well-being of staff and an organization-as-a-whole. Judith Herman reminds us that traumatic transference and countertransference are unavoidable in trauma therapy, and will inevitably have some impact on the therapeutic relationship (1992). Countertransference is when the professional projects their own unresolved issues upon their client. Traumatic countertransference (TC) is when this happens within the context of the unresolved trauma of the professional entangling with the unresolved trauma of the client (Herman, 1992). TC is similar to vicarious trauma, secondary trauma, and CF, but unlike the others it is viewed as a shorter-term response to a single client or group (McCann & Pearlman, 1990). TC often fuels VT, STS, CF, and burnout, though it is primarily contained to psychotherapy relationships (Pearlman & Saakvitne, 1995). Within the context of trauma-focused services and agencies, TC often fuels and VT, STS, and CF, which in turn increase risks for burnout (see Figure 11.1).

The figure above depicts the significant role that TC can play in the development of VT, STS, CF, and burnout in staff. As such, it would be wise for leaders and staff to consider the presence and potential risks of TC in their work. It is important also to note that these processes are not usually linear as depicted in this simplification. Many will experience VT, STS, or CF without experiencing TC or burnout. Similarly, many professionals experience TC or burnout without also experiencing CT, STS, or CF. On the other hand, burnout is also likely to contribute to additional TC, VT, STS, and CF.

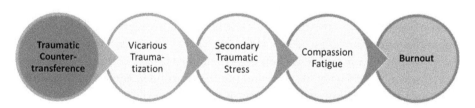

Figure 11.1 Simplified process of traumatic countertransference fueling burnout.

When it comes to these issues, perhaps Benjamin Franklin's old saying is particularly true – an ounce of prevention is worth a pound of cure (Kaklauskas & Greene, 2020). Kanno and Giddings (2017) summarize the research literature and offer multiple suggestions to organizational leaders to mitigate the adverse effects of TC, VT, STS, CF, and burnout. They suggest the following:

1) Provide ongoing and consistent supervision for staff, especially newer clinicians who are at higher risk
2) Cultivate peer support for staff within the organization
3) Reduce or rotate direct service hours if possible
4) Provide trainings and education on trauma for staff
5) Empower staff to address their own trauma through counseling or personal growth avenues

Most of these five suggestions are implementable in any agency. It is interesting to note that nearly all of these suggestions (except number three) have a specifically social and relational component. Herman (1992) suggests that "just as no [trauma] survivor can recover alone, no therapist can work with trauma alone" (p. 141). This sentiment is further depicted in the poignant article, *In the Belly of the Beast: Traumatic Countertransference*, by Richard Beck and Bonnie Buchele (2005) which emphasizes the importance of consultation and support. While TC, VT, STS, CF, and burnout are serious work hazards, especially for trauma therapists, there are also potential benefits of working with trauma survivors and ways that the work can promote personal and professional growth.

How do I navigate my own experience of traumatic countertransference and vicarious trauma?

How can I create habits or structures that prevent burnout for myself and others in my agency?

Vicarious Posttraumatic Growth

Vicarious posttraumatic growth (VPTG) is the phenomenon of professionals who work with trauma survivors to experience growth as a result of their work. This growth emerges in the professional's personal life as well as their professional growth. VPTG has been demonstrated in research with a wide variety of professionals including therapists, social workers, lawyers, educators, interpreters, case managers, nurses, doctors, and other healthcare workers. VPTG appears to manifest in the same five domains of posttraumatic growth (Calhoun & Tedeschi, 2014) (see Figure 11.2).

VPTG emerges in different ways for different people. When I reflect on my own experience, I can pinpoint various examples of VPTG from my work. Some of these examples include an increased sense of my own strengths such as my ability to bounce back, to tolerate pain, to help others make sense of tragedy, and my ability to offer insight, wisdom, and empathy. I also notice VPTG in my enhanced relationships with others – I have come to place more value in my marriage, my gratitude for my parents, and my appreciation for my friends and colleagues through hearing the many stories of relational trauma of my clients. My work with clients has fortified a steadfast sense of spiritual purpose and meaning in my career.

What are the specific ways that I have experienced vicarious posttraumatic growth as a result of my work?

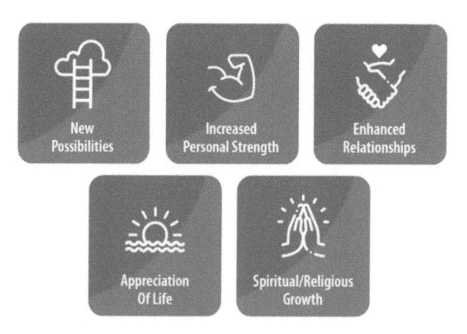

Figure 11.2 Five domains of posttraumatic growth (republished from Giacomucci, 2021, p. 170).

VPTG is much more common than many might expect. In one study of trauma counselors, over 70% reported VPTG in various forms including living life more fully, treating others with more kindness, and being more emotionally present or expressive in their personal lives (Arnold et al., 2005). Much of the research literature about cultivating VPTG, proposes the same or similar suggestions outlined above by Kanno and Giddings (2017). A systematic review on VPTG (Manning, de Terte, & Stephens, 2015) highlights that VPTG increases through specific behaviors and interpersonal variables (depicted in Figure 11.3) – specifically through engaging in supervision, peer support, self-care, and personal therapy (Arnold et al., 2005; Barrington & Shakespeare-Finch, 2013; Brockhouse et al., 2011; Linley & Joseph, 2005, 2007; Satkunanayagam et al., 2010; Splevins et al., 2010; Tehrani, 2010).

Various studies also discovered other variables that were positively related to VPTG, which include a sense of satisfaction and compassion satisfaction, competence, value in one' work, humor, empathy, optimism, positive affect, professional self-esteem, time, and witnessing trauma growth in clients (Brockhouse et al., 2011; Carmel, 1997; Gibbons, Murphy, & Joseph, 2011; Manning, de Terte, & Stephens, 2015; Stamm, 2005; Taubman-Ben-Ari & Weintroub, 2008). Furthermore, Linley and Joseph (2007) uncover that therapists with humanistic and transpersonal theoretical orientations are more likely to experience VPTG, whereas cognitive behavioral training was inversely related with VPTG. Some studies also discovered that professionals

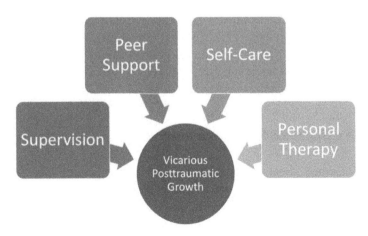

Figure 11.3 Behavioral and interpersonal variables contributing to vicarious posttraumatic growth.

with a trauma history themselves who are in personal therapy tend to report higher rates of VPTG (Brockhouse et al., 2011; Cosden et al., 2016; Linley & Joseph, 2007), which further supports SAMHSA's trauma-informed guidance of employing folks in recovery within agencies.

VPTG and STS would appear to be opposite responses to vicarious trauma, and many believe that they exist within an inverse relationship to each other – that STS would decrease while VPTG increases. VPTG describes a positive impact from vicarious trauma while STS describes an adverse impact. However, the research on their relationship is conflicting. Some studies demonstrate no relationship between VPTG and STS, some studies show a positive relationship between them, and other studies suggest a curvilinear relationship – that VPTG increases with STS until it reaches a certain point, after which STS continues to increase but VPTG levels off (Cleary et al., 2022; Manning, de Terte, & Stephens, 2015). The most recent meta-analysis on the topic reveals a small, significant positive relationship between VPTG and STS (Cleary et al., 2022). The relationship between VPTG and STS remains largely unclear, and more research is needed. Nevertheless, the objective for trauma-informed leaders and organizations is to help support their staff in reducing the adverse impacts of TC, VT, STS, CF, and burnout, while cultivating VPTG.

One of the most common measures employed in this context is the Professional Quality of Life scale (ProQOL) which is a 30-item, self-assessment tool measuring burnout, STS, and compassion satisfaction. This assessment is available for free at www.ProQOL.org. Other commonly used self-assessment tools include the Maslach Burnout Inventory, the Copenhagen Burnout Inventory, the Secondary Traumatic Stress Scale, the Posttraumatic Growth Inventory, and the PCL-5 PTSD Checklist. Many of these assessments are available for free online and can be employed by individuals or organizations to assess and evaluate changes over time (though some of these assessments require a fee and/or license to use).

SAMHSA's Guidance for Trauma-Informed Organizations

Trauma-informed organizations are focused on addressing the impact of trauma but also "promote positive well-being for the survivors of trauma receiving services, trauma caregivers, and the organizational leaders" (Handran, 2015, p. 3). Trauma-informed care philosophies do not only apply to our approach to clients but also the approach to staff, leaders, community partners, and the larger community. Trauma-informed organizations and systems carefully create structures that support staff in cultivating vicarious posttraumatic growth while addressing and mitigating the potential adverse impacts of TC, vicarious trauma, STS, CF, and burnout. A humanistic, empathetic, inclusive, ethical, and nonviolence approach is extended to all. Arledge and Wolfson (2001) emphasize that "in a trauma-informed system the human dimension should always be at the forefront, with consideration given to the whole person, regardless of whether the person is a consumer, a clinician, or a program administrator" (p. 91).

Trauma-informed organizations implement the four R's and six principles of trauma-informed care within the ten agency domains outlined by SAMHSA (2014a, 2014b) (see Table 11.1).

Table 11.1 SAMHSA's trauma-informed philosophy outlined in the four "R"s, six principles, and ten agency domains

The four "R"s	1. Realizes trauma has extensive impacts
	2. Recognizes symptoms of trauma or traumatic stress
	3. Responds through policies, procedures, and practices
	4. Resists retraumatization in all aspects of the work
The six principles	1. Safety
	2. Trustworthiness and transparency
	3. Peer support
	4. Collaboration and mutuality
	5. Empowerment, voice, and choice
	6. Cultural, historical, and gender issues
The ten agency domains	1. Governance and leadership
	2. Policy
	3. Physical environment
	4. Engagement and involvement
	5. Cross-sector collaboration
	6. Screening, assessment, and treatment
	7. Training and workforce development
	8. Progress monitoring and quality assurance
	9. Financing
	10. Evaluation

Trauma-informed organizations are constantly evolving, growing, and adapting to new research, best practices, and needs of clients, staff, and communities. Each of the four R's and six principles must be critically considered in each agency domain. It may seem easy enough for an administrator to reflect on this, but it really requires honest assessment, input, and ongoing evaluation from leadership, staff at all levels, clients, community partners, and other stakeholders. SAMHSA (2014b, pp. 160–161) offers a ten staged process for organizations to follow when beginning or continuing their journey toward the implementation of trauma-informed care:

1) Make a commitment to becoming a trauma-informed organization
2) Create an infrastructure to begin, support, and guide changes
3) Involve participants from across the organization including clients, staff, and community members
4) Assess current agency policies, procedures, and operations to determine how much they aid or inhibit trauma-informed approaches
5) Create a plan to further implement trauma-informed care in the organization
6) Develop collaborations with staff, clients, community members, and other service providers in different sectors
7) Follow through on putting the plan into action
8) Reassess implementation of the plan, its validity, and its relevance regularly
9) Use measures to improve the quality and effectiveness of approaches to meet needs
10) Implement practice that promote sustainability, including training, education, supervision, peer support, feedback, and the distribution of resources

Becoming, and maintaining a trauma-informed approach within an entire organization or system takes considerable time and effort. "Trauma-informed" is not just a marketing buzzword to carelessly slap onto a marketing brochure. It is a long-term commitment and dedication requiring action and more action. Furthermore, SAMHSA (2014b) provides 16 strategies within their implementation guide for behavioral health administrators to consider when developing a trauma-informed organization:

- Strategy #1: Show Organizational and Administrative Commitment to TIC
- Strategy #2: Use Trauma-Informed Principles in Strategic Planning
- Strategy #3: Review and Update Vision, Mission, and Value Statements

- Strategy #4: Assign a Key Staff Member to Facilitate Change
- Strategy #5: Create a Trauma-Informed Oversight Committee
- Strategy #6: Conduct an Organizational Self-Assessment of Trauma-Informed Services
- Strategy #7: Develop an Implementation Plan
- Strategy #9: Develop a Disaster Plan
- Strategy #10: Incorporate Universal Routine Screenings
- Strategy #11: Apply Culturally Responsive Principles
- Strategy #12: Use Science-Based Knowledge
- Strategy #13: Create a Peer Support Environment
- Strategy #14: Obtain Ongoing Feedback and Evaluations
- Strategy #15: Change the Environment to Increase Safety
- Strategy #16: Develop Trauma-Informed Collaborations

The strategies outlined above are described in more detail on pages 161–171 in SAMHSA's (2014b) *Trauma-Informed Care in Behavioral Health Services*, *TIP 57* (freely accessible online at https://www.ncbi.nlm.nih.gov/books/NBK207201/). These strategies provide a roadmap for leaders in developing trauma-informed organizations and can be used as a comprehensive guide.

Which of these 10 stages could my organization benefit from revisiting?

Which of these 16 strategies could my organization benefit from revisiting?

The Sanctuary Model and Creating PRESENCE

SAMHSA's publications on trauma-informed organizations include frequent references to the work of Sandra Bloom, MD, and the Sanctuary Model (including the pages references above articulating the 16 strategies for trauma-informed organizations in SAMHSA, 2014b). The Sanctuary Model is a trauma-informed systems approach developed by Bloom and colleagues between 1985 and 1991 in a Philadelphia psychiatric hospital (Bloom, 2013). The Sanctuary Model has evolved over the past few decades into a highly regarded operationalization of the trauma-informed philosophy within treatment centers, residential programs, therapeutic communities, hospitals, agencies, cities, and society (Bloom, 2012, 2013). It was developed through the integration of attachment theory, the neurobiology of trauma, and the importance of community (Bloom, 1997, 2008). It is based on seven commitments which are each approached as interdependent facets that collectively provide a foundation for all relationships and interactions between staff, clients, and leadership: (1) nonviolence; (2) emotional intelligence; (3) social learning; (4) open communication; (5) democracy; (6) social responsibility; and (7) growth and change (Bloom & Farragher, 2013). Sanctuary Model proposes Safety, Emotions, Loss, and Future (S.E.L.F.) as a "compass for recovery" that provides a comprehensive curriculum and foundation for interventions, groups, services, community meetings, and staff meetings (Bloom, 2008, 2013). S.E.L.F. represents four simple concepts disrupted by trauma and four domains or phases that organizations guided by the Sanctuary Model utilize to guide their decision-making, treatment plans, organizational changes, and service provision (Bloom & Farragher, 2013). Programs around the world have implemented Sanctuary Model into their organizations.

With the success of Sanctuary Model and the continued emergence of research and best practices, Dr. Bloom has recently initiated the next evolution of her work called "Creating PRESENCE" (2021). PRESENCE is an acronym that articulates the core values of her philosophy and practice:

- Partnership and Power
- Reverence and Restoration
- Emotional Wisdom and Empathy
- Safety and Social Responsibility
- Embodiment and Enactment
- Nature and Nurture
- Culture and Complexity
- Emergence and Evolution

This new program was developed in response to the COVID-19 pandemic to create an online implementation of trauma-informed philosophy within organizations and systems in a self-paced course. PRESENCE was created building on Blooms previous work with the intent of making the training more affordable and accessible.

In my opinion, the brilliance of Bloom's work is in her conceptualization of parallel processes in agencies and her teaching of organizations as complex, adaptive, emergent, and alive entities (Bloom & Farragher, 2013). As a group worker, I compare this to group work's concept of the "group-as-a-whole" – that the group is not just a bunch of individuals, but also a collective and dynamic entity that forms from the synergy of all of the parts of the group. The same group-as-a-whole phenomenon emerges within organizations which are also groups. Just as an individual's past trauma and loss impacts their behavior, emotions, defenses, relationships, well-being, beliefs, values, perspectives, and sense of self, so too does the past trauma and loss of an organization-as-a-whole (Bloom, 2007; Bloom & Farragher, 2013). Bloom (2013) writes that "organizations are not machines, but are living complex systems and as such are every bit as vulnerable to the impact of trauma and chronic stress as the people who receive and deliver service" (p. 14). In *Destroying Sanctuary: The Crisis in Human Service Delivery Systems* (2013), Bloom and Farragher describe many of the ways that organizations, as living entities, are vulnerable to trauma, loss, and chronic stress – including social defense mechanisms (denial, coercion, avoidance, scapegoating, etc.), organizational hyperarousal, organizational stress, loss of emotional management, organizational learning disabilities and amnesia, communication problems, conflict, organizational alexithymia, abuse of power, organizational injustice, learned helplessness, unresolved grief, and organizational trauma reenactments.

Organizations are living entities that are impacted by trauma in similar ways as individuals (Bloom & Farragher, 2013). Just as individuals unconsciously utilize defense mechanisms to manage anxiety and threat, so do organizations at the collective level. This manifests in an organization's collective denial, avoidance, dissociation, projection, coercion, and scapegoating of others. Chronic organizational stress and crisis can disrupt safety and develop into a state of organizational hyperarousal. Acute and chronic stress in individuals often causes a rupture in memory and learning capacities – the same phenomenon emerges in chronically stressed organizations. This fuels an inability of organizations to consider the complexities of problems or solutions and to develop reactive decisions, policies, or practices which fuel further fragmentation, lower morale, and conflict. Similarly, to how a trauma survivor's emotional regulation is impacted, organizations who have experienced trauma, loss, and chronic stress also experience a disruption of emotional regulation, containment, and stability which can lead to poor quality services, miscommunication, conflict, violence, and an inability to address or discuss the agency problems – organizational alexithymia. When the organization-as-a-whole loses its safety, stability, communication, integration, and ability to process emotions and ideas, it leads to further deterioration through conflict, organizational injustice, and trauma reenactments (Bloom & Faragher, 2013). The organization itself becomes stuck in the roles of perpetrator, victim, and abandoning authority and loses its ability to help trauma survivors heal. These "destructive processes routinely occur within and between organizations that mirror or 'parallel' the trauma-related processes for which our clients seek help" (Bloom, 2013, p. 15).

What are the traumas, losses, defenses, or other collective problems that my organization experiences?

Bloom highlights the potential parallel processes that emerge between clients, staff, leaders, and the organization-as-a-whole. She utilizes the following definition of parallel process from Smith, Simmons, and Thames (1989), "when two or more systems – whether these consist of individuals, groups, or organizations – have significant relationships with one another, they tend to develop similar thoughts, feelings, and behaviors" (p. 13). When working with individuals experiencing trauma, grief, rage, dissociation, defenses, helplessness, oppression, and conflict, it is inevitable that staff will be impacted and may develop similar thoughts, feelings, and behaviors – perhaps these parallel processes manifests in STS, CF, and burnout for professionals. When there is conflict between staff, it is more likely that there will be conflict with or between clients – this is particularly true in residential and inpatient settings. When staff avoid their trauma and grief, it is likely to promote avoidance of trauma and grief in clients. When leaders dehumanize their staff, there is a higher likelihood of staff dehumanizing their clients. If staff feel unsafe, they will struggle to establish safety with clients. The list of potential parallel processes can go on and on. The hopeful thing to drive home is that parallel processes can also emerge through healthy behaviors, positive change, resilience, growth, and recovery. When staff feel empowered by their leaders, they are more able to empower their clients. When staff feel safe, supported, and securely attached within their organization, they are better able to promote safety, support, and secure attachment with clients. When leaders and organizations attend to race, gender, culture, and identity with culturally responsive actions, staff are better able to attend to the same issues with their clients. Organizations-as-a-whole that are healthy, adaptive, and ethical generate (and retain) staff who are healthy, adaptive, and ethical – who, in turn, are able to promote health, adaptability, and ethics within their clientele.

What are parallel processes that sometimes emerge in my own organization between leaders, staff, and clients?

In trauma therapy, we move through three phases of the clinical map: (1) safety, strengths, containment, psychoeducation, and stability; (2) trauma processing; and (3) integration, posttraumatic growth, and future visioning.

A trauma therapist and client work together to assess unresolved trauma and loss from the past while considering how it impacts the individual's present-day behavior and personality structure. Treatment goals are established and refined in a collaborative process. Safety is established through empathy, relationship, strengths, containment, boundaries, and psychoeducation. Coping skills and resources are provided to the client to promote psychosocial stability. The emotions, sensations, negative cognitions, and memories related to past trauma are examined and processed. New insights, perspectives, and transformations are integrated while posttraumatic growth is cultivated. These three phases of the clinical map and the work of the trauma therapist with an individual client are a parallel process for the recovery journey of an organization-as-a-whole. A traumatized organization needs a trauma-informed leader or an outside consultant to guide it through its journey of recovery.

A traumatized organization that has not begun to address its own collective trauma, dysfunction, loss, secondary trauma, burnout, and attend to the needs of its staff is in no condition to be providing trauma-informed services, and especially not trauma-focused treatments. Just as individual therapists must engage in their own self-care, do their own personal growth, and manage their own TC, so too must organizations. Staff experiencing burnout are more likely to experience retraumatization in the workplace while contributing to the retraumatization of clients. Bloom and Farragher (2013) remind us that "burnout may then be the result of repetitive or chronic exposure to vicarious traumatization that is unrecognized and unsupported by the organizational setting" (p. 346). This conceptualization of burnout shifts some of the responsibility for mitigating and addressing burnout away from the individual worker and upon the collective organization. Trauma therapists and trauma-focused programs or providers are especially prone to burnout and vicarious trauma. Trauma-informed organizations demonstrate an ongoing commitment to attending to the burnout and STS of its staff. Bloom exclaims that "trying to implement trauma-specific clinical interventions without first implementing trauma-informed cultural change is like throwing seeds on dry land" (Menschner & Maul, 2016, p. 2). This poignant quote reminds us that programs offering trauma-focused services must first attend to developing a trauma-informed organization while addressing the potential negative impacts of the work upon staff. This is not only an ethical responsibility but also promotes organizational well-being and sustainability of the program. In the context of this psychodrama book, it is also worth noting Dr. Bloom's consistent positive regard for the benefits of psychodrama and drama therapy which were incorporated in her psychiatric hospital program (Bloom, 2000, 2013; Bloom & Farragher, 2013; Giacomucci, 2021; Weber & Haen, 2005).

Sociometry, Psychodrama, and Sociodrama in Organizations

The experiential methods of sociometry and psychodrama offer organizational leaders, trainers, supervisors, and educators powerful processes that can be used to promote peer support through experiential learning. One of the secondary benefits of psychodrama training is the personal growth and enhanced team cohesion that emerges in the process due to the emphasis on experiential teaching and "learn by doing." In my own experience providing psychodrama trainings or using experiential methods to teach trauma-informed principles at treatment centers and organizations, one of the common themes that emerges in feedback from staff and leaders alike is that the training process helped to enhance the connection and cohesion within the team or department who attended, as well as a sense of personal growth. The action-based methods illuminate relational patterns and socio-dynamics within organizations, between individuals, which tend to reflect larger societal and cultural patterns. The organizational group is a micro-cosm of society. Working in action, especially through sociometric processes, allows us to uncover these sociodynamics, appropriately respond to them, and strengthen working relationships. Psychodrama and experiential training sessions are a much different experience than sitting and listening to an educator lecture from a PowerPoint. Instead, they bring the content to life through action methods that emphasize experiential, relational, embodied, and engaging learning (Giacomucci & Skolnik, 2021).

Interestingly, the provision of psychodrama/experiential trainings within an agency also directly or indirectly address each of the five recommendations outlined earlier by Kanno and Giddings (2017) for reducing burnout and STS: (1) supervision, (2) peer support, (3) reduce/rotate direct service hours, (4) training and education, and (5) personal growth or counseling. Psychodrama trainings involve experiential demonstrations and action learning structures which develop cohesion and meaningful connections within the group. Peer support is cultivated in the process of learning. The training event includes inherent learning objectives and content that is taught through sociometric and psychodramatic means. Sociometry and psychodrama are process oriented so they can be used to teach any content. The nature of psychodrama trainings creates personal growth opportunities for participants through psychodrama demonstrations. Ongoing psychodrama training series regularly involve supervised practice segments or supervision sessions during the training to help develop or refine the implementation of experiential processes or the training series content into the work of those attending. The logistics of hosting a training event or training series is an opportunity to reduce or rotate direct service hours as staff will likely need role relief from their regular job duties to attend the training session(s). Therefore, the very act of hosting psychodrama trainings within an agency is likely to address all five of the suggestions by Kanno and Giddings (2017) for addressing burn-out and STS. These five recommendations also share considerable overlap with the four behavioral and interpersonal variables from Manning and colleagues' systematic review (2015) that were highlighted for their capacity to promote VPTG.

Psychodrama and sociometry have been used in organizational development since the beginning – one of Jacob Moreno's first jobs after finishing his medical degree was working as the chief physician of a fabric factory in Austria while serving as the public health officer of the town (Nolte, 2014). Moreno employed his sociometric and psychodramatic ideas in various organizations, industry, and government or military agencies (Moreno, 2019). Contemporary psychodramatists frequently are contracted to utilize their various skills to improve organizational functioning – including sociometry to explore and enhance the functioning of organizational groups and relationships, sociodrama and psychodrama to implement role training, problem solving, and social skills building, as well as experiential teaching methods for providing educational content in engaging ways to staff (de Souza, Dias, & Cubo, 2022; Faisandier, 2010; Giacomucci, 2019, 2021; Giacomucci & Skolnik, 2021; Jones, 2001; Nolte, 2014; von Ameln & Becker-Ebel, 2020).

Experiential sociometry tools have a variety of applications in organizational settings. Spectrograms can be used to explore and assess an organizational team based on various criteria. For example, in a training on VPTG at an addictions treatment center, I utilized the following series of spectrograms to assess the group-as-a-whole while promoting critical self-reflection:

- How consistent are you at engaging in your own self-care?
- How often do you feel burnout, vicarious trauma, or overwhelming stress related to the work?
- How much would you say that the work has prompted you to grow as a person and professional?

With each prompt the staff organized themselves on an imaginal line between opposite walls of the group room ranging from most to least, followed by discussion with each other about why they self-assessed to be where they are on the spectrogram. This series of spectrograms not only helped participants with self-reflection, peer support, and connections but also helped the clinical director and supervisors on the team to see which staff may need additional support regarding work stress, vicarious trauma, and burnout. Spectrograms are one of the simplest sociometric processes that can be easily implemented into any group, community, educational, or organizational setting (Giacomucci, 2020; Giacomucci et al., 2018) (see Chapter 4 for more examples).

Another experiential process that is particularly useful in organizations is the Circle of Strengths. This process uses props (usually scarves) to concretize strengths within the group, individual peers, self, clients, and the organization. There are various ways that it can be modified for different topics or purposes, but it is primarily used with strengths. In my experience, and based on the feedback from various clients, students, and colleagues, this process appears to cultivate group cohesion quicker than any other process that I am aware of.

> One of the first times that I employed this in an organizational setting was on a board of directors meeting for an organization that had recently begun to experience significant internal conflict among board members and leadership. The president approached me for help in leading a warm-up as a board member who was newer to the board and respected by board members on both sides of the conflict. There was fear that the conflict may escalate and lead to further fragmentation within leadership, so the president wanted to help establish more safety and connection at the start of the meeting. I immediately chose the Circle of Strengths for its power in helping participants establish safety and recognize strengths within the group. I asked board members to choose a scarf from my collection to represent a strength that they personally bring to the organization and to name it, placing it on the floor in front of them. Then, I positioned everyone into dyads and had them each choose a scarf to represent a strength they experience in their partner that could help with the difficulties in the organization. They each took turns presenting the strengths to their partner, honoring them for the positive qualities they bring to the organization. Next, I asked everyone to choose a scarf to represent a strength they experience in the organization-as-a-whole to present to the group. In this process, each person reflected back to the group, the positive qualities and aspects of the organization. I then facilitated the concretization of the organizations values and mission and added it into the circle of strengths which helped each person reconnect to, and prioritize, the purpose and mission of the organization. While the board meeting ended up still being emotionally charged, conflictual, and difficult, we were able to come together as a board and make difficult decisions about the future of the organization. It is hard to measure how much impact this process had on the organization, but this organization, which many of us feared might collapse, is now in a much healthier place a few years later.

Another use of sociometry in organizations, and perhaps one of the most helpful methods of exploring trauma-informed principles in organizations, is the use of the floor check (see Chapter 4 for a comprehensive overview of floor checks). The trauma-informed principles floor check involves placing pages of paper with each of the six trauma-informed principles throughout the room (safety, trustworthiness and transparency, peer support, collaboration and mutuality, empowerment, voice, and choice, and cultural, historic, and gender issues). After some brief psychoeducation on each of the principles, I offer a series of reflective questions, inviting participants to come stand by the principle that answer the question for them individually. Examples prompts could include:

- Which principle do you feel you most embody in your work personally?
- Which principle do you feel you have the most room to grow into in your work?
- Which principle do you feel the organization has the most room to grow in?
- Which principle do you feel the organization does the best at embodying already?
- Which principle do you feel your team has already grown in the past year?

With each question, a new arrangement of clustered participants emerges, and a few minutes are offered for those standing at the same place to share with each other in small groups about their choice. This promotes critical self-reflection on the implementation of these principles into one's work and areas for continued growth for individuals and the organization. This process also inherently involves some group-as-a-whole assessment about staff's perception of how trauma-informed principles are being implemented in the agency and where the areas of growth are. This is a simple, yet profoundly helpful process that I have used in various treatment centers, conferences, professional societies, board meetings, non-profit agencies, universities, and other corporate settings. In utilizing this process with agencies, I also find it valuable to connect the six trauma-informed principles to the core values of the organization or profession at hand to demonstrate that these frameworks are usually already considered within organizations (though often with different language).

Sociometry processes will be easier to implement in organizational settings than psychodrama or sociodrama as they require less spontaneity, vulnerability, and less training or experience from the facilitator. However, a skilled psychodramatist can utilize various role-playing structures to promote growth, new insight, connection, and change within organizations. One simple structure that I have come to utilize often in ongoing training series at organizations is enacting difficult interactions between clients and staff. The following example comes from ongoing training I have offered for therapists and support staff at a residential recovery center:

> After the group is properly warmed-up, I invite them to highlight some of the more difficult client interactions that they have been experiencing. We agree on one situation as a group and choose participants to reenact the scene. In this scene, a staff member, Andrew, is trying to motivate a resident named Mike to get out of bed, to clean his room, and to partic- ipate in the structured program. The resident is depressed and becomes increasingly combative as the staff member becomes increasingly frus- trated. After enacting the scene, I pause the action and ask participants to offer doubling statements for the staff member – "what do you think is going on internally for this Andrew in this situation?". Participants offer doubling statements ranging from "I am so frustrated at this resident, why can't he just get out of bed", to "I have so many other important job responsibilities, I don't have time to deal with this", to "I'm afraid that Mike isn't going to make it and will get kicked out or leave, and poten- tially die from their addiction if something doesn't change soon." With each statement Andrew and the group felt more and more validated by each other. Then, I ask for doubling statements for Mike which included "I am so depressed, I'm not sure that I want to live", to "I have tried other recovery programs and they didn't work for me, I don't have much hope or motivation that it will work this time either", to "I feel threatened by men in positions of authority telling me what I have to do because it activates feelings from childhood when my father was physically abusive to me". After the group has accessed new insights through doubling, we shift to role training and exploring new ways of responding to the client in the same situation. In this part, we reenact the original scene multiple times with participants stepping into Andrew's role to experiment and practice new, trauma-informed responses to the Mike. After a series new responses demonstrated in this context, the group shifts to sharing about the process and their experiential learning.

Using this psychodramatic process, the staff have a chance to articulate and explore interactions with clients that are a source of stress and frustration. The group validates each other's experiences while deepening their under- standing of what may be fueling the dysfunctional behaviors in the scene. Doubling offers new insight of underlying fueling factors while the role train- ing provides an integration of spontaneity and new responses to this old, reoc- curring situation. This structure for supervision group sis further described by Giacomucci (2021), Hinkle (2008), and von Ameln and Becker-Ebel (2020). The above scene could have been expanded further to explore transference and countertransference between the client and staff member.

The doubling statements began to illustrate the potential transference that the client had toward the staff member as his abusive father. Considering that the client was likely experiencing transference, it is also likely that the staff member was reciprocating with their own countertransference upon the client. If this was true for Andrew, the scene could have been deepened by enrolling Mike's father as well as the source of Andrew's countertransference – perhaps his own child who experiences depression or refuses to engage in his responsibilities at home. Providing an opportunity for Andrew to become more conscious of his own countertransference in the situation and express some of the unresolved feelings toward his own child, may help him show up in more helpful ways for the residents he works with. This level of work should only be done with cohesive groups who can tolerate the vulnerability of such a process and a skilled psychodrama facilitator. Working with countertransference can quickly lead into the personal trauma experiences of professionals which often needs to be reserved for therapy sessions rather than training events at one's workplace. The general structure described in the example above can be used psychodramatically with a specific situation and defining a specific client and staff interaction (such as the one described above between Andrew and Mike), or it can be used sociodramatically by defining the roles more collectively as "a staff member" and "a resident" and co-creating a situation that reflects commonly experienced interactions between the staff and clients.

Sociodramatic processes are often ideal for organizational session as they do not always require the same level of vulnerability that psychodrama often entails. Another example of sociodrama in this context comes from a presentation I have offered at various places including my local psychodrama collective and for a Turkish psychodrama training institute. This involves the use of multiple empty chairs to represent different sociodramatic roles.

> I started with two empty chairs to hold the roles of "a therapist experiencing burnout and secondary traumatic stress" and "a client experiencing PTSD". First, I invited participants to step into the empty chairs and provide doubling statements for each role, what may be going on beneath the surface for each individual in the therapeutic dyad. Participants doubled for the therapist with statements such as "I am so exhausted, I'm not sure I can be fully present with this client", "I'm overworked and numb", and "I am unsure if I am in a place where I can really help this person". Then we explored doubling statements from the client's role which included – "I am desperate for relief, but this therapist doesn't offer much help", "I really need validation and new skills but this therapist keeps talking about themself", and "nothing is changing for me, maybe I am going to be stuck dealing with PTSD for the rest of my life". Then, I

invited participants to talk directly to the therapist experiencing burnout to offer support and suggestions which resulted in a plethora of ideas and resources for the therapist to seek their own help. Having engaged with the topic of self-care, I initiated a role transition for the therapist to "a therapist experiencing vicarious posttraumatic growth" and invited additional doubling statements. The group spontaneously provided statements such as – "I can state my limits and boundaries and ask for help when I need it", "after seeking my own supervision and personal therapy, I feel more rejuvenated and competent to help my client", and "I am so grateful for the opportunity to serve others which has helped me grow as well". Then, we looked at messages to and from the "therapist experiencing vicarious posttraumatic growth" and the client which were infused with a new sense of presence, inspiration, and emotional connection. In the sharing portion of the group, participants connect with each other about the doubling statements that resonated most with them. There was a sense of connection and a shared bond about the difficulties and importance of maintaining self-care while showing up for clients who have experienced trauma. Participants shared about their own strategies for self-care and their own experiences of vicarious posttraumatic growth.

This sociodramatic process with multiple empty chairs provides participants with a chance to explore a shared topic without the personal vulnerability that psychodrama involves. Though participants were doubling and offering messages from a collective role, in most cases they were also using their own personal experience to inform their statements. While the sociodramatic roles provided aesthetic distance, it also allowed them to closely explore the themes and topics related to burnout, vicarious trauma, and VPTG while developing a stronger sense of community with their professional peers.

Another way that psychodrama can be employed in training sessions is for personal and professional growth. This method is often used in trainings that focus on teaching participants how to facilitate psychodrama through demonstrations of the method. In my ongoing monthly psychodrama training group at an addictions treatment center, we commonly use this method so that the clinical team can become more familiar with psychodrama as they begin to incorporate psychodrama interventions into their own groups. After a warming-up process, I invite staff to propose topics that they may need to work on for their own individual growth as a professional. In one specific session, multiple volunteers offer their topics and I facilitate a sociometric protagonist selection which results in a psychodrama protagonist with the topic of fear and a goal of developing more confidence in their work.

We begin to enroll supportive roles and strengths into the psychodrama scene. The protagonist chooses self-worth as the first strength and asks a fellow colleague to play the role. I instruct them to role reverse with self-worth and speak to themself from the voice of worthiness. In their dialogue with self-worth, they begin to access spontaneity and translate their sense of value from their personal life into their professional experience. Then, we move to interpersonal support, where the protagonist identifies a supervisor and the organization-as-a-whole as supportive roles that could help with confidence. They engage in a psychodramatic dialogue where the protagonist shares their work-related fears with their supervisor and is reversed roles to respond to themself as their supervisor. In this process, the protagonist gets to see themself through the eyes of their supervisor and provide affirmation, validation, and support. The supervisor naturally begins to remind the protagonist of the many ways that they already demonstrate confidence, especially when advocating for their clients. Then, they choose an auxiliary to play the role of the organization-as-a-whole, which provides them with a chance to explore their relationship with the entire agency and articulate the supportive messages that they hear from their team, clients, and leadership. Moving on, I invite them to consider which other roles could be helpful with the topic, offering a range of possibilities – God, confidence, resilience, competence, future self, a role model, or something else. The protagonist chooses the future self role and selects a peer to hold the role. I direct them in having a discussion with themself in the future, having developed a sense of professional confidence. They articulate multiple questions for their future self and ask for guidance with the fear they have been experiencing. They share about their fear of being inadequate for their clients, fears of making a mistake at work that might impact others, and fears of confrontations with other staff or clients. Before the auxiliary can respond, I have them reverse roles so the protagonist can answer their own questions in the role of their future self. They engage in a discussion with their self about the fear, about worthiness, and their value to their clients and the company. Multiple other participants double for the future self role offering additional validation, guidance, and support for the protagonist. They discuss strategies for coping with fear and developing confidence in the workplace. After the psychodrama scene, the group moves into the sharing phase and each staff member shares with the protagonist about their own difficulties with fear, worthiness, and confidence at work. The group rallies to support each other and validate that everyone experiences fear or imposter syndrome while sharing helpful tips for cultivating confidence going forward.

In this example, the protagonist became a representative of the group working on a sociometrically chosen topic of fear and confidence in the workplace. The psychodrama scene provided the protagonist with a meaningful affirmation of their worth and professional development while validating their fears. The connection with a future self-initiated a sense of hope and empowerment for the protagonist while prompting the rest of the group to connect with their own professional goals for the future. The process helped the supervisor see how they are experienced by the supervisee and provided information about which messages or types of support are must helpful for this staff member. It also illuminated for the rest of the team some of the fears that this individual, and others on the team, experience. The psychodramatic dialogue with the organization helped to summarize the collective support and worth that the individual receives from individual throughout the entire agency. The sharing portion of the group provided a sense of solidarity and activated an all-in-the-same-boat phenomenon that initiated ongoing peer support within the team. It is also interesting to note the potential parallel process in the intrapsychic and interpersonal themes that arise in a treatment team with those in the community of clients. This psychodrama scene is not so different from psychodrama scenes that might emerge in a client group as clients in residential treatment also struggle with a sense of self-worth, confidence, fear, and hope for the future. Staff who are committed to working on these issues for themselves will be better able to help their clients address similar issues related to their recovery.

Traditionally, psychodrama training involves learning by doing and is composed of doing psychodramas in training sessions with real issues and goals faced by participants. In an ongoing psychodrama training group, it is not uncommon for participants to be volunteering themselves as protagonist to explore personal issues, relationship problems, and even trauma or loss. While more intense and personal issues may emerge in psychodrama training and provide therapeutic opportunities for personal growth, it is also important that the trainer always prioritize learning, teaching, and education in a training group. One of my primary critiques of psychodrama trainers is that their trainings groups are often indistinguishable from therapy groups. A skilled psychodrama trainer can contain psychodrama demonstrations to personal work that relates to professional growth when necessary – and/or provide opportunities for personal growth around core personal issues during psychodrama demonstrations while bringing the group back into a training mindset after the sharing portion of the psychodrama. This requires adequate pacing as these types of psychodramas often take more time to enact and it is important that there is sufficient time for sharing but also processing the psychodrama from the role of trainer and trainees. This norm of doing personal work in psychodrama training sometimes scares professionals from engaging in psychodrama workshops so it is important that the trainer meets the group where they are at in terms of the norms, expectations, and appropriate level of personal disclosure based on the setting that the training is being held in. While some have articulated this as a limitation in psychodrama training, others experience it as a huge benefit of pursing psychodrama training as it inevitably also provides personal growth in addition to professional learning. In my own teaching, I find that (in general) guest lectures, university classes, and professional conference workshops need to have much more containment and boundaries while onsite trainings for organizational teams are often willing to be more vulnerable with each other. Ongoing training programs or multi-day psychodrama workshops afford more opportunities for deepening safety and connection, thus often include much more intense personal growth work during the training process.

Psychodrama and sociometry offer leaders, trainers, supervisors, and practitioners with dynamic tools that can be used as experiential teaching methods for trauma-informed care content. Experiential methods from psychodrama can be utilized in various ways to operationalize trauma-informed philosophy while addressing and mitigating burnout and vicarious trauma within staff. VPTG can be embodied, explored, and cultivated through the peer support, self-care, personal growth, and supervision/teaching offered in psychodrama training events. Psychodrama can be used to explore countertransference and promote resilience within organizations. The experiential teaching processes from sociometry and psychodrama not only offer action-based psychoeducational tools but also promote cohesion in organizational teams.

Conclusion

An organization is a living and dynamic entity that is impacted by trauma and loss in similar ways that individuals are. Working with trauma includes the risks of TC, vicarious trauma, STS, CF, and burnout. Trauma-informed leaders actively work to mitigate these work hazards and address vicarious trauma when it emerges. The same trauma-informed principles that we strive to embody in our work with clients are also equally relevant in professional relationships and organizational spaces. VPTG is celebrated and cultivated through organizational process such as consistent supervision, peer support, self-care, and supporting personal growth opportunities for staff. The guidance offered by SAMHSA can be implemented by organizational leaders for implementing and strategizing on how to further incorporate trauma-informed care into any agency. Experiential processes such as sociometry, psychodrama, and sociodrama can be employed to engage staff in various ways including around trauma-informed care content, assessing the organization-as-a-whole, enhancing social skills and relationships between staff, troubleshooting clinical or organizational difficulties, and promoting personal growth.

References

Adams, R. E., Boscarino, J. A., & Figley, C. R. (2006). Compassion fatigue and psychological distress among social workers: A validation study. *American Journal of Orthopsychiatry, 76*(1), 103–108.

Arledge, E., & Wolfson, R. (2001). Care of the clinician: Effective services for trauma survivors rely on addressing the support and care needs of clinicians and administrators. In M. Harris, & R. D. Fallot (Eds.), *Using trauma theory to design service systems* (pp. 91–98). San Francisco, CA: Jossey-Bass.

Arnold, D., Calhoun, L. G., Tedeschi, R., & Cann, A. (2005). Vicarious posttraumatic growth in psychotherapy. *Journal of Humanistic Psychology, 45*, 239–263. https://doi.org/10.1177/0022167805274729

Barrington, A. G., & Shakespeare-Finch, J. (2013). Working with refugee survivors of torture and trauma: An opportunity for vicarious post-traumatic growth. *Counselling Psychology Quarterly, 26*(1), 89–105.

Beck, R., & Buchele, B. (2005). In the belly of the beast: Traumatic counter-transference. *International journal of group psychotherapy, 55*(1: Special Issue), 31–44.

Bloom, S. L. (1997). *Creating sanctuary: Toward the evolution of sane societies.* New York: Routledge.

Bloom, S. L. (2000). Creating Sanctuary: Healing from systematic abuses of power. *Therapeutic Communities: The International Journal for Therapeutic and Supportive Organizations, 21*(2), 67–91.

Bloom, S. L. (2007). Loss in Human Service Organizations. In L. A. Vargas, & S. L. Bloom (Eds.), *Loss, Hurt, and Hope: The Complex Issues of Bereavement and Trauma in Children* (pp. 142–204). Newcastle-on-Tyne, UK: Cambridge Scholars Publishing.

Bloom, S. L. (2008). The sanctuary model of trauma-informed organizational change. *Reclaiming Children and Youth, 17*(3), 48–53.

Bloom, S. L. (2012). Trauma-organized systems. In C. R. Figley (Ed.), *Encyclopedia of trauma* (pp. 741–743). Thousand Oaks, CA: SAGE.

Bloom, S. L. (2013). *Creating sanctuary: Toward the evolution of sane societies (Revised).* New York: Routledge.

Bloom, S. L. (2021). *Creating presence: A trauma-informed online organizational approach for creating trauma – Responsive organizations.* www.creatingpresence.net.

Bloom, S. L., & Farragher, B. (2013). *Restoring sanctuary: A new operating system for trauma-informed systems of care.* New York: Oxford University Press.

Bride, B. E. (2007). Prevalence of secondary traumatic stress among social workers. *Social Work, 52*(1), 63–70.

Brockhouse, R., Msetfi, R. M., Cohen, K., & Joseph, S. (2011). Vicarious exposure to trauma and growth in therapists: The moderating effects of sense of coherence, organizational support, and empathy. *Journal of Traumatic Stress, 24*(6), 735–742. https://doi.org/10.1002/jts.20704

Calhoun, L. G., & Tedeschi, R. G. (Eds.). (2014). *Handbook of posttraumatic growth: Research and practice.* New York: Routledge.

Carmel, S. (1997). The professional self-esteem of physicians scale, structure, properties and the relationship to work outcomes and life satisfaction. *Psychological Reports, 80*(2), 591–602.

Cleary, E., Curran, D., Kelly, G., Dorahy, M. J., & Hanna, D. (2022). The meta-analytic relationship between secondary traumatic stress and vicarious posttraumatic growth in adults. *Traumatology.* https://doi.org/10.1037/trm0000373

Cosden, M., Sanford, A., Koch, L. M., & Lepore, C. E. (2016). Vicarious trauma and vicarious posttraumatic growth among substance abuse treatment providers. *Substance Abuse, 37*(4), 619–624.

Dale, M. (2008). Social workers owe it to themselves and clients to value a healthy lifestyle. The profession must prioritize self-care. *NASW News, 53*(10), 4.

de Souza, A. C., Dias, A. R., & Cubo, R. (2022). Brazilian organizational psychodrama: Paths, practices, and reflections. In H. J. Fleury, M. M. Marra, & O. H. Hadler (Eds.), *Psychodrama in Brazil* (pp. 287–300). Singapore: Springer.

Devilly, G. J., Wright, R., & Varker, T. (2009). Vicarious trauma, secondary traumatic stress or simply burnout? Effect of trauma therapy on mental health professionals. *Australasian Psychiatry, 43*(4), 373–385.

Faisandier, J. (2010). Thriving under fire: 'Bringing Moreno into the corporate training world'. *Australian and Aotearoa New Zealand Psychodrama Association Journal, 19*, 65–72.

Figley, C. R. (2002). *Treating compassion fatigue.* New York: Brunner-Rutledge.

Figley, C. R. (2013). *Compassion fatigue: Coping with secondary traumatic stress disorder in those who treat the traumatized.* New York: Routledge.

Giacomucci, S. (2019). Social group work in action: A sociometry, psychodrama, and experiential trauma group therapy curriculum. *Doctorate in Social Work (DSW) Dissertations,* 124. Retrieved from https://repository.upenn.edu/cgi/viewcontent.cgi?article=1128&context=edissertations_sp2

Giacomucci, S. (2020). Addiction, traumatic loss, and guilt: A case study resolving grief through psychodrama and sociometric connections. *The Arts in Psychotherapy, 67*, 101627. https://doi.org/10.1016/j.aip.2019.101627

Giacomucci, S. (2021). *Social work, sociometry, and psychodrama: Experiential approaches for group therapists, community leaders, and social workers.* Singapore: Springer Nature. https://doi.org/10.1007/978-981-33-6342-7

Giacomucci, S., Gera, S., Briggs, D., Bass, K. (2018). Experiential addiction treatment: Creating positive connection through sociometry and therapeutic spiral model safety structures. *Journal of Addiction and Addictive Disorders, 5,* 17. https://doi.org/10.24966/AAD-7276/100017

Giacomucci, S., & Skolnik, S. (2021). The experiential social work educator: Integrating sociometry into the classroom environment. *Journal of Teaching in Social Work, 41*(2), 192–202.

Gibbons, S., Murphy, D., & Joseph, S. (2011). Countertransference and positive growth in social workers. *Journal of Social Work Practice, 25*(1), 17–30.

Handran, J. (2015). Trauma-informed systems of care: The role of organizational culture in the development of burnout, secondary traumatic stress, and compassion satisfaction. *Journal of Social Welfare and Human Rights, 3*(2), 1–22.

Herman, J. L. (1992). *Trauma and recovery: The aftermath of violence—From domestic abuse to political terror.* New York: Basic Books.

Hinkle, M. G. (2008). Psychodrama: A creative approach for addressing parallel process in group supervision. *Journal of Creativity in Mental Health, 3*(4), 401–415.

Joinson C. (1992). Coping with compassion fatigue. *Nursing, 22*(4), 116–121.

Jones, D. (2001). Sociometry in team and organisation development. *British Journal of Psychodrama and Sociodrama, 16*(1), 10.

Kaklauskas, F. J., & Greene, L. R. (2020). Finding the leader in you. In F. J. Kaklauskas, & L. R. Greene (Eds.), *Core principles of group psychotherapy* (pp. 171–181). New York: Routledge.

Kanno, H., & Giddings, M. M. (2017). Hidden trauma victims: Understanding and preventing traumatic stress in mental health professionals. *Social Work in Mental Health, 15*(3), 331–353.

Kim, J. J., Brookman-Frazee, L., Gellatly, R., Stadnick, N., Barnett, M. L., & Lau, A. S. (2018). Predictors of burnout among community therapists in the sustainment phase of a system driven implementation of multiple evidence-based practices in children's mental health. *Professional Psychology: Research and Practice, 49*(2), 132–141.

Linley, P. A., & Joseph, S. (2005). Positive and negative changes following occupational death exposure. *Journal of Traumatic Stress, 18*(6), 751–758. https://doi.org/10.1002/jts.20083

Linley, P. A., & Joseph, S. (2007). Therapy work and therapists' positive and negative well-being. *Journal of Social and Clinical Psychology*, 385–403. https://doi.org/10.1521/jscp.2007.26.3.385

Manning, S. F., de Terte, I., & Stephens, C. (2015). Vicarious posttraumatic growth: A systematic literature review. *International Journal of Wellbeing*, 5(2), 125–139.

Mathieu, F. (2021). *Why it is time to stop using "Compassion Fatigue"*. https://www.tendacademy.ca/stop-using-compassion-fatigue/

McCann, I. L., & Pearlman, L. A. (1990). *Psychological trauma and the adult survivor: Theory, therapy, and transformation*. New York: Brunner/Mazel.

Nolte, J. (2014). *The philosophy, theory, and methods of J.L. Moreno: The man who tried to become god*. New York: Routledge.

Orrù, G., Marzetti, F., Conversano, C., Vagheggini, G., Miccoli, M., Ciacchini, R., … & Gemignani, A. (2021). Secondary traumatic stress and burnout in healthcare workers during COVID-19 outbreak. *International Journal of Environmental Research and Public Health*, 18(1), 337.

Pearlman, L. A., & Saakvitne, K. W. (1995). *Trauma and the therapist: Countertransference and vicarious traumatization in psychotherapy with incest survivors*. New York: WW Norton & Co.

Satkunanayagam, K., Tunariu, A., & Tribe, R. (2010). A qualitative exploration of mental health professionals' experience of working with survivors of trauma in Sri Lanka. *International Journal of Culture and Mental Health*, 3(1), 43–51. https://doi.org/10.1080/17542861003593336

Simionato, G., Simpson, S., & Reid, C. (2019). Burnout as an ethical issue in psychotherapy. *Psychotherapy*, 56(4), 470.

Simpson, S., Simionato, G., Smout, M., van Vreeswijk, M. F., Hayes, C., Sougleris, C., & Reid, C. (2019). Burnout amongst clinical and counselling psychologist: The role of early maladaptive schemas and coping modes as vulnerability factors. *Clinical Psychology & Psychotherapy*, 26(1), 35–46.

Simionato, G. K., & Simpson, S. (2018). Personal risk factors associated with burnout among psychotherapists: A systematic review of the literature. *Journal of Clinical Psychology*, 74(9), 1431–1456.

Smith, K. K., Simmons, V. M., & Thames, T. B. (1989). "Fix the Women": An intervention into an organizational conflict based on parallel process thinking. *The Journal of Applied Behavioral Science*, 25(1), 11–29.

Sodeke-Gregson, E. A., Holttum, S., & Billings, J. (2013). Compassion satisfaction, burnout, and secondary traumatic stress in UK therapists who work with adult trauma clients. *European Journal of Psychotraumatology*, 4(1), 21869.

Splevins, K. A., Cohen, K., Joseph, S., Murray, C., & Bowley, J. (2010). Vicarious posttraumatic growth among interpreters. *Qualitative Health Research, 20*(12), 1705–1716. https://doi.org/10.1177/1049732310377457

Stamm, B. (1995). *Secondary traumatic stress: Self-care issues for clinicians, researchers, and educators*: Lutherville: The Sidran Press.

Stamm, B. H. (2005). *The ProQOL manual: The professional quality of life scale: Compassion satisfaction, burnout, and compassion fatigue/secondary trauma scales*. Baltimore, MD: The Sidran Press.

Substance Abuse and Mental Health Services Administration. (2014a). *SAMHSA's concept of trauma and guidance for a trauma-informed approach*. HHS Publication No. (SMA) 14–4884. Rockville, MD: Substance Abuse and Mental Health Services Administration.

Substance Abuse and Mental Health Services Administration. (2014b). *Trauma-informed care in behavioral health services*. Treatment Improvement Protocol (TIP) Series 57. Rockville, MD: Substance Abuse and Mental Health Services Administration.

Taubman-Ben-Ari, O., & Weintroub, A. (2008). Meaning in life and personal growth among pediatric physicians and nurses. *Death Studies, 32*, 621–645.

Tehrani, N. (2010). Compassion fatigue: Experiences in occupational health, human resources, counselling and police. *Occupational Medicine, 60*, 133–138. https://doi.org/10.1093/occmed/kqp174

von Ameln, F., & Becker-Ebel, J. (2020). *Fundamentals of psychodrama*. Singapore: Springer Nature.

Weber, A. M., & Haen, C. (Eds.). (2005). *Clinical applications of drama therapy in child and adolescent treatment*. New York: Psychology Press.

Toward Trauma-Informed Ethics of Leadership in Group Therapy, Psychodrama, and Organizations

Chapter Summary

Leaders are in positions of power. They have the potential to promote well-being, purpose, and the provision of services to those in need, or the potential of causing significant harm to staff, clients, the community, and their profession. This chapter proposes trauma-informed principles as ethical principles for leaders of all types including group therapists, psychodramatists, organizational leaders, community leaders, supervisors, trainers, and educators. The importance of ethics, humility, relationships, vulnerability, and courage will be highlighted as it relates to leadership. Cultural responsiveness and humility will be revisited in the context of leadership in general. Suggestions for leaders will be articulated including prompts for critical reflection. Trends and new directions in trauma-informed care, group work, psychodrama, and leadership will be presented as we look to the future toward a culture of trauma-informed ethical leadership in all sectors.

Leadership as a Double-Edged Sword

Leaders have the power to cause great harm or promote incredible goodness within their organizations, communities, and society. We have countless examples of harmful leadership throughout history and probably also in our own personal experiences. There are various examples of noble and trauma-informed leaders in history as well, but for many, it is more difficult to identify role models for good leadership than it is to critique examples of

DOI: 10.4324/9781003277859-12

poor leadership. Brené Brown's popular book, *Dare to Lead* (2018), describes her own qualitative research on leadership where she consistently found that folks being interviewed had difficulty articulating what good leadership looks like, instead they were quick to describe examples of poor leadership. As leaders, it is important that we maintain awareness of both positive and negative qualities of leaders. We can't rely solely on avoiding shortcomings as a strategy in leadership – instead, we must also have a set of values and ideals that we strive to embody in our leadership while also being aware to not reenact harmful examples of leadership. Leaders need role models that we can look to for inspiration, for learning, and for guidance. In my own process of learning to be a leader, I frequently find myself reflecting on the role modeling of leadership from past supervisors, professors, and group therapists. Even beyond these role models, I also look to historical, archetypal, and fictional examples of leadership within world history, mythology, and pop culture – such as characters in movies or television shows.

Who can I look to and learn from as role models of trauma-informed leadership?

My own vision of a trauma-informed leader is constantly evolving but steadily includes a set of core functions:

- Serving a greater good – guided by personal ethics, professional codes, organizational values, and trauma-informed principles
- Providing protection, safety, and containment, especially in the face of chaos or threat
- Emphasizing the importance of relationships with gratitude and empowerment – helping others to be the best they can be
- Demonstrating wisdom and discernment collaboratively moving toward a shared vision
- Being human – practicing vulnerability, authenticity, humility, and continued personal growth
- Taking action to address social injustice and inequalities in one's organization, community, and society

Even in the process of writing this book, my sense of clarity about what it means to be a trauma-informed leader has shifted and grown. I expect it will continue to evolve as I continue to engage in personal growth and professional development.

Brené Brown offers us a simplified definition of what a leader is – "anyone who takes responsibility for finding the potential in people and processes, and who has the courage to develop that potential" (2018, p. 4). This definition resonates with me in that it explicitly highlights how good leaders create more leaders rather than creating followers. This fits with my personal experience of learning from mentors in that the best mentors I've had were the ones who helped me grow into my own leadership. Brené's definition of leadership is unique in that it also states that leaders take responsibility for finding and developing the potential in processes. Leaders cultivate the potential not only in people but also in systems and within their organizations. In the context of this book and trauma-informed care, we could expand this to include the processes of trauma-informed care, group therapy, and psychodrama.

Leadership is a double-edged sword. It can be incredibly fulfilling and meaningful to take on positions of leadership, but it also comes with a great and grave responsibility. Some have suggested that meaning in life can be found through the adoption of responsibility (Peterson, 2021). Many shy away from the responsibilities that come with leadership as it can be isolating, stressful, fearful, painful, and difficult. Being a leader is not easy. Leaders are often the target of negative projections from others, many of whom have had adverse experiences with people in power. Bloom (2013) articulates that:

> Leaders are subject to the constant attack and criticism of those who are led, while superhuman attributes are often unconsciously applied to the leader. Given all of our history, authority figures are understandably feared more than they are loved, needed more than they are appreciated or understood. The expectations put upon leaders are often quite unconscious and outside of the realm of negotiation or even conversation.
>
> (p. 189)

Leadership can be incredibly isolating and difficult at times. Dr. Bloom describes her own experience as medical director of a hospital program as mediating "between the real and the ideal" (2013, p. 189). Leaders are expected to uphold ideals, missions, and values that are often much more complicated to integrate into real world situations and systems. Limitations in resources, time, support, and systems can often create additional barriers to implementing ideas and ideals. Being in leadership requires strength, courage, vulnerability, wisdom, understanding, and grace. Trauma-informed care philosophy offers leaders with a set of core principles to guide decision-making and organizational culture. The six trauma-informed principles can serve as a supplement to any organizations' core values and to any individual's personal values.

What are the difficulties I've experienced as a leader?

What are the benefits that I've experienced stepping into leadership roles?

What are the projections that I put upon leaders in my organization, community, and society?

Toward a Trauma-Informed Ethics of Organizational Leadership

Leaders are often critiqued for their failures in leadership. Widespread corruption, greed, and abuse of power has left a bad taste in mouths of many when it comes to leadership. The ongoing corporate norm of choosing financial profit over the well-being of consumers, staff, and society has enraged many, especially when it occurs in the helping professions. These practices in social service fields have produced considerable moral distress for clients, families, staff, and leaders alike – "caring for others has gone from being a sacred obligation to a commodity that is delivered for the lowest possible dollar in service of the greatest amount of profit" (Bloom & Farragher, 2011, p. 320). Even non-profit and government organizations are guilty of these types of financial practices.

Leaders talk a big game but often fail to follow through on their commitments to the people they were put in place to serve. Many leaders have lost their integrity and trust. Instead of leading through ethics, leadership, competence, and inspiration, many leaders maintain their power through structures of control, fear, dependency, and abuse. There is exploitation where there should be empowerment. Unhealthy workplaces have a tendency to produce "toxic leaders" who govern through bullying, gaslighting, scapegoating, cronyism, and abuse of power (Lipman-Blumen, 2004). These dynamics are more likely to emerge in organizational leadership in times of crisis and trauma to the organization. This is particularly problematic in trauma-focused organizations where crisis and trauma are an everyday occurrence that staff are dealing with. Leaders may be propelled toward authoritarian behaviors that prevent true democratic participation in the organization, promote punitive punishments, disrupt relational connections, and lead to organizational rigidity (Bloom & Farragher, 2011). When leaders behave in this way, it is also likely to promote the emergence of a parallel process over time in which staff will treat clients with a similar sense of authoritarianism – disrupting connection and collaboration, employing punitive punishments, and engaging with rigidity and numbness (Bloom & Farragher, 2011).

Trauma-informed leaders practice humility rather than authoritarianism. The characteristic of humility tends to have different connotations based on culture and context but it is a foundation of trauma-informed leadership. My favorite definition of humility is that it is an honest and accurate appraisal of oneself. Being humble means that you don't minimize or exaggerate your abilities, accomplishments, or shortcomings. It is a form of action-based honesty. The outcome of a literature review of the research on humility in leadership suggests that humility is an interpersonal characteristic that conveys a) a willingness to accurately perceive oneself, b) appreciation of the strengths and achievements of others, and c) willingness to continue learning from others (Owens, Johnson, & Mitchell, 2013). A recent review and synthesis of the research on humble leadership demonstrates that it increases feedback-seeking behavior of staff, personal initiative and proactive behavior of staff, employee organizational citizenship behavior, ethical decision-making, engagement, commitment, resilience, trust, empathy, satisfaction, self-efficacy, well-being, and team/organizational performance (Kelemen, Matthews, Matthews, & Henry, 2022). The aforementioned definition of humility in leadership is interpersonal in nature. It implies that leaders must centralize the relational and social dynamics within their organizations and effectively cultivate organizational dynamics that promote movement toward common goals. Jones (2022) further articulates this through the lens of sociometry, sociodynamics, and group dynamics.

Angelo McClain, CEO of the National Association of Social Workers, recently published an article on humility in leadership where he states that "humble leaders have successfully tempered egotism and embraced a leadership perspective that seeks to elevate everyone, fostering within their organizations hope, efficacy, resilience, and optimism. These leaders believe in human development and are continuously trying to improve and learn" (2022, p. 48). Humility in leadership intersections with cultural humility which was discussed in Chapter 10. Trauma-informed leaders demonstrate humility in their relationships, self-awareness, appreciation for others, and a willingness to continue learning and growing.

How can I further demonstrate humility in my leadership?

In *Destroying Sanctuary* (2011), Bloom and Farragher suggest that chronic organizational stress and toxic leadership must be remedied with authentic empowerment, democratic participation in the organizational processes, collaborative leadership, the granting of autonomy to workers, and organizational justice. Trauma-informed leaders are ethical leaders who promote just workplaces and use ethical values as guides for managing complex workplace dilemmas. In a multi-level analysis of organizational justice in the workplace, Spell and Arnold (2007) conclude that "a socially constructed, collective view of justice has implications for understanding the psychological wellbeing of employees" (p. 746). The research on organizational injustice suggests that it is a source of lower workplace performance, stress, anger, anxiety, depression, medical illness, injuries, and even cardiovascular death for workers (Elovainio et al., 2003, 2004, 2005, 2006; Spell & Arnold, 2007; Tepper, 2001). Organizational justice is directly related to ethical leadership. Leaders are faced with unrelenting and ongoing ethical dilemmas in their work and groups. They are often the final judge of what is right and what is wrong. Bloom and Farragher (2011) summarize four main ethical paradigms that leaders are confronted, outlined in Table 12.1.

Trauma-informed leaders must account for each of these four paradigms of ethics in their governance while considering the complexities of their specific situation. This applies to leaders of all types – organizational leaders, group therapists, psychodramatists, educators, supervisors, and trainers. Bloom and Farragher (2013) suggest that "ethical conflicts are one of the most underestimated, but chronically unrelenting sources of stress in today's human service delivery environment" (p. 84). In my own experience as a leader, I find this to be true. As my organization grows to help more clients and its operation evolves with greater layers of complexity, I am faced with increasingly frequent ethical dilemmas involving patient care, child abuse, suicidality, staff well-being, legal liability, moral distress, financial risk, social justice, and encountering other professionals or agencies operating with unethical professional or business practices. These ethical dilemmas, especially when met with poor leadership and injustice are sure to fuel moral

Table 12.1 Four main ethical paradigms for leadership (articulated by Bloom & Farragher, 2011)

Ethics of justice	Concerned with fairness and equality, governed by laws, policies, and rules
Ethics that critique the ethics of justice	Concerned with questions of power, privilege, and marginalization related to who creates, benefits, and is silenced by the system and its policies
Ethics of caring	Concerned with the human and relational impact of decision-making
Codes of ethics	Vary between professions but outline boundaries of professional behavior, requirements for compliance, and mandatory reporting requirements

distress, helplessness, compassion fatigue, and burnout for leaders and the staff that work with them.

Trauma-informed leaders must address these issues with a firm commitment to ethics and self-care. While leaders are responsible for the organization, everyone who works at the organization, and everyone the organization provides services for, leaders must also prioritize their own well-being, self-care, and personal growth. We must continue to do our own work, to challenge our own biases, continue to heal from our own trauma, and work to maintain balance in our lives as leaders. Without maintaining our own well-being, it will be impossible to maintain the well-being of an entire organization and promote well-being for supervisees and clients. A similar case can be made for the importance of group therapists to engage in self-care. Leaders who continue to take part in their own personal work are likely to promote a parallel process of staff and clients continuing to engage in their personal growth work.

Trauma-informed leaders actively work to help their teams address the impact of vicarious trauma and burnout. They recognize that many of the difficult behaviors demonstrated by staff may also be fueled by unresolved trauma. They demonstrate courage and vulnerability while leading by example in their own self-care. Brené Brown reminds us that courage and vulnerability are interdependent on each other, and that "our ability to be daring leaders will never be greater than our capacity for vulnerability" (2018, p. 11). Trauma-informed leaders embody the six trauma-informed principles and actively work to prevent the retraumatization of staff or clients. They centralize the importance of human connection and authenticity while empowering others to be the best they can be. The same awareness, qualities, and practices that make an effective trauma-informed practitioner, also create a trauma-informed leader (Perry & Jackson, 2018). Trauma-informed leaders inspire others to become trauma-informed practitioners, supervisors, educators, and leaders.

How can I further inspire others through my leadership?

Toward a Trauma-Informed Ethics of Group Work

The ethics of leadership in organizations and the ethics of leadership in group therapy have much in common. Organizations are groups and many staff are also trauma survivors. Just as authoritarianism is important to avoid in organizational leadership, it also can have detrimental effects on outcomes in group therapy. Groups should be group-centered rather than leader-centered (CSAT, 2005; Giacomucci, 2021). SAMHSA's publication on group therapy leadership in substance abuse treatment suggests that the following qualities are important for group therapy leaders: consistency, active listening, firm identity, confidence, spontaneity, integrity, trust, humor, and empathy (CSAT, 2005). Group leaders should not only talk about principles of recovery but also role model these principles throughout the group (CSAT, 2005). This is echoed further in Lawrence Shulman's suggestion that "more is caught than taught" in group work (Shulman, 2009, p. 165). Role modeling healthy behavior, social interactions, and ethics are essential for group workers, just as they are for organizational leaders and individual practitioners.

The research literature about adverse and negative impacts of group psychotherapy is very limited, though some studies have suggested a 10%–16% negative outcomes rate for group participation across therapy groups, growth groups, and self-help groups (Dies & Teleska, 1985; Lieberman, Yalom, & Miles, 1973). Much of the group therapy literature on harms, risks, and adverse outcomes focus on the group leader's abuse of power, control, interpretation, leadership style, or interaction between members and the group (Lieberman et al., 1973; Maratos & Bledin, 2021; Roback, 2000). Other factors negatively impacting group therapy outcomes include countertransference, personality of the therapist or participants, inadequate pre-group assessment, selection error, attacks/rejections between participants, and individual characteristics of participants (Lieberman et al., 1973; Maratos & Bledin, 2021; Roback, 2000). Roback's (2000) review of adverse outcomes in group psychotherapy suggests that "the three major dynamics (leader, group, help-seeker) typically associated with facilitating positive outcome are also implicated in negative outcomes" (p. 120). These findings (and the serious lack of research in this area) further validate the importance of group leaders centralizing both ethical standards and trauma-informed principles in their work. Afterall, the primary purpose of codes of ethics and professional ethical standards are to protect clients and the public (Kaklauskas & Olson, 2020).

Riva and Cornish (2018) highlight that "group therapy ethics are considerably more complex than are the ethical concerns for individual psychotherapy, yet the amount of information on the ethics of group work is startlingly small" (p. 219). The nature of group therapy, which includes multiple strangers coming together for ongoing sessions, involves inherent risks related to confidentiality, privacy, safety, diversity, and boundaries that are not present in other types of therapy (Brabender & Macnair-Semands, 2022). There are a few published documents outlining best ethical practices in group work, including those by the Association of Specialists in Group Work (ASGW) (2021), American Group Psychotherapy Association (AGPA) and International Board for Certification of Group Psychotherapists (IBCGP) (2002), and the International Association of Social Work with Groups (IASWG) (2015). These ethical standards articulated by group work specific organizations help to fill in the gaps of other codes of ethics, such as those of the American Psychological Association (APA), American Counseling Association (ACA), and National Association of Social Workers (NASW), which do not provide thorough ethical guidance related to group work (Riva & Cornish, 2018). At the same time, the aforementioned group therapy ethical standards do not explicitly address the role of trauma in ethical group therapy practice; however, the ethical standards (and the best practices for group therapy published by the same organizations) reference almost all of SAMHSA's trauma-informed principles in different contexts not related to trauma. A synthesis of group therapy ethical standards with the standards for trauma-informed care provides practitioners with a solid framework for effective and ethical practice.

Riva and Cornish (2018) and Kaklauskas and Olson (2020) highlight multiple common group therapy ethical issues that group therapists should address, including: disclosures, documentation, boundaries, impaired professionals and self-care, confidentiality, dual and multiple relationships, voluntary vs involuntary participation, concurrent therapies, internet groups, standards of care, and competence of the group leader. Confidentiality is particularly complex in group work as the therapist is legally bound to confidentiality, but the other group attendees are not (MacNair-Semands, 2005; Woods & Ruzek, 2017). It is important to have this discussion with the group at the beginning of the group process for transparency. Each of these common ethical dilemmas in group therapy can be explored through the lens of trauma and trauma-informed care. In the list of common group therapy ethical issues above, we can clearly see the value of SAMHSA's trauma-informed principles (safety, trustworthiness and transparency, peer support, collaboration and mutuality, empowerment, voice, and choice, and cultural, historic, and gender issues) as guides for navigating these dilemmas while resisting retraumatization and promoting trauma recovery.

What are the common ethical issues that emerge in my own group work practice?

Ethical concerns increase when it comes to group teletherapy sessions as there are additional potential barriers to confidentiality, safety, and connection. A review of teletherapy ethical issues (Stoll, Müller, & Trachsel, 2020) highlights five primary areas of concern:

1) Confidentiality, privacy, and online security
2) Therapists' limited training/competencies in telehealth
3) Technology problems that disrupt communication
4) Lack of research support
5) Difficulties and risks related to emergency situations during teletherapy sessions

While group teletherapy presents some complex issues, it also offers unique benefits and opportunities that may be impossible for in person sessions. Yalom and Leszcz (2020) suggest that the group leader's responsibility includes establishing a safe, secure, and stable physical group space for in person groups translates to the leader's responsibility for ensuring a secure, safe, and stable online group environment.

Teletherapy is inherently aligned with trauma-informed principles in various ways. It offers trauma survivors with an opportunity to attend sessions from the comfort and safety of their home while mitigating confidentiality concerns of being seen walking into a treatment center. The widescale availability of online group offerings provides exponentially more choices and group options. This allows for the development of more homogeneous groups and groups offered by/for individuals of specific cultural, religious, racial, ethnic, gender, sexual orientation, age, or other identities. It also offers a more inclusive service option for those geographically isolated or limited in mobility or transportation. It is essential that group therapists examine their own competencies and limitations in facilitating teletherapy groups sessions and obtain additional training or consultation when necessary. While trauma-informed principles may be implicitly present in the provision of teletherapy groups, it is also imperative that practitioners explicitly consider the integration of trauma-informed principles in their facilitation (see Chapter 2 for comprehensive table outlining strategies for integrating trauma-informed principles in teletherapy groups).

The ASGW *Guiding Principles for Group Work* explicitly states that "ASGW views ethical processes as being integral to group work and views group workers as ethical practitioners" (2021, p. 3). This statement suggests that group workers centralize ethics in their standards, but in reality, group work ethical standards don't get mentioned very often in graduate education or post-graduate training. Instead, group therapy training programs prioritize theory and practice over ethical and legal considerations (Kaklauskas & Olson, 2020). In their chapter titled, *The Ethical Group Psychotherapist*, Kaklauskas and Olson (2020) suggest that group therapists often face challenging issues, such as trauma, abuse, substance use, illegal behavior, secrecy, bigotry, and oppression, which require the ability to think things through ethically, legally, clinically, and personally – as such, "the group therapist is uniquely prepared to address ethical dilemmas" (p. 143). Ethical standards, like trauma-informed principles or trauma awareness, must be put into action. A cognitive understanding is insufficient unless followed by praxis in the real world.

"A group is often more than the sum of its parts. At times, however, it may be less than the sum of its parts" (Roback, 2000, p. 117). As ethical group therapists, we must promote the former, while addressing the risks that lead to the latter. In the group therapy world, there continue to be groups that cause harm to participants – especially when groups are facilitated by practitioners who have insufficient training in group therapy or no awareness of trauma-informed principles. Competence is an ethical issue, especially when many professionals facilitating therapy groups have not received specialized training in group therapy (Brabender & Macnair-Semands, 2022). Group therapy is currently at a unique time in its history as its demand in practice has increased and new group therapy research studies have emerged supporting its efficacy. The APA recognized group psychotherapy as a specialty in psychology in 2018 while also approving the development of a new evidence-based group psychotherapy practice registry (Paxton & Harrison, 2022). These changes are likely to increase standards for group therapy and promote an increased interest in group therapy within practice, education, research, and organizations. The centralization of ethics ensures that group therapists can effectively continue to integrate and promote group therapy within all practice and educational spheres. For a comprehensive dive into group therapy ethics, see the newly published book, *The Ethics of Group Psychotherapy*, which includes various references, a quiz, discussion questions, vignettes, and role plays at the end of each chapter for further exploring the book content in training settings (Brabender & Macnair-Semands, 2022).

Toward a Trauma-Informed Ethics of Psychodrama

Ethics are particularly important in trauma-informed psychodrama practice. Psychodrama psychotherapy groups and psychodrama training tend to be very action-based, relational, and emotionally intense at times. The experiential component of both clinical practice and training creates increased opportunities for ethical dilemmas and issues to emerge than in talk therapy or didactic teaching events. Though trauma-informed principles are implicitly embodied in much of psychodrama's theories, philosophies, and methods, there has been few explicit attempts to integrate SAMHSA's trauma-informed principles into psychodrama practice or training. Many practitioners and trainers claim to practice or teach psychodrama in trauma-informed ways but do not reference or teach the six principles. One of the primary purposes of this book is to make the six trauma-informed principles more explicitly rooted within the psychodrama community.

There have been few publications on ethics in psychodrama. The American Society of Group Psychotherapy and Psychodrama (ASGPP) and the American Board of Examiners in Sociometry, Psychodrama, and Group Psychotherapy (ABE) currently require members to subscribe to the APA code of ethics. Various international psychodrama associations have published their own psychodrama codes of ethics such as the Federation of European Psychodrama Training Organizations (FEPTO), British Psychodrama Association (BPA), and The Australian and Aotearoa New Zealand Psychodrama Association (AANZPA). A published study in 1995 discovered that 94% of participating ABE certified psychodramatists were in favor of a formal code of ethics for psychodramatists, mandatory instructions on ethics in psychodrama training, and a section on ethical standards and issues in the psychodrama written examination (Kranz & Lund, 1995). In the same study, 55% of respondents indicated a belief that existing professional codes of ethics were insufficient for the unique complexities involved in psychodrama practice.

When it comes to online practice and teaching of psychodrama, there are additional ethical concerns, many of which mirror the same concerns related to group teletherapy which were already outlined. Very little has been written about the specific ethics of online psychodrama practice beyond content published by Daniela Simmons, current ASGPP President and Creator of Tele'Drama – an integration of Moreno's methods into telehealth formats (Simmons, 2022; Simmons & Wilches, 2022). Tele'Drama's website includes an abbreviated statement of ethics for online psychodrama participation which includes attention to safety, confidentiality, and risks of online participation. It emphasizes the importance of safety related to culture and identity due to the international nature of the organization. Simmons (2022) also addresses the importance of instructing participants not to video record or take photos of the session without explicit consent from all members. An editorial in the Brazilian Psychodrama Journal echoes concerns articulated by Simmons and highlights some additional concerns in online psychodrama such as the lost visibility of participants' bodies and the potential misattunement to somatic and movement-oriented aspects in the psychodrama process (Fleury, 2020).

Publications on psychodrama ethics seem to agree that psychodrama practice is unique compared to other therapy approaches due to its experiential nature and common inclusion of physical touch in role-playing (Kellerman, 1999; Moreno, 1994). Kellerman articulates that "the psychodramatic action-format, involving more emotional expression, more physical intimacy and more technical experimentation than other verbal approaches to psychotherapy, increases the need for safeguard for both participants and practitioners" (1999, p. 4). Kellerman (1999) advocates that all psychodramatists should be required to take a course specific to psychodrama ethics. He proposes seven principles for consideration in psychodrama code of ethics: responsibility, competence, welfare, advertisement, confidentiality, therapeutic relationships, and values. Moreno's early publication about a code of ethics for psychodrama positions ethics of psychodrama practice within the larger field of group psychotherapy (Moreno, 1962). While Moreno's code of ethics does include some standards for practitioners (confidentiality, do no harm, competence, research, choice, equality, financial cost, etc.) his code of ethics is also unique in that it suggests that the Hippocratic Oath should be extended to all patients in the group. This is based on his philosophy that each patient is a therapeutic agent for each other. While there has been little written about ethics in psychodrama, it is my firm believe that ethics is one of the most important areas of focus for the future of psychodrama.

What are the common ethical concerns that emerge in my own psychodrama practice or training?

My own experience in the psychodrama community and training institutes, I find that ethics and professionalism are sometimes lacking. Of course, there are ethical issues in every field, but I find them to be more complicated in the psychodrama world. In discussion with other colleagues in the field, I have heard them share concerns and aversion to psychodrama because of this same issue. Multiple of my graduate school professors articulate similar concerns when I mentioned psychodrama, particularly citing past psychodrama university courses, conference workshops, or training groups that were indistinguishable from therapy groups. This lack of differentiation and boundary between therapy and professional training in educational sessions is of concern (this piece was discussed in Chapter 11). It is an issue of ethics and professionalism. I find this to be one of the most significant barriers to psychodrama being accepted in the larger psychotherapy, group therapy, academic, and educational arenas.

Many psychodrama trainers argue that psychodrama cannot be adequately learned except through personal involvement and training groups that engage in real psychodramas with real personal issues. Yalom and Leszcz (2020) offer some guidance around this issue in the context of group therapy training that also applies to psychodrama training:

> There is a useful distinction to be made between a therapy group and a therapeutic group. *A training group, though it is not a therapy group, is therapeutic in that it offers the opportunity to learn about oneself.* By no means, though, is each member expected to do extensive therapeutic work. The basic contract of the group, in fact, its *raison d'être*, is training, not therapy. To a great extent, these goals overlap: a leader can offer no better group therapy training than that of an effective therapeutic group.
>
> (p. 658)

Psychodrama training needs to conform to the descriptions described above in training groups and needs to be conducted with additional boundaries in most other academic, university, or professional settings that do not involve an ongoing closed group (Giacomucci & Skolnik, 2021). See ASGPP's best practices document for more information on differentiating psychodrama therapy, training, and education (Giacomucci, 2020).

These problems can be traced back to Jacob Moreno who was not always one to emphasize professionalism and at times engaged in behavior that was ethically questionable at best. Some will say it was simply a sign of the times and that ethical norms and boundaries were much different in the 1940–1960s. While there may be some truth to this, I find that many contemporary psychodrama trainers seem to mirror some of Moreno's megalomania, lack of professionalism, and disregard for ethical standards or boundaries. I have seen several former students, trainees, or colleagues abandon psychodrama training due to unethical or harmful experiences with prominent trainers in the field. While there will always be examples of unethical practices in any field, my judgment is that this happens more frequently in the psychodrama community. I am a member of 12 different professional societies and of them, I find the psychodrama community to be most lacking in professionalism (though I also experience the psychodrama community as the most warm, creative, and enjoyable community I hold membership in). I challenge psychodramatists to do better. Again, I reiterate my 2019 call to action in ASGPP's national newsletter, *Psychodrama Network News*, urging psychodramatists to prioritize ethics and professionalism. A trauma-informed modality without a trauma-informed process for training professionals is fundamentally flawed.

In what ways can I further grow in my own professionalism and ethics?

How can I support and challenge my colleagues to uphold the highest standards of professionalism and ethics?

Furthermore, the psychodrama community in the United States has much room to grow when it comes to issues of diversity, social justice, and inclusion. Significant progress has been made in these areas in the past decade, but there is much more room to grow. While more psychodramatists are considering issues of diversity and social justice – and it is being centralized more often in the annual ASGPP conference and other international conferences, there remains a lacking literature base on anti-oppressive psychodrama practice (Fleury, 2021; Nieto, 2010) and clinical applications of psychodrama in specific marginalized communities. A trauma-informed psychodramatist embraces Moreno's vision of sociatry – healing for society – and assumes their co-responsibility for all of humankind while empowering others to honor their co-responsibility for humankind (Giacomucci et al., 2021). Psychodramatists (sociatrists) recognize that the structure of groups, organizations, communities, and societies are impacted by the sociodynamic effect, which leads to the unequal distribution of power, resources, money, opportunity, and social wealth. The objective of reversing this sociodynamic effect in all social groupings should be forefront and priority for psychodramatists and trauma-informed leaders (Giacomucci, 2017, 2019).

The integration of SAMHSA's six trauma-informed principles as ethical and clinical guides in psychodrama practice and training would provide a framework for psychodrama's reemergence as a popular and respected modality. Psychodrama was previously quite popular in the United States but fell from popularity in the 1980–2000s. It appears to be gaining traction again as a sought-after modality. This is demonstrated in multiple recent occurrences such as an increased number of psychodrama publications, special journal editions on psychodrama, psychodrama university courses, and an increase in psychodrama certification applicants. If psychodrama is to reemerge and maintain a respectable reputation in the field, it will need to be infused with a newfound commitment to ethics, trauma-informed care, professionalism, social justice, and empirical research. Psychodrama is currently at a major crossroad and its future is full of potentialities. Kellerman's guidance from over two decades ago continues to ring true, "The future of psychodrama rests on the careful selection and training of ethically minded practitioners" (1999, p. 15).

Conclusion: Trauma-Informed Leadership in Action

Trauma-informed leaders in group therapy, psychodrama, and organizations recognize the role of emotions and communication in their work. A leader communicating with calmness in an emotionally regulated manner can help regulate the anxiety and arousal of their team members or group members, whereas an anxious or angry leader will fuel more anxiety, depression, or aggression (Perry & Jackson, 2018). Trauma-informed leadership is more than just understanding trauma, it requires content knowledge but also attention to style and process (Manderscheid, 2009). Cognitive and intellectual knowledge of trauma is important, but only useful if it can be experientially operationalized in the real world. Trauma-informed leaders must translate theory, research, and principles into the complexities of practice, organizations, and society.

Trauma-informed philosophy has become exponentially more popular in the past decade. "Trauma-informed practice is sometimes regulated to a three-word slogan. This poses a genuine risk to it being dismissed as a fad, or watered down to a set of vague principles that cannot realistically impact on practice" (Perry & Jackson, 2018, p. 137). As trauma-informed leaders, we have a responsibility to the field and to our communities to teach others about the multifaceted nature of trauma-informed approaches in groups, psychodrama, organizations and beyond. Shulman reminds us that "more is caught than taught," so we must be role models demonstrating and embodying how to integrate SAMHSA trauma-informed principles into the real world. Becoming a better trauma-informed leader will require personal and professional growth work, in addition to an ongoing commitment to cultural responsiveness and humility. Awareness of trauma and trauma-informed principles alone is simply not enough. We must put our knowledge into action through changes in attitudes, behaviors, policies, and practices (Gerbrandt, Grieser, & Enns, 2021).

A culture of trauma-informed ethical practice must be maintained in all aspects of our work. As leaders of groups, organizations, and communities, we can offer corrective emotional experiences to clients, staff, and community members who may have experienced abuses of power in the past. Through ethical practice, we come to respect both the extraordinary healing potential and dangers inherent to our roles and our professional practices. Trauma-informed practitioners actively resist retraumatization and causing harm while promoting safety and healing for all involved. The centralization of ethics in group therapy and psychodrama are sure to help both approaches reemerge within the mental health and educational fields as respectable and highly desirable methods. The methods and philosophies articulated in group therapy and psychodrama provide leaders with the tools needed to engage groups in meaningful ways while promoting cohesion, connection, safety, peer support, collaboration, empowerment, and mitigating vicarious traumatization. SAMHSA's six trauma-informed principles, concretized as ethical imperatives, serve as guiding beacons for safe and effective practices in trauma-informed and trauma-focused group therapy and psychodrama.

Reading (or writing) a book on trauma-informed care is insufficient alone. We must take what we have learned and put it into action in our groups and our organization. This will require an ongoing commitment to growth, self-reflection, and learning. This will require us to cultivate our own systems of peer support, to address our own traumatic wounds, and care for our own vicarious traumatization. It will require community, courage, and commitment. Together, we can infuse our organizations and professions with trauma-informed principles and collectively enhance the quality of services and education for the next generation of clients, students, trainees, and workers.

How will I integrate my learning from this book into my work?

Who can support me in my development as a trauma-informed practitioner and/or leader?

What next steps can I take to be the best leader I can be?

References

American Group Psychotherapy Association (AGPA) & International Board for Certification of Group Psychotherapists (IBCGP). (2002). *AGPA and IBCGP guidelines for ethics.* New York: American Group Psychotherapy Association and International Board for Certification of Group Psychotherapists.

Association of Specialists in Group Work (ASGW). ASGW Guiding Principles for Group Work. ASGW. https://asgw.org/wp-content/uploads/2021/07/ASGW-Guiding-Principles-May-2021.pdf

Bloom, S. L. (2013). *Creating sanctuary: Toward the evolution of sane societies* (Revised). New York: Routledge.

Bloom, S. L., & Farragher, B. (2011). *Destroying sanctuary: The crisis in human services delivery systems.* New York: Oxford University Press.

Bloom, S. L., & Farragher, B. (2013). *Restoring sanctuary: A new operating system for trauma-informed systems of care.* New York: Oxford University Press.

Brabender, V., & MacNair-Semands, R. (2022). *The ethics of group psychotherapy: Principles and practical strategies.* New York: Routledge.

Brown, B. (2018). *Dare to lead: Brave work. Tough conversations. Whole hearts.* New York: Random House.

Center for Substance Abuse Treatment. (2005). *Substance abuse treatment: Group therapy.* Treatment Improvement Protocol (TIP) Series, No. 41. HHS Publication No. (SMA) 15-3991. Rockville, MD: Substance Abuse and Mental Health Services Administration.

Dies, R. R., & Teleska, P. (1985). Negative outcome in Group Psychotherapy. In D. Mays, & C. Franks (Eds.), *Negative outcome in psychotherapy* (pp. 118–142). New York: Springer.

Elovainio, M., Kivimäki, M., Steen, N., & Vahtera, J. (2004). Job decision latitude, organizational justice and health: Multilevel covariance structure analysis. *Social Science & Medicine, 58*(9), 1659–1669.

Elovainio, M., Kivimäki, M., Vahtera, J., Keltikangas-Järvinen, L., & Virtanen, M. (2003). Sleeping problems and health behaviors as mediators between organizational justice and health. *Health psychology, 22*(3), 287.

Elovainio, M., Leino-Arjas, P., Vahtera, J., & Kivimäki, M. (2006). Justice at work and cardiovascular mortality: A prospective cohort study. *Journal of Psychosomatic Research, 61*(2), 271–274.

Elovainio, M., van den Bos, K., Linna, A., Kivimäki, M., Ala-Mursula, L., Pentti, J., & Vahtera, J. (2005). Combined effects of uncertainty and organizational justice on employee health: Testing the uncertainty management model of fairness judgments among Finnish public sector employees. *Social Science & Medicine, 61*(12), 2501–2512.

Fleury, H. J. (2020). Psicodrama e as especificidades da psicoterapia on-line. *Revista Brasileira de Psicodrama, 28*(1), 1–4.

Fleury, H. J. (2021). O psicodrama confirma missão política da diversidade, equidade e inclusão. *Revista Brasileira de Psicodrama, 29*(3), 159–162.

Gerbrandt, N., Grieser, R., & Enns, V. (2021). *A little book about trauma-informed workplaces.* Winnipeg: Achieve Publishing.

Giacomucci, S. (2017). The sociodrama of life or death: Young adults and addiction treatment. *Journal of Psychodrama, Sociometry, and Group Psychotherapy, 65*(1), 137–143. https://doi.org/10.12926/ 0731-1273-65.1.137

Giacomucci, S. (2019). Social group work in action: A sociometry, psychodrama, and experiential trauma group therapy curriculum. *Doctorate in Social Work (DSW) Dissertations*, 124. Retrieved from https://repository.upenn.edu/cgi/viewcontent.cgi?article=1128&context=edissertations_sp2

Giacomucci, S. (2020). *Best practices for psychodrama in academia: The role transition from trainer to professor*. American Society of Group Psychotherapy & Psychodrama Professional Liaison Committee. Retrieved from https://asgpp.org/wp-content/uploads/2020/08/Best-Practices-Psychodrama-in-Academia.pdf

Giacomucci, S. (2021). *Social work, sociometry, and psychodrama: Experiential approaches for group therapists, community leaders, and social workers*. Springer Nature. https://doi.org/10.1007/978-981-33-6342-7

Giacomucci, S., Karner, D., Nieto, L. & Schreiber, E. (2021). Sociatry, psychodrama, and social work: Moreno's mysticism and social justice tradition. *Social Work with Groups, 44*(3), 288–303. https://doi.org/10.1080/01609513.2021.1885826

Giacomucci, S., & Skolnik, S. (2021). The experiential social work educator: Integrating sociometry into the classroom environment. *Journal of Teaching in Social Work, 41*(2), 192–202.

International Association of Social Work with Groups (IASWG). (2015). *Standards for social work practice with groups* (2nd ed.). New York City: IASWG.

Jones, D. (2022). *Leadership levers: Releasing the power of relationships for exceptional participation, alignment, and team results*. New York: Routledge.

Kaklauskas, F. J., & Olson, E. A. (2020). The ethical group psychotherapist. In F. J. Kaklauskas, & L. R. Greene (Eds.), *Core principles of group psychotherapy* (pp. 143–155). New York: Routledge.

Kelemen, T. K., Matthews, S. H., Matthews, M. J., & Henry, S. E. (2022). Humble leadership: A review and synthesis of leader expressed humility. *Journal of Organizational Behavior*. https://doi.org/10.1002/job.2608

Kellermann, P. F. (1999). Ethical concerns in psychodrama. *Journal of the British Psychodrama Association, 14*, 3–19.

Kranz, P. L., & Lund, N. L. (1995). Psychodramatists' opinions: Should the professional psychodrama community have a formal code of ethics? *Journal of Group Psychotherapy, Psychodrama & Sociometry, 48*(3), 91–95.

Lieberman, M. A., Yalom, I. D., & Miles, M. B. (1973). *Encounter groups: First facts*. New York: Basic Books.

Lipman-Blumen, J. (2004). *The allure of toxic leaders: Why we follow destructive bosses and corrupt politicians—And how we can survive them.* New York: Oxford University Press.

MacNair-Semands, R. (2005). *Ethics in group psychotherapy.* New York: American Group Psychotherapy Association.

Manderscheid, R. W. (2009). Trauma-informed leadership. *International Journal of Mental Health,* 38(1), 78–86.

Maratos, A., & Bledin, K. (2021). First do no harm? *Group Analysis.* Advanced Online Publication. https://doi.org/10.1177/05333164211020291

Mcclain, A. (2022, May). Humility in leadership helps elevate, empower others. *Social Work Advocates,* 5(2), 48.

Moreno, J. D. (1994). Of morals, ethics, and encounters. In P. Holmes, M. Karp, & M. Watson (Eds.), *Psychodrama since Moreno* (pp. 69–81). New York: Routledge.

Moreno, J. L. (1962). *Code of ethics for group psychotherapy and psychodrama: Relationship to the Hippocratic Oath.* Beacon, NY: Beacon House.

Nieto, L. (2010). Look behind you: Using anti-oppression models to inform a protagonist's psychodrama. In Leveton, E. (Ed.), *Healing collective trauma using sociodrama and drama therapy* (pp. 103–125). New York: Springer Publishing Company.

Owens, B. P., Johnson, M. D., & Mitchell, T. R. (2013). Expressed humility in organizations: Implications for performance, teams, and leadership. *Organization Science,* 24(5), 1517–1538.

Paxton, T., & Harrison, M. (2022). Introduction and update on the evidence-based group treatment website project. *The Group Psychologist,* Spring Issue. APA Division 49. Accessed at https://www.apadivisions.org/division-49/publications/newsletter/group-psychologist/2022/03/group-treatment-project

Perry, B., & Jackson, L. (2018). Trauma-informed leadership. In M. Frederico, M. Long, & N. Cameron (Eds.), *Leadership in child and family practice* (pp. 125–141). New York: Routledge.

Peterson, J. B. (2021). *Beyond order: 12 more rules for life.* New York: Penguin.

Riva, M., & Erickson Cornish, J. (2018). Ethical considerations in group psychotherapy. In M. Leach, & E. Welfel (Eds.), *The Cambridge handbook of applied psychological ethics* (pp. 218–238). Cambridge: Cambridge University Press.

Roback, C. (2000). Adverse outcomes in group psychotherapy: Risk factors, prevention, and research directions. *Journal of Psychotherapy Practice and Research,* 9(3), 113–122.

Shulman, L. (2009). *The skills of helping individuals, families, groups and communities* (6th ed.). Belmont: Cengage Learning.

Simmons, D. (2022). Ethical and procedural guidelines for TELE'DRAMA® (ONLINE) Training. Retrieved from https://www.teledrama.org/ethical-and-procedural-guidelines-for-telersquodrama-training.html

Simmons, D., & Wilches, A. (2022). TELE'DRAMA—International sociometry in the virtual space. *Zeitschrift für Psychodrama und Soziometrie, 21*(1), 119–129.

Spell, C. S., & Arnold, T. J. (2007). A multi-level analysis of organizational justice climate, structure, and employee mental health. *Journal of Management, 33*(5), 724–751.

Stoll, J., Müller, J. A., & Trachsel, M. (2020). Ethical issues in online psychotherapy: A narrative review. *Frontiers in Psychiatry, 10*, 993.

Tepper, B. J. (2001). Health consequences of organizational injustice: Tests of main and interactive effects. *Organizational Behavior and Human Decision Processes, 86*(2), 197–215.

Woods, J., & Ruzek, N. (2017). Ethics in group psychotherapy. In M. D. Ribeiro, J. Gross, & M. M. Turner (Eds.), *The college counselor's guide to group psychotherapy* (pp. 83–100). New York: Routledge.

Yalom, I. D., & Leszcz, M. (2020). *The theory and practice of group psychotherapy* (6th ed.). New York: Basic Books.

Index

Note: **Bold** page numbers refer to tables; *italic* page numbers refer to figures.

ACE *see* Adverse Childhood Experiences (ACE)
addiction 4–5, 82, 88, 104, 110, 111, 115, 157, 178, 249, 265, 268, 270
addiction treatment 3–4, 70, 89, 115, 120, 265, 270
Adverse Childhood Experiences (ACE) 14, 35
AGPA *see* American Group Psychotherapy Association (AGPA)
altruism 33, 34, 180, 195, 209
American Group Psychotherapy Association (AGPA) 9, 24, 42, 287
American Psychiatric Association 86
American Psychological Association (APA) 9, 24, 287, 289, 290
American Society of Group Psychotherapy and Psychodrama (ASGPP) 5, 6, 290, 292–293
amygdala 72
anti-oppressive 31, 106, 137, 222, 225, 227–231, 241, 243, 293
anxiety 3, 21, 50, 82, 137, 141, 199, 223, 224, 250, 261, 284, 294
APA *see* American Psychological Association (APA)
APA Division 49 for Group Psychology and Group Psychotherapy 9, 10
art therapy 118
ASGPP *see* American Society of Group Psychotherapy and Psychodrama (ASGPP)

ASGW *see* Association of Specialists in Group Work (ASGW)
assessment 15, 56–58, 109, 111–113, 122, 139–141, 144, 152, 233, 235, 238, 256, 258, 286
Association of Specialists in Group Work (ASGW) 9, 24, 287, 288
attachment theory 83, 259
Autobiography of a Genius (Moreno) 6
autonomy 86, 168, 206, 208–210, 212, 214, 216, 218, 230, 283

boundaries 20, 82, 83, 133, 142, 210, 263, 273, 286, 287, 291, 292
brain stem 72
Brown, Brené 20, 193, 280, 281, 285
burnout 19–20, 187, 190, 192, 226, 248–253, 252, 256, 257, 262–266, 270, 273, 285

Canon of Creativity 49, 50, *50*, 51
catharsis 33, 51, 52–53, 79, 80, 82, 91, 93, 94, 151, 169, 240
choice 13, 16, 17, 35, 37, 58, 105, 106, 109, 111, 113–117, 119, 122, 136, 142, 146, 150, 151, 160, 193, 195, 206–219, 227, 229, 241, 267, 287, 288, 291
circle of strengths 103, 106, 126–129, 183, 185, 266
clinical map 22–23, 25, 40, 44, 74, 83, 84–86, 88, 91, 104, 107, 110, 116, 119, 123, 134, 148, 167, 262, 263

closure 42, 52, 79, 80, 82, 90, 92, 94, 121, 149, 184, 185, 213, 240
code of ethics 45, 185, 198, 213, 290, 291
co-facilitation 5, 144, 197, 216
collaboration 16, 17, 31, 32, 34, 45, 69, 117, 146, 160, 163, 174, 180, 186, 190–203, 209, 211, 212, 229, 230, 233, 258, 259, 267, 282, 287, 295
collective trauma 3, 4, 17, 55, 58, 190, 222, 223–225, 227, 228, 231, 233, 234, 237, 242, 243, 263
community work 4, 8, 23, 104, 238
compassion fatigue 19, 192, 248–252, 285
concretization 80–81, 266
containment 13, 20, 23, 83, 84, 104, 105, 119, 133, 140, 141, 142, 148, 149, 151, 152, 216, 261–263, 273, 280
corrective emotional experience(s) 51, 68, 73, 87, 91, 156, 166, 179, 214, 295
countertransference 19, 20, 23, 32, 165, 236, 248, 252, 252–253, 268, 269, 273, 286
creativity 46, 47, 49–51, 50, 54, 76, 77, 87, 126, 164
cultural, historic, and gender issues 17, 21, **39,** 92, 117, 125, 146, 180, 193, 209, 222–243, 267, 287
culture 4, 8, 9, 15, 17, 18, 20, 25, 44, 54, 87, 129, 136–138, 169, 193–194, 206, 211, 222, 223–227, 230–236, 232, 238, 239, 242, 248, 260, 262, 279, 280, 281, 283, 290, 294

Dayton, Tian 47, 55–58, 60, 79, 82, 88–90, 104, 115, 116, 214
defense mechanisms 79, 82, 104, 108, 116, 175, 216, 261
depression 3, 82, 124, 159, 199, 224, 250, 269, 284, 294
director 5, 7, 12, 13, 48, 76–80, 82, 92–94, 106, 109, 116, 119, 149, 150, 162, 167–170, 214–217, 219, 238, 242, 266, 281
dissociation 21, 51, 79, 84, 86, 116, 175, 224, 261, 262
doubling 13, 55, 56, 77–79, 81, 82, 84, 90, 93, 94, 149, 151, 169, 177, 178, 200, 206, 216, 217, 219, 240, 241, 268–270
dyads 106–109, 116, 126, 147, 181, 182, 236, 266

ecomap 12, 57
empowerment 1, 4, 13, 16, 17, 31, 32, 37, 45, 68, 69, 117, 146, 148, 151, 156, 160, 176, 180, 186, 193, 195–198, 202, 206–219, 227, 229, 240, 267, 271, 280, 282, 283, 287, 295
empty chair 11, 80, 81, 89, 218, 240, 241, 269, 270
ethical standards 23, 91, 135, 140, 286, 287, 289, 290, 292
experiential teaching 117, 264, 265, 273
Eye-Movement Desensitization and Reprocessing (EMDR) 5, 46, 47, 182

floor check 89, 103, 104, 106, 114, 115–118, 185, 215, 267
Freud, Sigmund 45, 52, 109
future projection 13, 23, 73, 104, 177

genogram 12, 57
Gestalt Therapy 3, 81
grief 34, 81, 82, 88, 92–95, 115, 117, 120, 148, 201, 261, 262
group-as-a-whole 12, 32, 35, 36, 40–41, 106, 109, 114, 115, 118, 126, 128–129, 140, 143, 168, 186, 195, 199, 200, 202, 203, 209, 211, 215, 216, 260, 265, 267
group assessment 104, 113, 286
group cohesion 36, 41, 83, 88, 105, 106, 109, 123, 127, 141, 164, 179, 202, 266
group norms 137, 141–143, 145, 228

hands-on-shoulder sociometry 58, 104, 121–126, 185
healing centered engagement 222, 225–227
hippocampus 72
Hippocratic Oath 45, 185, 198, 291
hope 2, 3, 16, 20, 33, 51, 68, 74–76, 93, 120, 146, 148, 159, 174, 177, 178, 199, 209, 240, 249, 262, 268, 271, 272, 283
hypothalamus 72

International Association of Group Psychotherapy & Group Processes (IAGP) 9, 24
International Association of Social Work with Groups (IASWG) 24, 287
Interpersonal Neurobiology 35–36, 46, 72, 88

An Invitation to an Encounter 56
isolation 2–3, 34, 68, 141, 146, 175, 179, 182, 186, 187, 197, 199, 224

locogram 89, 103, 104, 106, 113–116, 122, 185, 215

mirror 11, 13, 22, 31, 33, 40, 55, 56, 77, 78, 79, 82, 84, 90, 149, 169, 176, 177, 186, 202, 228, 235, 240, 241, 261, 290, 292
Moreno, Jacob 6, 9, 10–13, *11*, 20, 25, 41–47, 49, 50, *50*, 52–54, *54*, 55–60, 71, 77–81, 91, 106, 121, 122, 182, 185, 198, 213, 236, *237*, 238, 240, 243, 265, 290–293
Moreno, Zerka 6, 44–46, 52, 56, 59, 81, 84, 87, 125, 176, 214, 237, *237*, 238
mutual aid 32–34, 36, 37, 68, 89, 106, 107, 112, 115, 127, 146, 174, 180, 181, 183–187, 199, 209, 215
mutual choice 17, 106, 122
mutuality 16, 17, 31–33, 35, 37, 45, 69, 106, 117, 146, 160, 180, 181, 186, 190–203, 208, 209, 211, 229, 230, 267, 287

neural integration 35, 85
neuroscience 14, 71–73

oppression 3, 4, 17, 111, 156, 190, 194, 223–225, 227, 228, 230, 231, 234, 240, 242, 262, 289

parallel process 19, 137, 143, 160, 192, 209, 212, 260, 262, 263, 272, 282, 285
peer support 3, 16, 17, 20, 31, 32, 37, 45, 68, 69, 105, 117, 125, 143, 146, 158, 160, 174–187, 193, 195–198, 202, 209, 211, 229, 233, 248, 252, 253, 255, 258, 264, 265, 267, 272, 273, 287, 295
perpetrator 52, 73, 79, 85, 86, 175, 176, 190–192, 203, 206, 218, 229, 233, 261
physical touch 122, 133, 142, 291
play 3, 21, 51, 52, 54, 73, 76, 81, 83, 87, 89–90, 92, 93, 124, 125, 139, 170, 184, 186, 197, 200–202, 217, 223, 239, 242, 252, 271, 289

Polyvagal theory 73, 218
posttraumatic growth 2, 20, 23, 55, 68, 69, 73–77, *75*, 86–88, 87, 104, 115, 117, 175, 182, 215, 248–273
post-traumatic stress disorder (PTSD) 13–15, 18, 21, 22, 24, 25, 31, 34, 44, 50, 68–95, 117, 134, 146, 151, 156, 157, 164, 174, 179, 210, 223, 225, 249, 250, 256, 269
prescriptive roles 84–86, **85**
psychodramatic journaling 82, 89
psychodramatic letter writing 82, 89
psychodrama training 5, 6, 89, 115, 165, 168, 264, 265, 269, 270, 272–273, 289, 290, 292
psychology 3, 9, 10, 12, 45, 57, 83, 176, 226, 289
PTSD *see* post-traumatic stress disorder (PTSD)

racism 59, 81, 191, 211, 223, 232, 235, 238, 239, 241
Relational Trauma Repair (RTR) Model 68, 88–92, 115
rescuer 85
resilience 4, 16, 19, 51, 93, 111, 117, 124, 128, 148, 165, 180, 181, 197, 213, 262, 271, 273, 283
retraumatization 2, 4, 7–8, 14, 16, 20, 23, 25, 32, 33, 79, 91, 135–136, 167, 186, 193, 222, 230, 234, 236, 263, 285, 287, 295
role atom 83–84
role reciprocity 53, 86, 184, 201, 202, 217, 240
role reversal 13, 55, 56, 77, 79–82, 93, 94, 112, 150, 177, 200, 216, 240, 241
role theory 49, 53–55, *54*, 55, 83, 86
role training 13, 73, 83, 87, 88, 90, 174, 177, 216, 217, 219, 239, 242, 265, 268
RTR Model *see* Relational Trauma Repair (RTR) Model

safety 4, 16, 17, 22, 23, 35–37, 39, 42, 45, 51, 68, 69, 73, 78–80, 83–85, **85**, 87, 88, 92, 94, 103–106, 109, 117, 119, 124–126, 128, 133–152, 156–158, 160–162, 164, 165, 167, 168, 177, 179–181, 183, 186,

193, 195, 197, 198, 202, 206, 207,
209–211, 216, 218, 224, 229, 235, 239,
240, 249, 260–263, 266, 267, 273, 280,
286–288, 290, 295
Sanctuary Model 248, 259–263
sculpting 81–82, 89, 90, 169, 170
secondary traumatic stress 19, 182, 197,
248–252, 256, 269
shame 34, 68, 109, 116, 146, 177, 178, 194,
201, 224, 228, 229
social atom 57, 57, 58, 89, 90, 103,
169, 170
social justice 5, 20, 222, 227, 234, 238, 243,
284, 293, 294
social networks 11, 12, 59, 103, 238
social work education 3, 6, 117–118
sociatry 5, 11, 12, 44, 222, 237, 238,
243, 293
sociodrama 11, 13, 81, 222, 236–243, 237,
264–273
sociodynamic effect 21, 58, 59, 123,
125, 293
sociogram 12, 58, 59, 59, 103, 106,
121–126, 182, 185
sociometric test 12, 58, 59, 121,
122, 182
sociometric theory 12, 57, 57–60, 59
sociostasis 125
soliloquy 13, 80, 82
spectrogram 84, 89, 103, 104, 106, 109–113,
122, 166, 167, 185, 239, 265, 266
spiritual 6, 8, 13, 15, 44–46, 74, 87, 109,
114, 117, 124, 128, 148, 215, 224,
236, 254
spontaneity 7, 11, 46, 47, 49–53, 50, 75, 77,
79, 80, 86, 87, 95, 164, 167, 168, 199,
239, 242, 267, 268, 271, 286
step-in sociometry 84, 103, 104, 106,
118–122, 185, 199
strengths-based 14, 71, 83, 92, 109, 112,
126, 129, 147–149, 152, 225
supervision 2, 6, 9, 23, 25, 91, 103, 112, 128,
174, 181, 248, 251–253, 255, 258, 264,
268, 270, 273
surplus reality 46, 47, 63, 73, 80, 86, 88, 95,
123, 124, 214
symbolic representation 72, 109

tele 58, 94, 122, 123, 167, 168, 184,
201, 202
telehealth 37, 39, 288, 290
Theater of Spontaneity 11, 52
therapeutic factors 33–36, 40, 104, 146, 179,
180, 195, 209, 231
Therapeutic Spiral Model 5, 23, 68, 78,
83–88, 85, 87, 90, 103, 109, 149
training 2, 5–10, 12, 13, 21, 22, 37, 39,
73, 83, 87–92, 103, 112, 115, 125, 163,
165, 168, 174, 177, 181, 216, 217, 219,
233–235, 238–240, 242, 248, 251, 253,
255, 258, 260, 264, 265, 267–270, 272,
273, 288–294
transference 32, 58, 162, 165, 218, 236, 248,
252, 268, 269
transparency 16, 17, 32, 37, 38, 80, 117,
125, 138, 143, 146, 156–170, 195, 209,
211, 229, 230, 238, 267, 287
trauma-based roles 55, 79, 80, 83, 84, 86,
148, 151
trauma-informed leadership 2, 19–21,
136–138, 161, 174, 190, 196–198, 203,
206, 211–213, 222, 256, 263, 273, 279,
280, 283–285, 293, 294–295
trauma-informed principles 1, 2, 4, 13, 16–18,
18, 20–25, 31–33, 37, 38–39, 44, 45, 69,
81, 91, 92, 94, 103, 104–106, 105, 108, 111,
117, 121, 125, 129, 133–135, 146, 156, 157,
160, 165, 176, 180, 185, 186, 191, 193, 195,
196, 209–212, 214, 218, 222, 224–226, 229,
232–236, 238, 243, 248, 258, 264, 267, 273,
279–281, 285–290, 293–295
traumatic grief 92, 94, 95
trauma triangle 85, 86, 87
trustworthiness 16, 17, 38, 45, 69, 105, 106,
117, 146, 147, 156–170, 180, 186, 193,
195, 267, 287
12-step 89, 180

universality 33, 106, 121, 146, 179, 186,
195, 209

van der Kolk, Bessel 10, 14, 47, 71, 72,
105, 207
vicarious posttraumatic growth 2, 20, 182,
248–273

vicarious trauma 2, 14, 19, 20, 25, 74, 81,
    142, 187, 226, 248–273, 285, 295
victim 47, 70, 79, 85, 86, 139, 175, 176,
    179, 190–192, 194, 203, 206, 207, 208,
    210, 261
voice 16–17, 37, **38,** 45, 53, 55, 93, 105,
    117, 146, 147, 150, 160, 184, 193, 195,
    206–219, 229, 230, 267, 271, 287

warm-up/warming-up 11, 48–51, 58, 76, 81,
    83, 88, 91, 92, 104, 106, 109, 112, 113,
    118, 119, 121, 128, 129, 143, 147–149,
    168, 183, 199, 215, 216, 239, 240, 270, 266

Yalom, Irvin 9, 10, 33–35, 40, 52, 69, 104,
    139, 141, 146, 151, 164, 165, 179, 180,
    186, 195, 209, 230, 231, 286, 288, 292

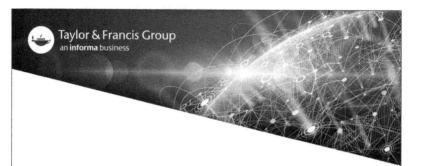

For Product Safety Concerns and Information please contact our EU
representative GPSR@taylorandfrancis.com
Taylor & Francis Verlag GmbH, Kaufingerstraße 24, 80331 München, Germany

www.ingramcontent.com/pod-product-compliance
Ingram Content Group UK Ltd.
Pitfield, Milton Keynes, MK11 3LW, UK
UKHW021450080625
459435UK00012B/439